Intraoperative Radiation Therapy

Editors

Ralph R. Dobelbower, Jr.

Professor and Chairman
Department of Radiation Therapy
Medical College of Ohio
Toledo, Ohio

Mitsuyuki Abe

Professor and Chairman
Department of Radiology
Faculty of Medicine
Kyoto University
Kyoto, Japan

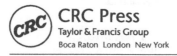

CRC Press
Taylor & Francis Group
Boca Raton London New York

CRC Press is an imprint of the
Taylor & Francis Group, an **informa** business

CRC Press
Taylor & Francis Group
6000 Broken Sound Parkway NW, Suite 300
Boca Raton, FL 33487-2742

© 1989 by Taylor & Francis Group, LLC
CRC Press is an imprint of Taylor & Francis Group, an Informa business

First issued in paperback 2019

No claim to original U.S. Government works

ISBN 13: 978-0-367-45097-7 (pbk)
ISBN 13: 978-0-8493-6846-2 (hbk)

Visit the Taylor & Francis Web site at
http://www.taylorandfrancis.com

and the CRC Press Web site at
http://www.crcpress.com

Library of Congress Cataloging-in-Publication Data
Intraoperative radiation therapy.
    Includes biliographies and index.
    1. Cancer--Intraoperative radiotherapy.   I. Dobelbower,
Ralph R.   II. Abe, Mitsuyuki, 1932-   . [DNLM:
1. Intraoperative Care. Neoplasms--radiotherapy.
QZ 269 I59]
RD652.I57 1989   616.99'40642   88-835187
ISBN 0-8493-6846-4

Library of Congress Card Number 88-835187

PREFACE

The introduction of megavoltage radiations has brought about significant improvements in the cure rate of malignant diseases. However, a continuing obstacle to definitive radiotherapy is the difficulty of delivering cancerocidal doses to tumors surrounded by critical organs. Also, the improvement in the overall survival achieved by megavoltage beams has recently reached a plateau. In this situation, a great deal of interest is now being expressed in the use of intraoperative radiation therapy (IORT), a procedure whereby a dose of radiation is delivered to a surgically exposed tumor or tumor bed while normal organs are shifted from the field. This provides the possibility of overcoming certain limitations of conventional radiotherapy.

The idea of IORT is not new. Descriptions of X-ray irradiation during surgery appeared in the early 1900s. The purpose of IORT at that time was to deliver a sufficient dose of radiation to deep-seated tumors with beams of limited penetration then available.

With the advent of electron beam therapy there has been new interest in IORT. With this modality, depth of beam penetration is sharply limited, allowing greater sparing of normal tissue and thereby improving the therapeutic ratio of local control vs. complications. Because of the generally encouraging results obtained by IORT, its use has spread in Japan and the U.S. At present, a number of institutions around the world are planning to use this technique.

The purpose of this book is to review the entire subject of IORT. It is our hope that this book will serve as a comprehensive reference for institutions planning to develop IORT facilities and to give radiation and surgical oncologists updated information on this rapidly developing field.

ACKNOWLEDGMENT

The authors acknowledge Mr. Mark Calcamuggio for his editorial comments and Miss Sandra K. Price for clerical preparation of this publication.

THE EDITORS

Ralph R. Dobelbower, Jr., M.D., Ph.D., F.A.C.R., is Professor and Chairman of the Department of Radiation Therapy at the Medical College of Ohio at Toledo. He holds a joint appointment as Professor of Neurological Surgery at that institution.

Dr. Dobelbower graduated in 1962 from the Pennsylvania State University with a B.S. in physics and also earned an A.B. degree from that institution in 1963. He received his medical training at the Jefferson Medical College of Philadelphia, graduating with an M.D. degree in 1967. In 1975, he earned a Ph.D. degree in physiology from Thomas Jefferson University. Dr. Dobelbower interned at the Balboa U.S. Naval Hospital in San Diego, CA, in 1967 and 1968 and served as a lieutenant commander in the Medical Corps of the U.S. Navy until 1971. After completing residency training in radiation therapy and nuclear medicine at the Thomas Jefferson University Hospital in 1974, Dr. Dobelbower was appointed as instructor of radiation therapy and nuclear medicine at that institution. He was promoted to the rank of Assistant Professor in 1975 and to Associate Professor in 1979.

From 1974 through 1979, Dr. Dobelbower served as Assistant to the Director of the Patterns of Care Study in Radiation Therapy. From 1970 through 1975, he was a Clinical Fellow of the American Cancer Society, and from 1975 through 1979, he served as a Junior Clinical Fellow of the American Cancer Society. From 1977 to 1979, Dr. Dobelbower served on the Advisory Committee of the Gwynedd-Mercy College School of Radiation Therapy Technology, and since 1980 has been the Medical Advisor of the Radiation Therapy Technologist Training Program at the Michael J. Owens Technical College.

In 1980, Dr. Dobelbower established the Division of Radiation Oncology at the Medical College of Ohio. In 1985, he was named Professor and Founding Chairman of the Department of Radiation Therapy.

Dr. Dobelbower is a member of the American Association for Cancer Research, the American Association of Physicists in Medicine, the American College of Radiology, the American Endocurie Therapy Society, the American Radium Society, the American Society of Therapeutic Radiology and Oncology, the Children's Cancer Study Group, the Council of Affiliated Regional Radiation Oncology Societies, the Eastern Cooperative Oncology Group, the North American Hyperthermia Group, the Pan-American Medical Association, the Radiation Research Society, the Radiation Therapy Oncology Group, and the Radiological Society of North America. He serves on the editorial board of the *International Journal of Pancreatology*.

Dr. Dobelbower founded the Northwest Ohio Society of Radiation Oncologists and served as its first president in 1982 and 1983. He was a founding member of the Simon Kramer Society and has served as its vice president since 1981. Dr. Dobelbower is chairman of various studies in the Eastern Cooperative Oncology Group and several intergroup studies.

Among other honors, Dr. Dobelbower was called to deliver the Second Annual Marting Lecture in 1986. He has been a member of the Society of Sigma XI since 1975. In 1985, he was made an honorary member of the Chicago Radiological Society. In 1987, he was awarded the medal of the Faculte de Medecine de Montpellier as well as the medal of the Facolta di Medicinae Chirurgia di Universitas Catholica Sacri Cordis Jesu in Rome.

Dr. Dobelbower has over 60 scientific publications to his credit. He has been the recipient of several research grants from the National Institutes of Health and the American Cancer Society. In 1986, he organized the First International Symposium on Intraoperative Radiation Therapy. He has delivered over 70 invited lectures at national and international meetings. His current major research interests include treatment of gastrointestinal neoplasms and intraoperative radiation therapy.

Dr. Dobelbower is recognized as the world's foremost authority on the treatment of cancer of the pancreas with radiation therapy.

Mitsuyuki Abe, M.D., F.A.C.R., is Professor and Chairman of the Department of Radiology, Faculty of Medicine, Kyoto University. After completing his basic medical education at Kyoto University in 1959, Dr. Abe studied radiology at that institution until 1962 when he commenced a fellowship at Universität Freiburg, completing his specialty training in 1964. He then served as a Junior Clinical Instructor in the Department of Radiology at Kyoto University until 1967 when he was promoted to Instructor of Radiology. In 1977, he was appointed Professor and Chairman of the Department of Radiology, Faculty of Medicine, Kyoto University.

Dr. Abe has served on numerous national and international committees and societies. Since 1981, he has been a member of the Executive Committee of the Japan Society for Cancer Therapy. Since 1982, he has been the principal advisor of the U.S.-Japan Cooperative Research Program as well as the Director of the Japan Radiosensitization Research Association. In 1984, he was the organizer of The First Annual Meeting of the Japanese Society of Hyperthermic Oncology, and he has served on the Executive Committee of that organization until the present time. Since 1985, he has served on the Executive Committee of the International Society of Radiation Oncology.

Dr. Abe is co-editor of 5 books dedicated to radiation medicine (a total of 63 volumes). He currently serves on the editorial boards of six national and two international scientific journal. In addition, since 1974, he has been Chief Editor of the *Japanese Journal of Hyperthermic Oncology*.

Dr. Abe has received numerous honors including the Japanese Medical Association Award in 1979. In 1983, he was presented the Philipp-Franz-von Siebold Prize by the President of the Federal Republic of Germany. In 1987, he was made an honorary fellow of the American College of Radiology. In 1988, he was awarded an Honorary Doctor's degree of Essen University of the FRG, and commendation of the Minister of State for Science and Technology in Japan.

Dr. Abe has been an active lecturer on oncologic and radiologic topics. On at least 30 occasions, he has been called upon to speak abroad in 7 different countries and in 3 different languages.

Dr. Abe has authored or co-authored over 350 publications in the scientific literature: 233 in Japanese and 118 in English and German. His current research interests are intraoperative radiation therapy and hyperthermic oncology.

Dr. Abe is regarded as the world's foremost authority on intraoperative radiation therapy for gastric cancer.

CONTRIBUTORS

Mitsuyuki Abe, M.D.
Professor and Chairman
Department of Radiology
Faculty of Medicine
Kyoto University Medical School
Kyoto, Japan

Ebrahim Ashayeri, M.D.
Associate Professor
Department of Radiotherapy
Howard University Hospital
Washington, D.C.

Farideh R. Bagne, Ph.D, J.D.
Associate Professor
Department of Radiation Therapy
Medical College of Ohio
Toledo, Ohio

Robert W. Beart, M.D.
Professor and Chairman
Department of Surgery
Mayo Clinic
Scottsdale, Arizona

E. Bodner, M.D.
Professor and Chairman
2nd Department of Surgery
University Hospital
Innsbruck, Austria

Donald G. Bronn, M.D., Ph.D.
Assistant Professor
Department of Radiation Therapy
Medical College of Ohio
Toledo, Ohio

Felipe A. Calvo, M.D., Ph.D.
Director
Department of Radiation Oncology
Clinica Universitaria
Pamplona, Spain

Mariad A. Crommelin, M.D.
Department of Radiation Oncology
Catharina Hospital
Eindhoven, The Netherlands

Gregorio Delgado, M.D.
Division of Gynecologic Oncology
Georgetown University School of Medicine
Washington, D.C.

Ralph R. Dobelbower, Jr., M.D., Ph.D.
Professor and Chairman
Department of Radiation Therapy
Medical College of Ohio
Toledo, Ohio

Carlos Dy, M.D.
Department of Oncology
Clinical University of Navarra
Pamplona, Spain

John D. Earle, M.D.
Chairman and Professor
Division of Radiation Oncology
Mayo Clinic
Rochester, Minnesota

Ahmed Eltaki, M.D.
Department of Radiation Therapy
Medical College of Ohio
Toledo, Ohio

Luis A. Escude, M.S.
Director
Physics Section
Clinica Universitaria
Pamplona, Spain

Jennifer Fieck
Department of Radiation Oncology
Mayo Clinic
Rochester, Minnesota

H. Frommhold, M.D.
Professor and Chairman
Department of Radiation Therapy
University Hospital
Innsbruck, Austria

Peter G. Garrett, M.D.
Staff Radiation Oncologist
Department of Radiation Therapy
Methodist Hospital of Indiana
Indianapolis, Indiana

Karl S. Glaser, M.D.
General Surgeon
2nd Department of Surgery
University of Innsbruck
Innsbruck, Austria

Alfred L. Goldson, M.D.
Professor and Chairman
Department of Radiation Oncology
Howard University Hospital
Washington, D.C.

Samuel H. Greenblatt, M.D.
Associate Professor
Department of Neurological Surgery
Medical College of Ohio
Toledo, Ohio

Leonard L. Gunderson, M.D.
Professor and Vice-Chairman
Department of Radiation Oncology
Mayo Clinic
Rochester, Minnesota

Ronald Hamaker, M.D.
Otolaryngology
Head and Neck Surgery
Methodist Hospital
Indianapolis, Indiana

Gerald E. Hanks, M.D.
Vice-Chairman and Professor
Department of Radiation Oncology
Fox Chase Cancer Center
University of Pennsylvania
Philadelphia, Pennsylvania

Takehisa Hiraoka, Ph.D.
Associate Professor
1st Department of Surgery
Kumamoto University Medical School
Kumamoto, Japan

Paul E. Hodel, M.D.
Assistant Professor
Department of Anesthesiology
Medical College of Ohio
Toledo, Ohio

Harald J. Hoekstra, M.D., Ph.D.
Division of Surgical Oncology
University Hospital of Groningen
Groningen, The Netherlands

D. Ann Hollon, R.N. R.T. (T)
Technological Administrator
Department of Radiation Therapy
Medical College of Ohio
Toledo, Ohio

Kenneth R. Kase, Ph.D.
Professor and Director
Department of Radiation Oncology
University of Massachusetts Medical
 Center
Worcester, Massachusetts

Moneer A. Khalil, M.D.
Acting Assistant Chief
Department of Radiation Medicine
Roswell Park Memorial Institute
Buffalo, New York

Krystyna D. Kiel, M.D.
Assistant Professor
Department of Radiation Oncology
Northwestern Memorial Hospital
Chicago, Illinois

Toby Kramer, M.D.
Assistant Professor
Department of Therapeutic Radiology
Rush Presbyterian St. Luke's Medical
 Center
Chicago, Illinois

**Ramachandra Murty Krishnamsetty,
 M.D.**
Radiation Oncologist
Merle M. Mahr Cancer Center
Trover Clinic
Madisonville, Kentucky

Alvaro Martinez
Division of Radiation Oncology
Mayo Medical School
Mayo Clinic
Rochester, Minnesota

John T. Martin, M.D.
Professor and Chairman
Department of Anesthesiology
Medical College of Ohio
Toledo, Ohio

J. Kirk Martin, Jr., M.D.
Chairman
Department of Surgery
Mayo Clinic
Jacksonville, Florida

Masao Matsutani, M.D.
Chairman
Department of Neurosurgery
Tokyo Metropolitan Komagome Hospital
Tokyo, Japan

Tadayoshi Matsuda
Department of Radiation Therapy
Tokyo Metropolitan Komagome Hospital
Tokyo, Japan

Keiichi Matsumoto
Vice Director
Department of Urology
Yokosuka National Hospital
Yukosuka, Japan

D. M. Mehta, M.D.
Department of Radiation Oncology
University Hospital of Groningen
Groningen, The Netherlands

Hollis W. Merrick, III, M.D.
Associate Professor
Department of Surgery
Medical College of Ohio
Toledo, Ohio

Andrew J. Milligan, Ph.D.
Associate Professor
Department of Radiation Therapy
Medical College of Ohio
Toledo, Ohio

Yoshimasa Miyauchi, Ph.D.
Professor
1st Department of Surgery
Kumamoto University Medical School
Kumamoto, Japan

David M. Nagorney, M.D.
Assistant Professor
Department of Surgery
Mayo Medical School
Rochester, Minnesota

Ikuo Nakamura, M.D.
Professor and Chairman
Department of Radiological Technology
College of Medical Science
Kumamoto University
Kumamoto, Japan

George L. Nardi, M.D.
Visiting Surgeon
Department of Surgery
Massachusetts General Hospital
Boston, Massachusetts

Takehiro Nishidai, Ph.D.
Lecturer
Department of Radiology
Faculty of Medicine
Kyoto University
Kyoto, Japan

J. Oldhoff
Department of Surgery
University Hospital of Groningen
Groningen, The Netherlands

Colin G. Orton, Ph.D.
Professor
Department of Radiation Oncology
Wayne State University School of
  Medicine and Harper-Grace Hospitals
Detroit, Michigan

John I. Pearce, M.Sc.
Department of Radiation Medicine
Roswell Park Memorial Institute
Buffalo, New York

Edmund S. Petrilli, M.D.
Clinical Associate Professor
Georgetown University School of
  Medicine
Washington, D.C.

Richard W. Piontek, M.S.
Assistant Professor
Department of Radiation Therapy
Hitchcock Medical Center
Dartmouth College
Hanover, New Hampshire

Newell O. Pugh, J., M.D.
Chief and Director
Departments of Radiation Therapy and
  Cancer Center
Methodist Hospital of Indiana
Indianapolis, Indiana

Mark Rayport, M.D., Ph.D.
Professor and Chairman
Department of Neurological Surgery
Medical College of Ohio
Toledo, Ohio

Tyvin A. Rich, M.D.
Associate Professor
Department of Clinical Radiotherapy
M.D. Anderson Cancer Center
Houston, Texas

David L. Roseman, M.D.
Professor
Department of General Surgery
Rush Medical College
Chicago, Illinois

David B. Ross, M.D.
Staff Radiation Oncologist
Department of Radiation Therapy
Methodist Hospital of Indiana
Indianapolis, Indiana

William U. Shipley, M.D.
Radiation Therapist and Associate
  Director, MGH Cancer Center
Department of Radiation Medicine
Massachusetts General Hospital
Boston, Massachusetts

Mark I. Singer, M.D.
Otolaryngology
Head and Neck Surgery
Methodist Hospital
Indianapolis, Indiana

Herman Suit, M.D.
Department of Radiation Medicine
Massachusetts General Hospital
Boston, Massachusetts

Masaji Takahashi
Professor
Department of Oncology
Chest Disease Research Institute
Kyoto University
Kyoto, Japan

Yoshiaki Tanaka, M.D.
Department of Radiation Therapy
Tokyo Metropolitan Komagome Hospital
Tokyo, Japan

Seiki Tashiro, Ph.D.
Associate Professor
1st Department of Surgery
Kumamoto University Medical School
Kumamoto, Japan

Joel E. Tepper, M.D.
Professor and Chairman
Department of Radiation Oncology
University of North Carolina
Chapel Hill, North Carolina

Manfred Url, Dr. Phil.
Radiation Physicist
Universitat Klinik fur Strahlentherapie
Innsbruck, Austria

J. Vermeij, M.D., Ph.D.
Department of Radiation Oncology
University Hospital of Groningen
Groningen, The Netherlands

Andrew L. Warshaw, M.D.
Visiting Surgeon
Department of Surgery
Harvard Medical School
Massachusetts General Hospital
Boston, Massachusetts

Harvey B. Wolkov, M.D.
Medical Director
Department of Radiation Oncology
Radiation Oncology Center
Mercy General Hospital
Sacramento, California

William C. Wood, M.D.
Chief
Division of Surgical Oncology
Massachusetts General Hospital Cancer
  Center
Boston, Massachusetts

TABLE OF CONTENTS

Chapter 1

HISTORY OF INTRAOPERATIVE RADIATION THERAPY

Mitsuyuki Abe

TABLE OF CONTENTS

I. HISTORICAL BACKGROUND OF INTRAOPERATIVE RADIATION THERAPY

The beginnings of intraoperative radiation therapy (IORT) can be traced back about 80 years. In 1907, intraoperative irradiation was first described by Beck[1] for a patient with advanced pyloric cancer; 2 years later, he reported on the clinical experiences with IORT with X-ray for seven patients with inoperable gastric cancers and one with colon cancer in which he pulled the tumors into the abdominal wounds in order to irradiate them directly.[2] Beck said in his paper, "As the mountain does not come to Mohammed, Mohammed must go to the mountain. In other words, if the tubal light does not reach the deep-seated structures, the structures must be brought to the tube." In 1915, Finsterer[3] reported the clinical results of inoperable carcinomas of the stomach and colon which were treated in a similar fashion.

These techniques may be classified as IORT in the broad sense that radiotherapy was performed during surgical procedures. However, the practice of IORT at that time was different from that of the IORT currently performed; the purpose then was to deliver a dose to deep-seated tumors with the low-energy radiation beams then available.

Between the late 1930s and 1950s, a number of papers on IORT using orthovoltage X-ray were published. In 1937, Eloesser[4] reported the use of IORT with 200-kilovolt peak (kVp) X-rays in six patients with advanced gastric and rectal tumors. In 1940, Pack and Livingston,[5] and in 1941, Goin and Hoffman,[6] reported on patients with bladder cancers treated by IORT. They opened the bladder, reduced the tumor to the level of the bladder wall by fulguration, and then irradiated. Henschke and Henschke[7] developed high dose rate intraoperative contact X-ray irradiation using a technique of scanning with a cone 2.5 cm in diameter and reported this (they called it "operative irradiation") in 1944. In 1947, Fairchild and Shorter[8] published the clinical results of 15 patients with unresectable gastric cancers treated by IORT with 950 to 1542 rad from a 250-kVp X-ray unit. Some of these patients received postoperative external beam irradiation with cumulative doses of 970 to 2541 rad. Of the 15 patients treated in this fashion, 1 lived 2 years and 2 lived 15 months after treatment. In 1953, Barth[9] reported a technique in which the tumor was operatively laid open and then exposed to short-distance irradiation. Barth and Meinel[10] further developed this technique and published in 1959 the clinical results of intraoperative contact irradiation in carcinomas of the lung and esophagus, and intracranial and mediastinal tumors using 150 kVp X-rays. In that same year, Lutterbeck[11] described his clinical experience with intraoperative contact X-ray irradiation of bladder cancer.

The authors listed above had some encouraging early results, but it is difficult to estimate the real benefit of IORT performed back then because the long-term follow-up data were not published. Before 1960, IORT (with orthovoltage X-rays) had been used as a palliative treatment for advanced cancer and to give high doses to deep-seated tumors.

II. CURRENT IORT

Modern intraoperative radiation therapy was begun by Abe and co-workers using a megavoltage machine in 1964. The advent of megavoltage radiotherapy made it possible to deliver a sufficient dose to any location in the body, significantly improving the cure rate of malignant diseases. However, a cancerocidal dose of external beam irradiation cannot be given if the tumors are located near radiosensitive structures. On the other hand, during surgery the possibility always exists that microscopic disease will be left behind, even after what is believed to be a curative operation. To overcome these limitations of radiotherapy and surgery, IORT was developed.[12-14] In IORT, normal organs can be shifted out of the beam path and, hence, a sterilizing dose can safely be given to surgically exposed tumors or cells which are hard to eliminate with a surgical procedure. The above-mentioned problems, which both radiotherapy and surgery have by nature, can thus be resolved simultaneously by IORT.

From this point of view, Abe et al.[14] defined IORT as a treatment modality in which resectable lesions are removed surgically and the remaining cancer nests are sterilized by irradiation during a surgical procedure. They have treated a variety of malignant diseases by IORT[12-18] and reported that IORT is best performed with an electron beam, since a specific beam energy can be chosen to produce the desired depth of tissue penetration with sharp fall-off of radiation dose with increasing depth in tissue, thereby avoiding the problems caused by exposure of normal tissues beneath the tumors.[12] It has been demonstrated that some patients who underwent noncurative surgery with incomplete excision of neoplasms could be cured by intraoperative electron beam irradiation to the unresectable tumor remnants.[13] Because of the encouraging results obtained through IORT, its use has spread in Japan. The institutions in which this radiotherapy is performed increased to a total of 38 in 1985. To date, more than 1500 patients have been treated with IORT in Japan.

IORT was first introduced in the U.S. by Henschke and Goldson[19] in 1975. They developed an integrated facility in which the entire surgical-radiotherapeutic procedure could be carried out and treated their first case using a Varian® 18-meV linear accelerator on November 26, 1976.[20,21] This arrangement of using a radiation therapy room as an operating suite made IORT very easy to perform — patients could now have the whole procedure in one room. Based on the experiences in Japan and at Howard University, a number of other institutions started clinical trials of IORT in the U.S. The Massachusetts General Hospital (MGH) was the second center to begin IORT (1978),[22] followed by the National Cancer Institute (1979),[23,24] Mayo Clinic (1981),[25] the New England Deaconess Hospital (NEDH) division of the Joint Center for Radiation Therapy (1982)[26] and the Medical College of Ohio (1983). Between 1976 and 1982, nearly 300 patients were treated in the U.S.

Intraoperative radiation therapy with electron beams has opened the way to treatment of deep-seated tumors adjacent to critical organs. This new form of radiotherapy has also widened the scope of radiotherapy by permitting curative treatment of radioresistant tumors without affecting normal structures, such as skin.

A. IORT IN JAPAN

The importance of IORT was demonstrated by Abe[28] in a comparative study of 194 gastric cancer patients treated by gastrectomy with and without IORT. Patients were treated with surgery alone or surgery plus IORT depending upon the day they were admitted to the Kyoto University Hospital. In the IORT group, patients received gastrectomy followed by IORT to unresectable remnants or the lymph node groups around the celiac axis, splenic artery, and hepatic artery, which most frequently contain metastatic cancer and are the hardest to eliminate with surgical procedures. When the posterior wall of the stomach was grossly adherent to the pancreas, this portion was also encompassed by the IORT field. A single dose of 20 to 40 Gy was delivered, depending upon the residual tumor volume. The 5-year survival rates of patients treated by operation alone were 93.0% for stage I, 54.5% for stage II, 36.8% for stage III, and 0% for stage IV. The 5-year survival rates of patients treated by surgery plus IORT were 88.1% for stage I, 77.0% for stage II, 44.6% for stage III, and 19.5% for stage IV.

The special advantage of IORT over conventional radiotherapy or surgery is that the former can provide higher tumor control with less functional damage. This was demonstrated by Matsumoto et al.[29] in patients with bladder cancer; they reported the results of 116 patients treated by IORT at the National Cancer Center in Tokyo. The tumor was exposed by opening the bladder, and a single dose of 25 to 30 Gy was delivered with 4 to 6 meV electrons to the tumor with a 1.5-cm margin. Additional fractionated external beam irradiation (30 to 40 Gy covering the whole bladder) was given in order to prevent heterotropic recurrence.

The 5-year survival rate for T1 lesions was 96.3%; for T2, 61.6%; and for T3 and T4 combined, 7.4%. Bladder function was preserved in every patient. Heterotropic recurrence in the bladder was observed in 19.3% of patients within 5 years, which was significantly low when compared to the results of other treatment modalities (such as transurethral resection, surgery alone, or conventional external beam radiotherapy) employed at the National Cancer Center.

These encouraging results have promoted wide use of IORT for a variety of malignant diseases in Japan. A total of 59 patients with biliary tract cancer have been treated at 12 Japanese institutions;[17] 16 of the 59 patients are alive after single doses of IORT (25 to 40 Gy), with the longest survival being 18 months. In approximately 90% of the patients, recanalization of the obstructed portion of the bile duct was achieved because of the tumor regression. Takahashi et al.[30] reported the clinical results of 14 patients with locally advanced prostatic cancer who were treated by IORT with or without external beam irradiation. A treatment cone was inserted directly on the tumor using a perineal approach. The electron energy used for IORT ranged from 10 to 14 meV, depending upon the tumor volume. Of five patients treated by IORT alone, four received a single dose of 30 to 35 Gy and achieved local control, while one received 28 Gy and failed. Nine patients with more advanced prostatic cancer were treated by IORT with a dose of 20 or 25 Gy in conjunction with external beam irradiation to a dose of 50 Gy, which included the primary tumor and the pelvic lymph nodes. All nine patients achieved local control. Of the 14 patients, 9 are alive with no evidence of disease; the longest survival being 5 years and 7 months; 3 are alive with metastases, and 2 are dead of metastases. It is worthy of note that no serious complication involving the bladder, urethra, or rectum is found in the surviving patients.

Since pancreatic cancer rarely yields to curative measures, regardless of the modality of treatment, IORT has been applied to this disease. From 1980 through 1984, 302 patients with pancreatic cancer entered a multi-institutional cooperative study in Japan on the treatment of pancreatic cancer. These patients were divided into three groups: Group 1 consisted of patients treated by IORT, with a single dose of 20 to 40 Gy; Group 2 included patients treated by IORT in combination with external beam radiotherapy (in this group a single dose of 20 to 30 Gy was followed by additional external beam irradiation to cumulative doses of 30 to 50 Gy, depending upon tumor size and performance status of the patients); Group 3 consisted of patients who underwent operation alone. Of the 302 patients, 272 were evaluable for analysis. Of the 272, 122 belonged to Group 1, 47 to Group 2, and 103 to Group 3. In stages I, II, and IV, no difference in median survival was found in the three groups. However, the median survival of stage III patients treated by IORT plus external beam radiotherapy was 12 months; this was significantly better than that of the same stage patients treated by operation alone (5.5 months) or IORT without external beam radiotherapy (5.5 months).[31] From these results, it can be seen that IORT alone is insufficient to produce long-term control for large pancreatic tumors, yet a combination of IORT with external beam irradiation is adequate for such tumors. This is supported by MGH data from pancreatic cancer patients treated by IORT combined with external beam irradiation.[32]

Intraoperative radiation therapy may be particularly applicable for radioresistant tumors such as soft tissue sarcoma and glioblastoma. Abe and Takahashi[18] treated patients with soft tissue tumors by IORT in an attempt to achieve good local control with less cosmetic and functional loss; 11 patients with benign soft tissue tumors and 14 with soft tissue sarcoma were treated. The patients referred for IORT had disease that was recurrent or inoperable, or amputation of the affected limb had been recommended. As much tumor tissue as possible was removed and the skin incision was wide so that the lesions were sufficiently covered by the treatment cone without including the skin. A single dose of 30 to 45 Gy was delivered directly to the known or suspected residual lesions. The local control rate achieved was 88.0%.

Glioblastoma is also known to be highly radioresistant and is hardly ever eliminated by conventional therapy. Matsutani et al.[33] applied IORT to patients with localized glioblastoma located in the superficial regions of the brain. The patients received a combination of fractionated external beam irradiation with cumulative doses of 30 to 40 Gy, followed 4 weeks later by a craniotomy with necrotic tumor removal and IORT with a single dose of 10 to 20 Gy to the residual tumor or tumor bed. This yielded significantly better results (2-year survival rate: 68.6%) than those having surgery alone.

B. IORT IN THE U.S.

As mentioned previously, IORT in the U.S. was first started by Goldson and co-workers[20] at Howard University Hospital in 1976. Initially, they used IORT for the therapeutic and prophylactic treatment of paraaortic lymph nodes in patients with cancer of the uterine cervix.[34] A total of 22 patients with this disease treated by IORT survived from 1 to 50 months with a median of 12 months.[35] Later they applied IORT to the treatment of other abdominal tumors[36] and intracranial malignancies.[37] Between 1978 and 1981, 19 patients with advanced pancreatic cancer were treated by IORT with a single dose ranging from 15 to 30 Gy. Because this was a pilot study and 10 of the 19 patients had liver metastasis, the median survival was only 5.5 months. Post-mortem examination revealed that a single dose of 15 to 30 Gy was not sufficient to eliminate all cancer cells. From this finding, Goldson et al. wrote that IORT will play its most important role when it is combined with external beam radiotherapy.

At MGH, the second American center to use IORT, investigators used this technique as a means of delivering boost dosage to the tumor as a supplement to external beam irradiation. The reason is that there are several advantages to a combined external beam-IORT approach over IORT alone: (1) improvement in local control because of a decreased risk of marginal recurrence, and (2) less risk of normal tissue damage.

In 1978, a pilot study of IORT in combination with external beam irradiation was started at MGH;[32] 12 patients with localized but unresectable carcinoma of the pancreas were treated. The IORT dose ranged from 15 to 18 Gy, and the average preoperative external beam irradiation was 19.24 Gy, with an average dose of 26.43 Gy delivered postoperatively for a mean total external beam dose of 45.67 Gy. Chemotherapy was given to 6 of the 12 patients. The median survival was 15 months,[32] which compares favorably to the median survival of 10.5 months seen in patients treated at the MGH between 1961 and 1971 for resectable pancreatic cancer.[38]

The most encouraging results have been achieved in patients with colorectal cancer. Gunderson et al.[39] reported data from 32 patients who received standard treatment with external beam irradiation to doses of 45 to 50 Gy, as well as surgery, but in addition, had an IORT boost dose of 10 to 15 Gy to the remaining tumor or tumor bed. For 16 patients who presented with unresectable primary lesions, the addition of IORT resulted in a total absence of local recurrence with a minimum 20-month follow-up, and the survival rate was statistically better than for the group treated with only external beam irradiation and surgical resection.[40]

Similar optimistic results have been obtained in patients with soft-tissue sarcomas, where it is difficult to deliver a sufficient dose by external beam irradiation alone. At MGH, patients with retroperitoneal sarcoma were treated by preoperative irradiation to doses ranging from 45 to 50 Gy followed by IORT with doses of 15 to 20 Gy to the tumor bed. Local control was obtained in 13 of 15 patients with retroperitoneal and extremity sarcomas.[41,42]

The U.S. National Cancer Institute began evaluating IORT in 1978 as a potential adjunct to surgical resection of advanced malignant tumors in the abdomen.[43] A total of 20 patients with advanced tumors all considered unlikely to be cured by conventional treatments, and which included gastric cancer, pancreatic cancer, retroperitoneal sarcomas, and osteosarcoma of the pelvis, underwent gross tumor resection followed by IORT with a dose of 20 Gy. Local tumor control was achieved in 11 of the 16 surviving patients with a median follow-up period of 18 months.

At the Mayo Clinic, the general approach and policy are basically the same as at the MGH — IORT administered as a boost dose in combination with external beam irradiation. From 1981 to 1983, 47 patients with a variety of abdominal and soft-tissue tumors which were residual after resection, recurrent or unresectable for cure were treated by IORT with a single dose of 10 to 20 Gy plus fractionated external beam irradiation with doses of 45 to 50 Gy. Local failure in the radiation field was substantiated in only 2 of the 47 patients (4%).[25] In addition, investigators at the Mayo Clinic are exploring the use of IORT in pediatric oncology. Kaufman[44] reported clinical results from two children with malignant tumors in the abdomen treated by IORT, and suggested that IORT may be useful in the pediatric age group, too.

At NEDH, a 300-kVp X-ray machine has been placed in an operating room. This approach has the following advantages: (1) it is possible to install an orthovoltage unit in a surgical suite because of relatively modest shielding requirements, (2) placement of the IORT unit within an operating room eliminates transporting anesthetized patients, and (3) disruption of routine radiotherapy in the radiotherapy department can be avoided. However, definite disadvantages of IORT with orthovoltage X-rays compared to electron beams are nonhomogenous dose distribution, especially when the tumor is large, and a higher level of exposure of normal tissues under the tumor. Between 1982 and 1983, 38 patients with a variety of advanced abdominal tumors were treated by 300-kVp X-ray IORT with or without external beam irradiation.[26] The IORT dose was 12.5 Gy for smaller tumors and 17.5 Gy for larger ones. The dose of fractionated external radiotherapy ranged from 45 to 50.4 Gy. At surgery, 29 patients had unresectable tumors and 9 had the tumor resected. A total of 17 patients (45%) are alive and 6 have no evidence of disease with a follow-up of 4 to 18 months. Local failure in 27 patients treated with IORT plus external beam radiotherapy was seen in 56%, but this varied from 11% (1/9) for patients with resected disease to 78% (14/18) for patients with unresected disease. Rich et al.[26] emphasized that the use of orthovoltage IORT for boost therapy may be valid, especially when combined with surgical resection and external beam irradiation.

Dobelbower et al.,[45] at the Medical College of Ohio, which began IORT in 1983, suggested that IORT may be particularly useful in tumors which have recurred after conventional radiotherapy because they can be treated by IORT without affecting previously irradiated normal structures.

C. IORT IN OTHER COUNTRIES

Austria and Germany have an old history of IORT. In Austria, IORT was started as early as 1910,[3] and in Germany it was performed in the 1940s. Both countries contributed much to the development of IORT techniques.[3,7,9,10,46] Unfortunately, however, recent publication on IORT in these countries is very limited. Sabitzer and co-workers[47] at Landeskrankenhaus in Klagenfurt, Austria, reported in 1983 one patient with pancreatic cancer treated by IORT with 17.5 Gy, followed by external beam irradiation to a dose of 44 Gy over 4.5 weeks. Since May 1984, Frommhold[48] at University Clinic in Innsbruck has treated 12 patients with pancreatic cancer with 20 to 25 Gy IORT in combination with 20 to 40 Gy external beam irradiation. The University Clinic of Navarra, Spain, started IORT in September 1984, and since then the Clinic has treated over 200 patients with malignant diseases by IORT.[49] Vermeij, et al.[50] are planning to construct an IORT facility at Groningen University Hospital, Holland.

III. FUTURE PROSPECTS

During the past 20 years, substantial data on modern IORT for treating various malignancies has been accumulated from many institutions. The results of IORT alone or in combination with external beam irradiation have indicated that IORT with single high doses can be delivered to tumors with tolerable acute and late morbidity, thereby improving the therapeutic ratio and producing greater local tumor control. Intraoperative radiation therapy data on gastric cancer at Kyoto University, bladder cancer at the National Cancer Center in Tokyo, and colorectal cancer at MGH suggest that improvement in local control by IORT reflects in an increase in the 5-year survival figure in selected diseases.

The disadvantages of IORT are that an adequate dose must be given in one session, which makes choosing the proper dose level difficult, and the tumor volume which can be eliminated by a single dose of irradiation is relatively small. In other words, the indications for IORT are restricted. The former problem must be resolved from analysis of accumulated clinical results of IORT. Regarding the latter problem, hypoxic cell sensitizers may make it possible to extend the indications for and also improve the effectiveness of IORT. This is because IORT provides a unique situation in that radiosensitizers can be delivered regionally to the tumor-bearing area by intra-arterial infusion. Therefore, a drug dose necessary to get sufficient radiosensitization may be given, even though it may be too toxic for systemic use. The use of hypoxic cell sensitizers combined with IORT may be particularly favorable, since the drugs seem to be most effective when they are given in combination with a large, single-dose irradiation rather than with fractionated doses. Another possibility is the use of hyperthermia, since it may be relatively easy to raise the temperature selectively in the surgically exposed tumor area.

Recently, great interest has been paid to the use of pions or heavy ions in radiotherapy because of their physical and biological advantages over photon radiotherapy. The advantage of dose distribution of these particles is especially attractive in treating deep-seated tumors near critical organs. However, the enormous complexity and cost of the machinery seriously limit their wide use. Intraoperative radiation therapy will continue to play an important role in the treatment of locally advanced refractory cancers in which improvement in local control can translate into improvement in long-term survival.

REFERENCES

1. **Beck, C.,** Über Kombinationsbehandlung bei bösartigen Neubildungen, *Berl. Klin. Wochenschr.*, 44, 1335, 1907.
2. **Beck, C.,** On external Roentgen treatment of internal structures (eventration treatment), *N.Y. Med. J.*, 89, 621, 1909.
3. **Finsterer, H.,** Zur Therapie inoperabler Magen-und Darmkarzinome mit Freilegung und nachfolgender Röntgenbestrahlung, *Strahlentherapie*, 6, 205, 1915.
4. **Eloesser, L.,** The treatment of some abdominal cancers by irradiation through the open abdomen combined with cautery excision, *Ann. Surg.*, 106, 645, 1937.
5. **Pack, G. and Livingston, E.,** *Treatment of Cancer and Allied Diseases*, Vol. 1, Hoeber, New York, 1940, 253.
6. **Goin, L. S. and Hoffman, E. F.,** The use of intravesical low voltage contact Roentgen irradiation in cancer of the bladder, *Radiology*, 37, 545, 1941.
7. **Henschke, G. and Henschke, U.,** Zur Technik der Operationsbestrahlung, *Strahlentherapie*, 74, 228, 1944.
8. **Fairchild, G. C. and Shorter, A.,** Irradiation of gastric cancer, *Br. J. Radiol.*, 20, 511, 1947.

9. **Barth, G.,** Erfahrungen und Ergebnisse mit der Nahbestrahlung operativ freigelegten Tumoren, *Strahlentherapie,* 91, 481, 1953.
10. **Barth, G. and Meinel, F.,** Intraoperative Kontakttherapie in den grossen Körperhöhlen, *Strahlentherapie,* 109, 386, 1959.
11. **Lutterbeck, E. F.,** Contact Roentgen radiation of bladder tumors, *J. Urol.,* 82, 90, 1959.
12. **Abe, M., Fukuda, M., Yamano, K., Matsuda, S., and Handa, H.,** Intra-operative irradiation in abdominal and cerebral tumours, *Acta Radiol.,* 10, 408, 1971.
13. **Abe, M., Yabumoto, E., Takahashi, M., Tobe, T., and Mori, K.,** Intraoperative radiotherapy of gastric cancer, *Cancer,* 34, 2034, 1974.
14. **Abe, M., Takahashi, M., Yabumoto, E., Onoyama, Y., Torizuka, K., Tobe, T., and Mori, K.,** Techniques, indications and results of intraoperative radiotherapy of advanced cancers, *Radiology,* 116, 693, 1975.
15. **Abe, M., Yabumoto, E., Nishidai, T., and Takahashi, M.,** Trials of new forms of radiotherapy for locally advanced bronchogenic carcinoma-irradiation under 95% O_2 plus 5% CO_2 inhalation, *Strahlentherapie,* 153, 149, 1977.
16. **Abe, M., Takahashi, M., Yabumoto, E., Adachi, H., Yoshii, M., and Mori, K.,** Clinical experience with intraoperative radiotherapy of locally advanced cancers, *Cancer,* 45, 40, 1980.
17. **Abe, M. and Takahashi, M.,** Intraoperative radiotherapy: the Japanese experience, *Int. J. Radiat. Oncol. Biol. Phys.,* 7, 863, 1981.
18. **Abe, M. and Takahashi, M.,** Klinische Erfahrungen mit der intraoperativen Strahlentherapie von local fortgeschrittenen Karzinomen, *Strahlentherapie,* 158, 585, 1982.
19. **Henschke, U. and Goldson, A. L.,** Personal communication, 1975.
20. **Goldson, A. C.,** Preliminary clinical experience with intraoperative radiotherapy, *J. Natl. Med. Assoc.,* 70, 483, 1978.
21. **Goldson, A. L.,** Past, present and prospects of intraoperative radiotherapy (IOR), *Semin. Oncol.,* 8, 59, 1981.
22. **Gunderson, L. L., Shipley, W. U., Suit, H. D., Epp, E. R., Nardi, G., Wood, W., Cohen, A. M., Nelson, J., Battit, G., Biggs, P. J., Russell, A., Rockett, A., and Clark, D.,** Intraoperative irradiation, A pilot study combining external beam photons with "boost" dose intraoperative electrons, *Cancer,* 49, 2259, 1982.
23. **Tepper, J. and Sindelar, W.,** Summary of the workshop on intraoperative radiation therapy, *Cancer Treat. Rep.,* 65, 9, 1981.
24. **Tepper, J., Sindelar, W., and Glatstein, E.,** Phase I study of intraoperative radiation therapy combined with radical surgery for intra-abdominal malignancies, *ASCO Proc.,* 21, 395, 1980.
25. **Gunderson, L. L., Martin, J. K., Jr., Earle, J. D., Byer, D. E., Voss, M., Fieck, J. M., Kvols, L. K., Rorie, D. K., Martinez, A. M., Nagorney, D. M., O'Connell, M. J., and Weber, F. C.,** Intraoperative and external beam irradiation with or without resection: Mayo pilot experience, *Mayo Clin. Proc.,* 59, 691, 1984.
26. **Rich, T. A., Cady, B., McDermott, W. V., Kase, K. R., Chaffey, J. T., and Hellman, S.,** Orthovoltage intraoperative radiotherapy: a new look at an old idea, *Int. J. Radiat. Oncol. Biol. Phys.,* 10, 1957, 1984.
27. **Gunderson, L. L., Tepper, J. E., Biggs, P. J., Goldson, A. L., Martin, J. K., McCullough, E. C., Rich, T. A., Shipley, W. U., Sindelar, W. F., and Wood, W. C.,** Intraoperative ± external beam irradiation, in *Current Problems in Cancer,* Vol. 7, Hickey, R. C., Ed., Year Book Medical Publishers, Chicago, 1983, 1.
28. **Abe, M.,** Intraoperative radiation therapy for gastrointestinal malignancy, in *Clinical Management of Gastrointestinal Cancer,* DeCosse, J. J. and Sherlock, P., Eds., Martinus Nijhoff, Boston, 1984, chap. 13.
29. **Matsumoto, K., Kakizoe, T., Mikuriya, S., Tanaka, T., Kondo, I., and Umegaki, Y.,** Clinical evaluation of intraoperative radiotherapy for carcinoma of the urinary bladder, *Cancer,* 47, 509, 1981.
30. **Takahashi, M., Okada, K., Shibamoto, Y., Abe, M., and Yoshida, O.,** Intraoperative radiotherapy in the definitive treatment of localized carcinoma of the prostate, *Int. J. Radiat. Oncol. Biol. Phys.,* 11, 147, 1985.
31. **Abe, M.,** Intraoperative radiotherapy for carcinoma of the stomach and the pancreas, in 16th Plenary Session Proceedings, ICR, Hawaii, 1985, 207.
32. **Wood, W. C., Shipley, W. U., Gunderson, L. L, Cohen, A. M., and Nardi, G. L.,** Intraoperative irradiation for unresectable pancreatic carcinoma, *Cancer,* 49, 1272, 1982.
33. **Matsutani, M., Matsuda, T., Nagashima, T., Kono, T., Hoshino, T., and Terao, H.,** Surgical treatment and radiation therapy for glioblastoma multiforme with special reference to intraoperative radiotherapy, *Jpn. J. Cancer,* 30, 201, 1984.
34. **Goldson, A. L., Delgado, G., and Hill, L. T.,** Intraoperative radiation of the paraaortic nodes in cancer of the uterine cervix, *Obstet. Gynecol.,* 52, 713, 1978.

35. **Goldson, A. L.,** Update on 5 years of pioneering experience with intraoperative electron irradiation, in *Proc. 9th Varian Clinic Users Meet.,* Session II, Varian, Palo Alto, 1982, 21.

36. **Goldson, A. L., Ashaveri, E., Espinoza, M. C., Roux, V., Cornwell, E., Rayford, L., McLaren, M., Nibhanupudy, R., Mahan, A., Taylor, H. F.,Hemphil, N., and Pearson, O.,** Single high dose intraoperative electrons for advanced stage pancreatic cancer: phase 1 pilot study, *Int. J. Radiat. Oncol. Biol. Phys.,* 7, 869, 1981.

37. **Goldson, A. L., Streeter, O. E., Jr., Ashaveri, E., Collier-Manning, J., Barber, J. B., and Fan, K. J.,** Intraoperative radiotherapy for intracranial malignancies, A pilot study, *Cancer,* 54, 2807, 1984.

38. **Tepper, J., Nardi, G., and Suit, H. D.,** Carcinoma of the pancreas: review of Massachusetts General Hospital's experience from 1963 to 1973, *Cancer,* 37, 1519, 1976.

39. **Gunderson, L. L., Cohen, A. C., Dosoretz, D. D., Shipley, W. U., Hedberg, S. E., Wood, W. C., Rodkey, G. V., and Suit, H. D.,** Residual, unresectable, or recurrent colorectal cancer: external beam irradiation and intraoperative electron beam boost ± resection, *Int. J. Radiat. Oncol. Biol. Phys.,* 9, 1597, 1983.

40. **Dosoretz, D. E., Gunderson, L. L., Hedberg, S., Hoskins, B., Blitzer, P. H., Shipley, W., and Cohen, A.,** Preoperative irradiation for unresectable rectal and rectosigmoid carcinomas, *Cancer,* 52, 814, 1983.

41. **Tepper, J. E., Wood, W. C., Cohen, A. M., Shipley, W. U., Orlow, E., Hedberg, S. E., Warshaw, A. L., Nardi, G. L., and Biggs, P. J.,** Intraoperative radiation therapy, in *Important Advances in Oncology 1985,* Devita, V. T., Jr., Hellman, S., and Rosenberg, S. A., Eds., Lippincott, Philadelphia, 1985, chap. 12.

42. **Suit, H. D., Mankin, H. J., Wood, W. C., and Proppe, K. H.,** Preoperative intraoperative, and postoperative radiation in the treatment of primary soft tissue sarcoma, *Cancer,* 55, 2659, 1985.

43. **Sindelar, W. F., Kinsella, T., Tepper, J. E., Travis, E. L., Rosenberg, S. A., and Glatstein, E.,** Experimental and clinical studies with intraoperative radiotherapy, *Surg. Gynecol. Obstet.,* 157, 205, 1983.

44. **Kaufann, B. H., Gunderson, L. L., Evans, R. G., Burgert, E. O., Jr., Gilchrist, G. S., and Smithson, W. A.,** Intraoperative irradiation: a new technique in pediatric oncology, *J. Pediatr. Surg.,* 19, 861, 1984.

45. **Dobelbower, R. R., Jr., Ahuja, R. K., Thomford, N. R., Mondalek, P. M., Neisler, J. W. H., Milligan, A. J., Phibbs, G. D., Merrick, H. W., Greenblatt, S. H., and Howard, J. M.,** Intraoperative electron beam therapy, 16th General Program, ICR, Hawaii, 1985, 362.

46. **Fuchs, G. and Uberall, R.,** Die intraoperative Rontgentherapie des Blasenkarzinoms, *Strahlentherapie,* 135, 280, 1968.

47. **Sabitzer, H., Manfreda, D., Millonig, H., Primik, F., Redtenbacher, M., and Schneider, F.,** Chirurgischradiologisch kombiniertes Therapieverfahren beim Pankreaskarzonoma-Falldemonstration-Zukunftsaspekte, *Wien. Klin. Wochenschr.,* 95, 523, 1983.

48. **Frommhold, H.,** Personal communication, 1985.

49. **Calvo, F. A.,** Personal communication, 1987.

50. **Vermeij, J., Oldhoff, J., and Crommelin, M. A.,** Personal communication.

Chapter 2

THE RATIONALE FOR INTRAOPERATIVE RADIOTHERAPY

Ralph R. Dobelbower, Jr.

TABLE OF CONTENTS

I. INTRODUCTION

In many oncologic clinical situations the dose of radiation that can be safely delivered to a tumor is restricted by the limited radiation tolerance of adjacent normal tissue. By avoiding delivery of high doses to these tissues, we can improve the therapeutic ratio of local control to complication. The therapeutic ratio is a measure of radiocurability and can be described by the following relationship:

$$\text{Therapeutic ratio} = \frac{\text{normal tissue tolerance dose}}{\text{tumoricidal dose}}$$

where the normal tissue tolerance dose and the tumoricidal dose must be individually defined for the specific tumor and tissue in question.

The goal of definitive (curative) radiotherapy is to produce local tumor eradication without unacceptable complications. The radiotherapist tries to use a dose and technique of irradiation which will maximize tumor control and minimize the risk of clinically significant complications. When the therapeutic ratio is greater than one (i.e., when the tumoricidal dose is less than the normal tissue tolerance dose), cure without complication is possible, but when the therapeutic ratio is less than one (i.e., when the tumoricidal dose exceeds the normal tissue tolerance dose), treatment to curative dose levels is not possible without significant risk of complication.

Unfortunately, the therapeutic ratio appears to be somewhat less than one in a number of clinical situations; unresectable adenocarcinoma of the pancreas, malignant mesothelioma, cancer of the biliary tree, glioblastoma multiforme, etc. To improve the cure rate in the treatment of any tumor, one must be able to modify either the aggressiveness or the efficacy of the treatment without significantly increasing the complication rate. The rationale for this approach is illustrated in Figure 1. In this figure, the curves describing the tumor control probability and the probability of normal tissue complication as a function of radiation dose have similar shapes (but may have different slopes) and will generally be displaced from one another on the dose axis. The relative position of these curves in any given circumstance determines the therapeutic ratio, which becomes increasingly favorable as the curve for tumor control is located further to the left of the curve for normal tissue tolerance (i.e., the therapeutic ratio increases). In other circumstances, when the curve for tumor control is located to the right of the normal tissue complication curve, the therapeutic ratio is equal to a value less than unity. Note, however, that if normal tissue damage or complications are to be avoided altogether, the radiation dose cannot exceed A, but in this case, tumor control probability is low. By accepting a relatively low probability of normal tissue injury, the radiation dose can be increased to B, where the tumor control probability is significantly improved. Further increase of radiation dose above C, where tumor control probability is very high, will only result in an increased complication rate. Such an increase of dose beyond C will result in a less favorable therapeutic ratio without concommitant increase in local tumor control. Often there is considerable overlap on the dose axis of the upper range of the tumor control curve and the lower range of the normal tissue injury curve. Under these circumstances, the radiotherapist must make a value judgment as to what level of normal tissue injury is acceptable in return for an improved probability of tumor control. Thus, it is theoretically possible to achieve local control of any tumor if a high enough radiation dose is delivered to the local site. In practice, however, one can deliver only the dose that is tolerated by the normal tissues in the treatment area.

Thus, in order to improve the cure rate or the therapeutic ratio in the treatment of any tumor, we must be able to modify either the aggressiveness or the efficacy of the treatment without significantly increasing the complication rate. This is demonstrated schematically

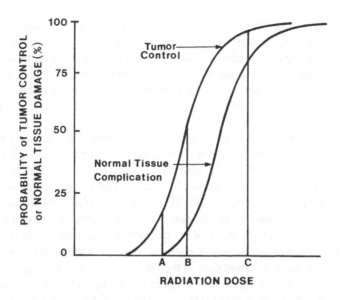

FIGURE 1. Probability of tumor control and normal tissue complication as functions of radiation dose. (A) Dose for low probability of local tumor control with minimal risk of normal tissue complication. (B) Dose for moderate likelihood of local tumor control with low risk of normal tissue complication. (C) Dose for maximum probability of local tumor control with high risk of normal tissue complications. (Modified from Withers, H. R. and Peters, L. J., in *Textbook of Radiotherapy*, Fletcher, G., Ed., Lea & Febiger, Philadelphia, 1980, 144. With permission.)

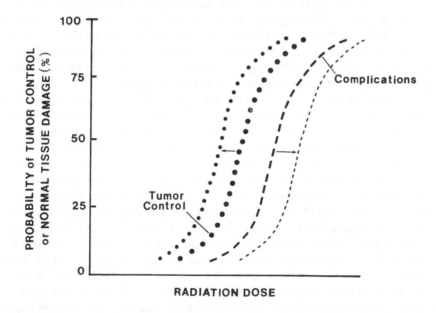

FIGURE 2. Probability of tumor control (· ·) and normal tissue complications (– – –) as functions of radiation dose. The therapeutic ratio (see text) is improved as the tumor control curve shifts to the left or the complication curve shifts to the right along the radiation dose axis.

in Figure 2. With increasing doses of radiation, the likelihood of local tumor control increases, but the likelihood of complication may also increase. In order to improve the therapeutic ratio, an agent or technique must either move the tumor control curve to the left and increase the efficacy of treatment or move the complication curve to the right and decrease complications. Under these circumstances, the radiotherapist must make a value judgement as to what level of normal tissue injury is acceptable in return for an improved probability of tumor control.

For improved tumor control with minimal complications, it is necessary to improve the therapeutic ratio by various manipulations: fractionation and protraction of radiation dose; radiosensitizers; adjuvants such as chemotherapy, immunotherapy, and hyperthermia; regional therapy; field shaping; multiple fields; intracavitary or interstitial placement of radioisotopes; shrinking field techniques; etc. The most successful of these manipulations aim at delivering the radiation dose on the disease and sparing adjacent normal tissue.

Intraoperative radiation therapy (IORT), in general, and intraoperative electron beam therapy (IOEBT), in particular, represent attempts to improve the therapeutic ratio by direct application of a large single radiation dose to the surgically exposed tumor, the partly resected tumor, or the bed of a resected tumor. This permits precise tumor dose localization while sensitive normal tissues, such as small bowel, are displaced from the path of the beam. This allows delivery of a higher radiation dose and hopefully will result in increased local tumor control without increased radiation complications.

II. ADVANTAGES AND DISADVANTAGES OF IORT

There are several biological disadvantages of IORT, including the use of a single dose which limits sublethal damage repair, repopulation, redistribution, and reoxgenation — processes which form the bases for enhancing the therapeutic ratio with conventional fractionated radiation therapy. The major advantage of IORT is exclusion of most normal tissue from the path of the radiation beam. However, a large, single radiation dose (15 to 30 Gy) may not sterilize tumor in all cases. Clearly, this depends on the bulk of the disease, and an adjunct may be needed. The philosophy in most cases has been to employ IORT as a boost treatment in addition to conventional external beam therapy.

With the combination of surgery and irradiation (IORT), one can direct a beam of radiation directly to a surgically exposed unresectable neoplasm or to the bed of a resected tumor after surgically displacing adjacent critical structures from the path of the beam. Since tumor may extend to the surface of exposed tissue to be irradiated, and since critical organs such as kidneys or spinal cord may be directly behind the tumor, the following dosimetric characteristics are important: high surface dose, uniform dose through the target volume, and fast fall-off of dose with tissue depth deep to the target volume. The radiation beam most commonly used for IORT is a megavoltage electron beam, since such beams provide reasonable dose homogeneity with rapid fall-off of dose beyond the treatment volume (Figure 3). By employing electron beams for IORT, one can avoid irradiation of structures deep to the target volume. As the volume to be irradiated is relatively small, and as the tissue irradiated is predominately tumor, doses on the order of 10 to 50 Gy can be delivered. Another advantage of IORT is that surgery is not delayed as it is with preoperative irradiation.

There are several potential advantages of using a combined external beam-IORT approach over IORT alone. By delivering external beam therapy after IORT, one may improve local tumor control by decreasing the risk of marginal or incisional recurrence as both areas may be included in the external beam fields.

Finally, the disadvantages of IORT are primarily radiobiological and practical. In general, fractionated radiation therapy is superior to single-dose treatment because tumors are composed of individual cells that differ in radiosensitivity according to position in the cell

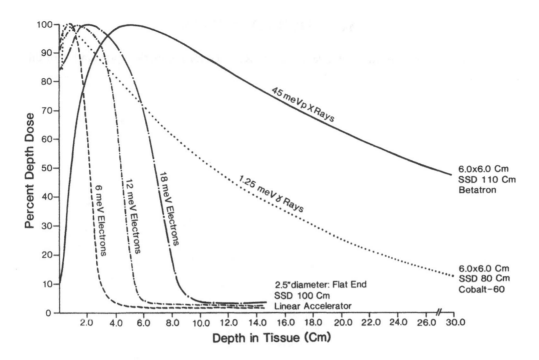

FIGURE 3. Percent radiation dose as function of depth in tissue for five radiation beams. Photons: 45-million electron volt peak (meVp) X-rays (———); 1.25-meVp γ-rays (· · ·). Electrons: 6 meV (– – – – –); 12 meV (·–··–·); 18 meV (·——·). In comparison to high-energy photon beams, electron beams provide (1) Relatively high surface dose, (2) Relatively uniform dose distribution to a certain depth, and (3) Rapid decrease of dose with increasing depth in tissue after a certain depth. The depth of electron penetration and dose deposition increases with increasing electron beam energy.

cycle and oxygen tension. With conventional fractionated radiation therapy, cells in relatively radioresistant phases of the cell cycle have an opportunity to progress into a more radiosensitive phase before subsequent radiation fractions are delivered. Also, with fractionated therapy, hypoxic cells may be reoxygenated between fractions, resulting in greater tumor responsiveness than with single-dose treatments.

Practical difficulties with IORT are related to integrating two modalities: surgery and radiation therapy. This is best accomplished in a single room, which necessitates either placing a radiation therapy machine in a surgical suite, or modifying a radiation therapy suite to meet operating room standards. Neither approach is simple, nor inexpensive. The alternative is to transport anesthetized patients with open surgical wounds from the surgical suite to the radiation therapy suite (and, in some instances, back to the surgical suite), which can produce measurable changes in vital physiologic functions. Trauma may be caused by transportation. Also, it may not be possible to adequately protect the patient or the equipment from significant incidental contamination with infectious agents while in transit. Conventional anesthesia equipment is not designed to operate while being jostled and transported. Operation under such conditions may result in unpredictable alterations in function. Accidental disconnection or malfunction of critical monitoring equipment during transportation is yet another potential hazard. For these reasons, IORT is best carried out in specially constructed suites where patient transport is minimal. However, many investigators have reported transporting anesthetized patients to and from radiation therapy facilities (in separate buildings in some instances) without catastrophe.

The subsequent chapters in this work report experiences and results from investigators around the world using IORT in attempts to enhance the therapeutic ratio in the treatment of malignant disease in various clinical situations.

ACKNOWLEDGMENTS

The author expresses his gratitude to Sandra K. Price for her clerical preparation of this manuscript.

Chapter 3

RADIOBIOLOGY OF LARGE RADIATION FRACTIONS

Andrew J. Milligan

TABLE OF CONTENTS

I. RADIOBIOLOGY OF LARGE RADIATION FRACTIONS

Few data exist in the recent literature describing the effects of large radiation fractions on either tumors or normal tissues. In a discussion of intraoperative radiation therapy (IORT), where radiation doses are typically delivered in one fraction, few reports accurately describe tissue responses. Since the field is relatively new, and radiobiological documentation of tissue responses have yet to be clarified, no sound theoretical basis exists for determining tissue tolerances to these high doses.

The general concept of tolerance is vague and can be interpreted differently within the radiotherapy community. Complications can run the gamut from death to minimal tissue injury with many different radiation effects considered complications by both the radiation therapy and radiation biology communities. However, it must be stressed that complications must be evaluated in any given clinical situation to establish a risk-benefit ratio. Essentially, the situation comes down to a choice between low tumor control rates with no complications vs. high tumor control rates with commensurate complications.[1]

Much of the data describing normal tissue complications and local tumor control from radiation therapy arises from the work of Stranquist in 1944.[2] He produced a series of isoeffect curves for a series of tissue and tumor endpoints: skin necrosis, cure of skin cancer, moist desquamation, dry desquamation, and erythema. He characterized the total dose of radiation required to effect each of these specific endpoints as a function of the time over which a radiation fractionation protocol was delivered (Figure 1). The responses are parallel, but not identical, for all tumor and normal tissues, indicating that different doses are required for achievement of different tissue endpoints. These data were generated for squamous cell carcinoma, and application of this information to other tumors, such as pancreatic adeno-carcinoma, may not be appropriate. It is essential that a series of curves be generated for each tumor histopathologic type.

In 1951, Cohen[3] published data exploring the biological dose factors in clinical radiation therapy. In the report, he explored the effect of various fraction numbers and sizes on tumor curability. He studied a series of 10 patients with epidermoid carcinoma receiving single doses of radiation therapy from 14 to 25 Gy. All the patients receiving single-dose radiation therapy were cured of their respective tumors, with the exception of one patient treated for a head and neck lesion with 14 Gy. Comparisons were made between tumor cure doses and skin necrosis doses. While achieving these cure rates, the acceptable skin tolerance dose was determined to be approximately 15 Gy, with the risk of normal tissue necrosis at this dose under 2%. For a single dose of radiation, the mean tumor control dose was approximately 15 Gy, which compared favorably to the skin tolerance dose. The probability of curing an irradiated tumor was estimated to be 90% at a tumor dose of 20 Gy.

In 1969, Field[4] reported early and late effects in the skin of rats following irradiation. He compared the effects of single X-ray doses to fractionated X-ray doses. A dose of 34.5 Gy was delivered in one fraction, and the skin reaction following treatment was observed for 40 weeks. He reported that after irradiation of the foot, erythema and swelling appeared within a few hours and lasted for a few days. At 7 d postirradiation, a second wave of erythema began with subsequent breakdown of the tissue after the larger radiation doses. The peak of this reaction was reached on day 17 or 18, with subsequent healing. Field reported that this wave of radiation damage was recognized as an early reaction to radiation. Following this early reaction, at 8 weeks posttreatment, the injury once again began to increase, with a further wave lasting much longer than the first with resultant necrosis of tissue at the larger doses. Field concluded that the relationship between early and late reactions in rat skin was the same for one, two, or five fractions of radiation. For all treatment regimens, once a critical dose was reached, late reactions resulting from irradiation of normal tissues increased with dose much more sharply than the early reactions. He concluded that early reactions were a sensitive measure of late radiation injury.

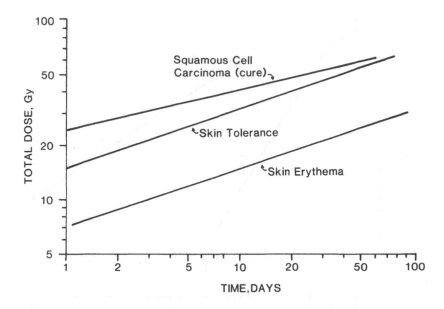

FIGURE 1. Isoeffect dose for specific endpoints (shown on figure) as a function of time over which radiation is delivered.

Ellis, in 1969,[5] described responses of various tissues to different fractionation schemes in an article exploring the usefulness of the nominal standard dose concept. In single-dose treatments, the control dose for squamous cell carcinoma was approximately 25 Gy, while the normal tissue tolerance for human skin was approximately 15 Gy. However, the corresponding difference between tumor and normal tissue decreased significantly for protracted radiotherapy. At a period of about 6 weeks, the typical control dose for human squamous cell carcinoma was approximately 60 Gy, while the normal tolerance dose for human skin was about 52 Gy. The differences between these doses were much less than those observed for single fractions.

In 1977, Ellis and Goldson[6] published a report of 35 patients treated with various fraction schemes for a variety of tumors. While the majority of these patients were treated with fractionated radiotherapy, a number of them received single large doses of radiation followed by additional fractionated radiotherapy. While the situation was not directly applicable to IORT, large initial radiation fractions of up to 8.5 Gy were employed. Under specific circumstances, once-a-week treatments were better than multiple fractions per week. They suggested that cells with higher extrapolation numbers responded to a smaller number of large fractions, leaving fewer cellular survivors than conventional protracted radiation doses. A small number of large dose fractions demonstrated the same cell-killing effect on normal connective tissue as conventional fractionation, but a greater cell-killing effect was observed on cells with higher extrapolation numbers, such as certain radioresistant tumors.

Since few data exist concerning the effects of single, high-dose radiation to specific organs, the most appropriate studies for examining differential tumor and normal tissue response are fractionation studies. With single, high-dose radiation therapy, the classical four "R's" of radiobiology need to be examined in terms of their response. These four R's include: (1) recovery from sublethal damage, (2) repopulation of the tumor and normal tissue, (3) reoxygenation of the tumor during treatment, and (4) redistribution of cells in the cell cycle. With single-dose radiotherapy, cells have no time to undergo these characteristic changes.[7] Nevertheless, examination of a variety of fractionation models may provide information as to the effects in both tumor and normal tissues resulting from single, high-dose radiation treatments.

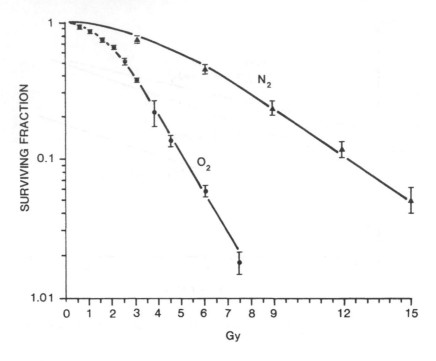

FIGURE 2.   Cellular survival vs. radiation dose for cells irradiated under oxygenated (O_2) conditions or hypoxic (N_2) conditions.

In the single, high-dose treatments, the principle which governs radiation response of the irradiated tissue is the radiation sensitivity of the irradiated tissues. By examination of tissue response to various fractionation protocols, extrapolation may be possible to single IORT doses to examine biological effects. Although shorter overall treatment times may be desirable to treat a growing tumor, the effects of large single-dose fractions are largely unknown.

It has become more clear over the past several years that large single doses produce higher complication rates than expected in normal tissues. This is due to the steeper relationship between effective dose per fraction to late radiation injury. One technique for assessing effects due to altered fractionation schemes has been the linear quadratic model of radiation response of tissue. Examining a typical radiation dose, cell survival curve (Figure 2), the dose response relationship can be described by:[8] $S = e^{-(\alpha D + \beta D^2)}$, where S = fractional survival, D = radiation dose, and α, β = constants determined from mathematical curve fitting.

The two constants of this linear quadratic model represent two phases of the cell survival curves. This initial gradual slope is controlled by the D portion of the mathematical model, and the latter, steeper portion of the survival curve is controlled by the D^2 portion of the model. One useful quantity to evolve from this model has been the ratio of α/β, which has the dimensions of cGy^{-1}. This quantity indicates the dose at which the cell-killing rate from the linear low-dose term is equal to the cell-killing rate from the dose-squared term. Characteristically, late-reacting tissues (i.e., tissues that demonstrate late radiation effects) are described by small α/β ratios, indicating survival curves which "bend over" at relatively low doses. Those cells that demonstrate survival curves with high α/β ratios indicate cells of early reacting tissues.

The effect of fractionation on tissues is characterized by the isoeffect relationship.[9] The relationship between total dose required to achieve isoeffect and dose per fraction suggests that tissues demonstrating delayed effects display steeper slopes than those for early acute effects. This relationship between early and late effects is described by the α/β ratio determined from the survival curves. For IORT, extrapolation of the fractionation curves to one fraction may provide insight into the differences in response between tissues; however, no justification has been provided for use of this technique for examining differences in tissue response to IORT doses. Regardless, this may be one mechanism by which comparison between radiation responses of tissues can be performed at high doses.

Overgaard et al.,[10] in 1985, reported a series of melanoma patients treated with two different fractionation schemes, 9 Gy for three fractions vs. 5 Gy for eight fractions. While no statistically significant difference was noted between the tumor responses of patients treated by these two different fractionation schemes, a difference was seen in the normal tissue reactions. Those patients treated with the 9 Gy fractions displayed a higher percentage of normal tissue complications. This pattern was also reported in a study by Jacobsson et al.,[11] in 1985, in which they examined dose-response curves for mouse bone regeneration after single doses of cobalt-60 irradiation. As radiation doses increased up to 18 Gy per fraction, normal tissue reactions increased as monitored by lip mucosal reaction. At doses of approximately 15 Gy per fraction, the average mucosal reaction was a severe reddening of the tissue. However, at doses of 18 Gy per fraction, the average reaction consisted of exudation or a crust covering about half of the mice lips. A dose-response curve for bone regeneration produced by Jacobsson et al. demonstrated a graded response in percent change in bone formation as a function of (single) radiation dose. They examined five radiation doses: 5, 8, 11, 15, and 26 Gy and investigated bone regeneration using a bone growth chamber. They observed that in a dose range of 5 to 8 Gy, bone regeneration was reduced by about 20% compared to nonirradiated controls. Between 8 and 11 Gy, they postulated that a small increase in radiation dose resulted in greatly reduced bone formation. At 11 Gy and above, the depression in bone formation, as compared to controls, was about 65 to 75%. Therefore, the crucial dose for bone regeneration was approximately between 8 and 11 Gy. Within that range, there was a critical relationship for normal tissue response.

Archambeau et al.,[12] in 1985, examined dermal microvascular morphology response after single radiation doses of 16.49, 22.31, and 26.19 Gy in swine skin. They described a series of events occurring at various times postirradiation. Moist desquamation occurred between 23 and 36 d following these single-dose X-ray exposures, with loss and subsequent repopulation of epidermal basal cells. Following this initial phase, a second breakdown occurred in tissue between 36 and 70 d, resulting in loss of endothelial cells in the vessels of the dermis. However, the qualitative morphology of the microvasculature remained unchanged from the time of irradiation until approximately 32 to 36 d posttreatment. This decrease in endothelial cell population resulted in a second breakdown of the epithelium. Archambeau[13] also described a difference in the time course of response of the endothelial population density and the epidermal population following single exposures to high doses. During the period of 28 to 32 d following irradiation, there were no changes in the endothelial cell population. During the time when no changes occurred in the endothelial population, the epidermal population decreased to a minimum and returned to control levels. This epidermal population change was due to the response of the cells and the recovery of those cells following irradiation. The second decrease in epidermal population occurred after 32 to 36 d following irradiation and was concurrent with a decrease in an endothelial cell population. This secondary epidermal loss was due to a decrease in the microvascular component of the tissue. The average turnover time of the microvascular component varied, ranging from months to years. If the changes observed in response to radiation hold for other endothelial components, this suggests that the average turnover time of the endothelial cells is approximately 1 month.

Thames et al.[14] examined tissue responses following varied dose fractionation schedules. The biologic effects were altered in response to various fractionation schemes and by using mathematical models for the linear quadratic formula; predictions were made describing the effects of high single doses of radiation on specific cell populations. Data suggested a dissociation of the acute and late radiation responses with changes in the dose per fraction. These differences were modeled and the quantity of the α/β was indicative of the response for each individual tissue. The α/β ratio for acute reactions was greater than the α/β ratio for late reactions. Therefore, examination of the survival curves of individual tissues suggested which tissues were more susceptable to the development of late effects following high-dose irradiation. The differences in dose survival curves for tumors and their normal tissue counterparts indicated that worsening of late effects might accompany increases in dose per fraction, with no change in acute reactions. This observation suggests that in the IORT setting, where high doses of radiation are delivered in one fraction, there is a decided disadvantage if both tumor and surrounding normal tissues are irradiated with equally high doses.

II. SUMMARY

From the radiobiology standpoint, it is clear that the high dose of radiation delivered by IORT techniques is not advantageous for eliminating tumors while preserving normal tissue. The normal tissues are at a higher risk for developing late complications as described by the α/β ratios, while the treatment of tumors with single-dose radiation therapy is not able to take advantage of factors such as reoxygenation for maximum tumor elimination. The fundamental advantage of IORT lies not in the radiobiological principles, but rather in the physical principle of the therapy. If radiation doses are delivered to tumors while sparing surrounding normal tissues, then differences in radiation sensitivity and response of these tissues become an insignificant point, since little or no radiation is delivered to the normal structures. While the radiobiologic principles are important to consider in the treatment of tissue with radiation, in this application the fundamental advantage lies in the physical principle of depositing energy within the tumor by accurate localization of the radiation dose. If significant normal structures receive as high a dose as the irradiated tumor, severe complications will result, allowing little or no advantage to this type of therapy.

REFERENCES

1. **Goitein, M. and Schultheiss, T. E.**, Strategies for treating possible tumor extension: some theoretical considerations, *Int. J. Radiat. Oncol. Biol. Phys.*, 11, 1519, 1985.
2. **Strandqvist, M.**, Studien uber die Kimulative Wirkung der Rontgenstrahlen bei Fraktionerung, *Acta Radiol.*, 55, 1, 1944.
3. **Cogen, L.**, Estimation of biological dosage, factors in clinical radiotherapy, in *Dosage Factors in Radiotherapy*, 1951, 180.
4. **Field, S. B.**, Early and late reactions in skin of fats following irradiation with X-rays or fast neutrons, *Radiology*, 92, 381, 1969.
5. **Ellis, F.**, Dose, time and fractionation: a clinical hypothesis, *Clin. Radiol.*, 20, 1, 1969.
6. **Ellis, F. and Goldson, A. L.**, Once a week treatments, *Int. J. Radiat. Oncol. Biol. Phys.*, 2, 537, 1977.
7. **Beck-Bornholdt, H.-P., Peacock, J. H., Biol, M. I., and Stephens, T. C.**, Kinetics of cellular inactivation by fractionated and hyperfractionated irradiation in Lewis lung carcinoma, *Int. J. Radiat. Oncol. Biol. Phys.*, 11, 1171, 1985.
8. **Thames, H. D., Withers, R. W., Peters, L. J., and Fletcher, G. H.**, Changes in early and late radiation responses with altered dose fractionation: implications for dose-survival relationships, *Int. J. Radiat. Oncol. Biol. Phys.*, 8, 219, 1982.
9. **Williams, M. V., Denekamp, J., and Fowler, J. F.**, A review of α/β ratios for experimental tumors: implications for clinical studies of altered fractionation, *Int. J. Radiat. Oncol. Biol. Phys.*, 11, 87, 1985.

10. **Overgaard, J., von der Maase, H., and Overgaard, M.,** A randomized study comparing two high-dose per fraction radiation schedules in recurrent or metastatic malignant melanoma, *Int. J. Radiat. Oncol. Biol. Phys.,* 11, 1836, 1985.

11. **Jacobsson, M., Jonsson, A., Albrektsson, T., and Turesson, I.,** Dose-response for bone regeneration after single doses of cobalt-60 irradiation, *Int. J. Radiat. Oncol. Biol. Phys.,* 11, 1963, 1985.

12. **Archambeau, J. O., Ines, A., and Fajardo, L. F.,** Correlation of the dermal microvasculature morphology with the epidermal and endothelial population changes produced by single X-ray fractions of 1649, 2231 and 2619 rad in swine, *Int. J. Radiat. Oncol. Biol. Phys.,* 11, 1639, 1985.

13. **Archambeau, J. O. and Bennett, G. W.,** Quantification of morphologic, cytologic and kinetic parameters of unirradiated swine skin: a histologic model, *Radiat. Res.,* 98, 254, 1984.

14. **Thames, H. D., Withers, H. R., and Peters, L. J.,** Tissue repair capacity and repair kinetics deduced from multifractionated or continuous irradiation regimens with incomplete repair, *Br. J. Cancer,* 49, 263, 1985.

Chapter 4

APPLICATION OF DOSE-EFFECT RELATIONSHIPS TO INTRAOPERATIVE RADIOTHERAPY

Colin G. Orton

TABLE OF CONTENTS

I. INTRODUCTION

The need for reliable dose-effect relationships in fractionated radiotherapy has increased significantly in recent years with the advent of a variety of innovative fractionation techniques, such as hyperfractionation, hypofractionation, accelerated fractionation, high dose rate fractionated remote afterloading, single fraction intraoperative radiotherapy (IORT), and many forms of dynamic fractionation. Unfortunately, there are many problems associated with the use of the two most commonly cited dose-effect relationships: the time-dose factor, TDF (or NSD/CRE), and the linear-quadratic, L-Q, models. Some of these problems are reviewed in this chapter.

A. THE TDF MODEL

The principal advantage of the TDF model is simplicity. TDFs calculated for different parts of a course of radiotherapy as linearly additive (unlike NSDs and CREs) and account for the effects of all three parameters: time, dose, and fractionation.[1] There is provision for the calculation of TDFs for brachytherapy and for combined brachytherapy/fractionated therapy modalities.[2] Finally, the scale of TDFs is convenient; a TDF of 100 being roughly equivalent to normal connective tissue tolerance.[3]

The disadvantages of the TDF method are, however, numerous. The exponents used in the TDF equation appear to be appropriate only for certain tissues and organs and for certain endpoints, either acute or late effects, rarely both.[4-11] Also, even when the TDF equation applies, it is only useful over a restricted range of values of time, dose, and fractionation.[12,13] It is probable that the TDF equation is not a good approximation for the large single doses used in IORT. This, however, is thought by some people to not be a problem with the L-Q model.

B. THE L-Q MODEL

The L-Q model is based upon the apparent linear-quadratic shape of cell survival curves, for which there is some radiobiological and physical support.[14-20] The analogue of TDF in the L-Q model is the extrapolated response dose (ERD).[16] This model is relatively simple to use, although many of the publications written about it make ERDs seem almost as difficult to use as was the case in the early days of the CRE concept.[21] Most authors have failed to point out that, like their counterpart TDFs, ERDs are linearly proportional to the number of fractions and, hence, are also linearly additive.

Many of the disadvantages of the L-Q model are similar to those of TDFs. The important parameter α/β is known only approximately and for only a few human tissues and organs.[16] The appropriate values of α/β depend upon the endpoint observed (early or late effects), and these are not known for most human tissues.[16] Finally, in order to account for the effects of overall treatment time upon proliferation, an additional "time" factor has to be incorporated into the L-Q equation.[16] This not only greatly complicates its use, but adds one more "unknown and untested" parameter to the model. However, in IORT, the use of single doses precludes any problems of ignoring overall treatment time, unless a supplementary course of fractionated therapy is given.

One further problem with the L-Q method which applies equally to the TDF concept (and almost all other dose-effect models) is that no provision is made for application to inhomogeneous dose distributions.

C. INHOMOGENEOUS DOSE DISTRIBUTIONS

It is rare in IORT that a single organ or tissue will be irradiated uniformly throughout. Yet, most dose-effect relationships allow for the use of only a single value for this tissue "dose". It is unclear whether it is most appropriate to use the maximum, the minimum, the mean, or the modal dose for this value. Indeed, in many instances the dose distribution varies so much across the tissue or organ that it is probable that none of these values are appropriate.

What is needed is some type of "integral" dose-effect model similar to the integral-response models recently introduced by several investigators for the calculation of probabilities of complication.[22-25] Two such models are presented in this chapter, one based upon the TDF concept, and the other upon the L-Q method. At the same time, many of the problems of these two models cited earlier have been corrected in a consistent and unified manner, thus making it easy to compare the results obtained by the application of the two methods. These models are presented in the following two sections.

II. THE INTEGRAL TDF MODEL

Before proceeding to discuss the handling of inhomogeneous dose distributions, it is expedient to first review the derivation of a variable-exponent TDF equation which effectively eliminates several of the problems cited earlier and incorporates some of the advantages in a uniform manner. More detailed discussions of this variable-exponent model have been presented elsewhere, so only a brief review will be given here.[26,27]

A. VARIABLE-EXPONENT TDF EQUATION

Many investigators have proposed the use of different exponents for the TDF (or NSD/CRE) equation,[4-11] but none have done so in a unified way. Consequently, a wide variety of TDF values have resulted, apparently unrelated in any systematic way to tissue tolerance. Many inherent advantages of the TDF concept are lost. The following "unified" variable-exponent TDF equation[26-27] maintains these advantages, even after the addition of a "volume" correction factor, which is an essential component of the integral TDF concept to be described later:

$$TDF = K_1 N d^\delta (T/N)^{-\tau} v^\phi \tag{1}$$

where N = number of fractions, d = dose per fraction, T/N = average time in days between fractions, δ, τ, and ϕ are tissue-specific exponents, v is the partial volume of tissue irradiated and is a fraction of some reference volume ($v = 1$), and K_1 is a scaling factor which makes TDF = 100 for the reference volume ($v = 1$) of tissue irradiated to tolerance.

It should be realized that not only are the values of the parameters δ, τ, ϕ, and K_1 dependent upon the specific tissue irradiated, they are probably also dependent upon the endpoint observed, e.g., early or late effects.

An example of the use of this model will be presented later and compared to solutions obtained by the other models to follow.

B. THE ITDF EQUATION

In order to integrate the effects of inhomogeneously irradiating different partial volumes of a tissue or organ to different doses, it is necessary to divide the volume of the tissue of interest into partial volume elements Δv_i, which are not necessarily equal in size nor are they necessarily small, but within which the dose per fraction, d_i, is constant. Then, since the TDF calculated using Equation 1 for each volume element ($= TDF_i$) is a linear function of $(\Delta v_i)^\phi$, it is apparent that values of $(TDF_i)^{1/\phi}$ are linearly additive. Hence, if this "integral" TDF is ITDF,[28]

$$(ITDF)^{1/\phi} = \sum_i (TDF_i)^{1/\phi}$$

or

$$ITDF = \left[\sum_i (TDF_i)^{1/\phi} \right]^{\phi}$$

which leads to the equation

$$ITDF = K_1 \left[\sum_i \{N_i d_i^\delta (T_i/N_i)^{-\tau}(v_i)^\phi\}^{1/\phi} \right]^{\phi} \qquad (2)$$

Note that in most practical applications it is only the dose per fraction, d_i, that will be different in each partial volume element of an inhomogeneous dose distribution; so N_i and (T_i/N_i) will be constant and the ITDF equation is simplified.

An example of the use of Equation 2 will be presented later, after presentation of the integral L-Q model.

III. THE INTEGRAL L-Q MODEL

As was the case with TDFs, it is necessary to introduce a volume correction factor into the L-Q equation in order to apply it to inhomogeneous dose distributions. Furthermore, it is expedient to also incorporate a scaling factor in order to avoid generating a wide variety of extrapolated response doses whose magnitude depends upon the α/β values used and bears no simple relationship to tissue tolerance. The conventional ERD equation is[16]

$$ERD = Nd\left(1 + \frac{d}{\alpha/\beta} \right)$$

where α/β is a tissue-specific parameter which may be different for early and late reactions.

In order to avoid confusion, a new term, the linear-quadratic factor (LQF), will be used for the modified, scaled, and volume-dependent ERD equation,[27] where

$$LQF = k_1 Nd\left(1 + \frac{d}{\alpha/\beta} \right)v^\phi \qquad (3)$$

where k_1 is a scaling factor which makes LQF = 100 for the reference volume ($v = 1$) of tissue irradiated to tolerance.

As before, an example of the use of this equation will be given later.

A. THE ILQF EQUATION

Using the same nomenclature as for the derivation of the ITDF model, the ILQF equation is[28]

$$ILQF = \left[\sum_i (LQF_i)^{1/\phi} \right]^{\phi}$$

or

$$ILQF = k_1 \left[\sum_i \left\{ N_i d_i \left(1 + \frac{d_i}{\alpha/\beta} \right)(\Delta v_i)^\phi \right\}^{1/\phi} \right]^{\phi} \qquad (4)$$

As before with the ITDF equation, this is simplified in most practical situations where N_i is constant for all volume elements.

The following IORT example will demonstrate the practical application of all four of the equations presented above.

IV. EXAMPLE: INTRAOPERATIVE THERAPY

A patient with recurrent pelvic disease has received whole pelvis irradiation in 28 treatments of 1.8 Gy/fraction. Both ureters were included in this volume. Further treatment is to be delivered intraoperatively with high-energy electrons. The treatment plan shows that, on average, one fifth of the ureters will receive the full 100% electron dose, one fifth will receive 80% of this dose, one fifth 60%, one fifth 40%, and one fifth 20%. What maximum electron beam dose (at the 100% level) can be delivered in a single fraction without exceeding ureteral tolerance, assuming that "tolerance" for total organ irradiation is reached in 35 daily fractions of 2.14 Gy/fraction?

A. TDF SOLUTION

Assuming that it is necessary to consider that both ureters are irradiated to the maximum dose, then the TDF for the IORT is

$$TDF_{IORT} = K_1 Nd^\delta (T/N)^{-\tau}$$

$$= K_1 d^\delta$$

since, for a single fraction, $N = 1$ and, for simplicity, (T/N) has been assumed to be also equal to unity.

The TDF parameters δ, τ, and ϕ are not known for ureteral irradiation. For demonstration purposes, the published values for stroma of $\delta = 1.538$, $\tau = 0.169$, and $\phi = 0.18$ will be assumed to apply.[26,27] The value of K_1, determined by substitution of $d = 2.14$ Gy/fraction, $N = 35$, and $T/N = 1.33$ days/fraction in the TDF equation, is

$$K_1 = 0.931$$

The TDF to both ureters from the whole pelvis irradiation is

$$TDF_{WP} = 0.931 \times 28 \times 1.8^{1.538} \times (1.33)^{-0.169}$$

$$= 61.3$$

Then the residual TDF which can be delivered by a single dose of d Gy by IORT is given by

$$TDF_{IORT} = 100 - 61.3 = 38.7 = 0.931\ d^{1.538}$$

Solving for d gives

$$d = 11.28 \text{ Gy/fraction (large volume)}$$

However, if it is assumed that ureteral tolerance is governed by irradiation of only the small ($v = 0.2$) volume of the ureters irradiated to the maximum dose, then the TDF to this small volume from the whole pelvis irradiation is thus

$$\mathrm{TDF_{WP}} = 0.931 \times 28 \times 1.8^{1.538} \times (1.33)^{-0.169} \times (0.2)^{0.18}$$

$$= 45.9$$

Hence,

$$\mathrm{TDF_{IORT}} = 100 - 45.9 = 54.1 = 0.931 \, d^{1.538} \times (0.2)^{0.18}$$

which yields

$$d = 16.92 \text{ Gy/fraction (small volume)}$$

B. LQF SOLUTION

The value of k_1 is determined by substitution of $N = 35$, $d = 2.14$ Gy/fraction, and $\alpha/\beta = 2.5$ Gy (assumed) in the LQF equation

$$\mathrm{LQF} = 100 = k_1 \times 35 \times 2.14\left(1 + \frac{2.14}{2.5}\right)$$

Hence,

$$k_1 = 0.719$$

Then, assuming that both ureters are at risk to their entire volume as if irradiated throughout to the maximum dose, the LQF for the whole pelvis irradiation is

$$\mathrm{LQF_{WP}} = 0.719 \times 28 \times 1.8\left(1 + \frac{1.8}{2.5}\right) = 62.3$$

and the residual LQF which can be delivered in a single fraction d Gy of IORT is given by

$$\mathrm{LQF_{IORT}} = 100 - 62.3 = 37.7 = 0.719 \, d\left(1 + \frac{d}{2.5}\right)$$

The solution to this quadratic equation is

$$d = 10.26 \text{ Gy/fraction (large volume)}$$

On the other hand, if it is assumed that only the small, high-dose volume ($v = 0.2$) of ureteral tissue is at risk, then substitution in the LQF equation for the whole pelvis irradiation gives

$$\mathrm{LQF} = 0.719 \times 28 \times 1.8\left(1 + \frac{1.8}{2.5}\right) \times (0.2)^{0.18} = 46.6$$

Hence:

$$\mathrm{LQF_{IORT}} = 100 - 46.6 = 53.4 = 0.719 \, d\left(1 + \frac{d}{2.5}\right) \times (0.2)^{0.18}$$

Solving for d gives

$$d = 14.55 \text{ Gy/fraction (small volume)}$$

C. ITDF SOLUTION

Each of the 5 volume elements represented by $v = 0.2$ receives both the 28 treatments of 1.8 Gy/fraction plus the IORT electron beam dose. Then, if TDF_{100}, TDF_{80} ....TDF_{20} are the TDFs corresponding to the volumes of tissue ($v = 0.2$) irradiated to 100%, 80%...20% of the maximum electron dose, respectively,

$$ITDF = 100 = [TDF_{100}^{5.56} + TDF_{80}^{5.56} + ...TDF_{20}^{5.56}]^{0.18}$$

where:

$$TDF_i = 0.931 \times (0.2)^{0.18}[(28 \times 1.8^{1.538} (1.33)^{-0.169}) + d_i^{1.538}]$$

If d Gy is the IORT electron beam dose at the 100% level, then the values of d_i at the 80%, 60%...20% levels are 0.8 d, 0.6 d...0.2 d, and substitution of these in the IORT equation above yields

$$d = 15.01 \text{ Gy/fraction}$$

D. ILQF SOLUTION

Following the same procedures as with the ITDF solution,

$$ILQF = 100 = [LQF_{100}^{5.56} + LQF_{80}^{5.56} + ...LQF_{20}^{5.56}]^{0.18}$$

where

$$LQF_i = 0.719 \times (0.2)^{0.18}\left[28 \times 1.8\left(1 + \frac{1.8}{2.5}\right) + d_i\left(1 + \frac{d_i}{2.5}\right)\right]$$

Then insertion of the various values of d_i into the ILQF equation yields

$$d = 13.30 \text{ Gy/fraction}$$

V. DISCUSSION

The inability of the conventional TDF and L-Q models to account for the effect of inhomogeneous irradiation of tissues and organs can present significant difficulties when applied to typical treatment planning problems for IORT. If the *total volume* of the tissue which is at risk is considered to have been irradiated to the maximum dose without consideration being given to the fact that much of the tissue receives a lower dose, then the tissue tolerance dose will be underestimated. Conversely, to account for only the reduced volume of tissue which receives the maximum dose and to ignore the rest of the tissue which is irradiated to a lower dose will tend to overestimate the tolerance dose. This is illustrated in Table 1, which reviews various solutions to the example. It is readily evident that, by only considering the large volume of tissue irradiated, both the TDF and L-Q models underestimate the dose per fraction that can be delivered safely to this patient. This underestimation is highly significant. On the other hand, the table also illustrates the effect of ignoring all but the small volume of tissue irradiated to a high dose. The tolerance dose is overestimated, especially in this case when dose inhomogeneities are significant.

The use of the "integral" forms of the two-dose effect relationships remedies this situation. Although computations are increased in complexity, most problems which occur in clinical practice can be solved using a hand calculator, especially if simplified by reduction

TABLE 1
Solutions to the IORT Example Using Various Dose-Effect Relationships

TDF solution		LQF solution		ITDF	ILQF
Large volume	Small volume	Large volume	Small volume	solution	solution
11.28 Gy	16.92 Gy	10.26 Gy	14.55 Gy	15.01 Gy	13.30 Gy

into a few dose regions as in the example used to illustrate the models in this chapter. More complex problems can be solved on a mini computer with relatively simple algorithms. Treatment planning computers would be ideal for this, since they are already programmed to calculate dose distribution data. The ultimate program would use multiplane CT or MRI input and 3-D dose computational algorithms to obtain a voxel-by-voxel representation of the dose distribution throughout each organ or tissue at risk. This approach is similar to several "integral response" models which have been proposed by several investigators,[22-25] although none of these previous models have accounted for fractionation effects.

One final question. Which is the more accurate model, TDF of L-Q? This is a problem which has been debated extensively elsewhere, and no unequivocal answer can be given. The L-Q model suffers from the disadvantage that no attempt is made to account for the effect of overall treatment time, but it does appear to have firmer radiobiological roots, although even this has been disputed.[29] In contrast, the TDF model does try to account for overall treatment time (although the method has been frequently disputed also)[30-31] and is relatively simpler to use than the L-Q method, but it is only a good approximation within certain limits of N and d,[12-13] which are typically unspecified, but presumably exclude single fractions as used in IORT. With neither of the two models are the relevant parameters (δ, τ, ϕ, and α/β) known with any degree of confidence for most tissues. Hence, it is important to realize that at present, neither model is accurate and solutions obtained to clinical problems should be considered as rough estimates only. In practice, if there is no clinical experience available on which to base a decision and resort has to be made to a mathematical model, it is probably expedient to solve the problem by both the TDF and L-Q methods, accounting for dose imhomogeneities, if significant, and to utilize the solution which is the most conservative.

REFERENCES

1. **Orton, C. G. and Ellis, F. A.,** Simplification in the use of the NSD concept in practical radiotherapy, *Br. J. Radiol.,* 46, 529, 1975.
2. **Orton, C. G.,** Time-dose factors (TDFs) in brachytherapy, *Br. J. Radiol.,* 47, 603, 1974.
3. **Orton, C. G.,** Bioeffect dosimetry in radiation therapy, in *Radiation Dosimetry: Physical and Biological Aspects,* Orton, C. G., Ed., Plenum Press, New York, 1986, 1.
4. **Wara, W. M., Phillips, T. L., Sheline, G. E., and Schwade, J. G.,** Radiation tolerance of the spinal cord, *Cancer,* 35, 1558, 1975.
5. **Pezner, R. D. and Archambeau, J. O.,** Brain tolerance unit: a method to estimate risk of radiation brain injury for various dose schedules, *Int. J. Radiat. Oncol. Biol. Phys.,* 7, 397, 1981.
6. **Cohen, L. and Creditor, M.,** An iso-effect table for radiation tolerance of the human spinal cord, *Int. J. Radiat. Oncol. Biol. Phys.,* 7, 961, 1981.
7. **Field, S. B., Hornsey, S., and Kutsutani, Y.,** Effects of fractionated irradiation on mouse lung and phenomenon of slow repair, *Br. J. Radiol.,* 49, 700, 1976.
8. **Hornsey, S. and White, A.,** Isoeffect curve for radiation myelopathy, *Br. J. Radiol.,* 53, 168, 1980.
9. **Cohen, L. and Creditor, M.,** Iso-effect tables for tolerance of irradiated normal human tissues, *Int. J. Radiat. Oncol. Biol. Phys.,* 9, 233, 1983.

10. **Wara, W. M., Phillips, T. L., Margolis, L. W., and Smith, V.,** Radiation pneumonitis — a new approach to the derivation of time-dose factors, *Cancer,* 32, 147, 1973.
11. **Cohen, L. and Awschalom, M.,** Fast neutron radiation therapy, *Annu. Rev. Biophys. Bioeng.,* 11, 359, 1982.
12. **Ellis, F.,** Fractionation in radiotherapy, in *Modern Trends in Radiotherapy,* Vol. 1, Deeley and Wood, Eds., Butterworth, London, 1967, 34.
13. **Winston, B. M., Ellis, F., and Hall, E. J.,** The Oxford NSD calculator for clinical use, *Clin. Radiol.,* 20, 8, 1969.
14. **Fowler, J. F. and Stern, B. E.,** Dose-time relationships in radiotherapy and the validity of cell survival models, *Br. J. Radiol.,* 36, 163, 1963.
15. **Fowler, J. F. and Stern, B. E.,** Dose-rate effects: some theoretical and practical considerations, *Br. J. Radiol.,* 31, 389, 1960.
16. **Barendsen, G. W.,** Dose fractionation, dose rate and iso-effect relationships for normal tissue responses, *Int. J. Radiat. Oncol. Biol. Phys.,* 8, 1981, 1982.
17. **Douglas, B. G. and Fowler, J. F.,** The effect of multiple small doses of X-rays on skin reactions in the mouse and basic interpretation, *Radiat. Res.,* 66, 401, 1976.
18. **Chadwick, K. H. and Leenhouts, H. P.,** A molecular theory of cell survival, *Phys. Med. Biol.,* 18, 78, 1973.
19. **Kellerer, A. M., and Rossi, H. H.,** The theory of dual radiation action, *Curr. Top. Radiat. Res.,* 8, 85, 1972.
20. **Zaider, M. and Rossi, H. H.,** Microdosimetry and its application to biological processes, in *Radiation Dosimetry: Physical and Biological Aspects,* Orton, C. G., Ed., Plenum Press, New York, 1986, 171.
21. **Kirk, J., Gray, W. M., and Watson, E. R.,** Cumulative radiation effect. I. Fractionated treatment regimens, *Clin. Radiol.,* 22, 145, 1971.
22. **Dritschilo, A., Chaffey, J. T., Bloomer, W. A., and Marck, A.,** The complication probability factor: a method for selection of radiation treatment plans, *Br. J. Radiol.,* 51, 370, 1978.
23. **Wolbarst. A. B., Sternick, E. S., and Dritschilo, A.,** Optimized radiotherapy treatment planning using the complication probability factor (CPF), *Int. J. Radiat. Oncol. Biol. Phys.,* 6, 723, 1980.
24. **Wolbarst, A. B.,** Optimization of radiation therapy. II. The critical voxel model, *Int. J. Radiat. Oncol. Biol. Phys.,* 10, 741, 1984.
25. **Schultheiss, T. E. and Orton, C. G.,** Models in radiotherapy: definition of decision criteria, *Med. Phys.,* 12, 183, 1985.
26. **Orton, C. G. and Cohen, L.,** A variable exponent TDF model, in *Optimization of Cancer Radiotherapy,* Paliwal, B. R., Herbert, D. E., and Orton, C. G., Eds., American Institute of Physics, New York, 1985, 347.
27. **Orton, C. G. and Cohen, L.,** A unified approach to dose-effect relationships in radiotherapy. I. Modified TDF and linear quadratic equations, *Int. J. Radn. Oncol. Biol. Phys.,* 14, 549, 1988.
28. **Orton, C. G.,** A unified approach to dose-effect relationships in radiotherapy. II. Inhomogeneous dose distributions, *Int. J. Radn. Oncol. Biol. Phys.,* 14, 557, 1988.
29. **Herbert, D.,** Does the LQ model fit? Yes, but—, submitted.
30. **Fowler, J. F.,** What next in fractionated radiotherapy?, *Br. J. Cancer,* 49 (Suppl. VI), 285, 1984.
31. **Fowler, J. F.,** Non-standard fractionation in radiotherapy, *Int. J. Radiat. Oncol. Biol. Phys.,* 10, 755, 1984.

Chapter 5

PHYSICAL ASPECTS AND DOSIMETRIC CONSIDERATIONS FOR INTRAOPERATIVE RADIATION THERAPY WITH ELECTRON BEAMS

Farideh R. Bagne

TABLE OF CONTENTS

I. INTRODUCTION

Intraoperative radiation therapy (IORT) is a treatment technique whereby a large single dose of radiation is delivered to a tumor or tumor bed with minimal radiation to the surrounding normal structures. The standard radiation modality for IORT is megavoltage electrons, although superficial and orthovoltage X-rays have also been used for this purpose. The equipment for generating the electrons are betatrons, microtrons, or linear accelerators, with the majority of institutions utilizing modified units for IORT. Recently, dedicated machines have been designed with a number of desirable features: multidirectional head rotation, lower shielding requirements (by generating electrons only), lower cost, and novel monitoring aspects.

Regardless of the type of accelerator used, the physical aspects of IORT with electron beams are unique. First, the entire therapeutic dose is delivered in a single fraction, thus treatment documentation and verification is more important and more difficult than for conventional multifraction treatment. Second, the physical parameters necessary for treatment planning, including beam energy, applicator shape and size, source-tumor distance, and bevel angle of the applicator are not known until immediately before the actual patient irradiation; as a result, pretreatment planning is virtually impossible. Third, because of variations in the extent and anatomical location of the tumor, a variety of applicators with differing shapes, bevel angles, and geometries must be calibrated for clinical use. This requirement combined with the available electron energies of accelerators necessitate generation of massive amounts of physical data. Consequently, methods must be devised to reduce the quantity of the required data without sacrificing the accuracy in dose delivery. Finally, irradiation under operating conditions creates certain difficulties in patient dose monitoring.

This chapter describes the required equipment and treatment facility for IORT. It then considers the needed dosimetric parameters and establishes criteria for electron beam characterization. Additionally, the treatment planning documentation and verification aspects are discussed. Also, this chapter presents the patient dose monitoring techniques currently available for IORT. While emphasis is placed on the IORT facility of the Medical College of Ohio (MCO), the physical and technical considerations, if not the associated data, are generally applicable to other IORT facilities.

II. TREATMENT FACILITY

This section describes an example of a treatment facility where the existing radiation therapy room and equipment have been modified for IORT with electron beams. For information on dedicated IORT units, the reader is referred to the published data.

A. RADIATION TREATMENT/OPERATING ROOM

The IORT facility of the MCO is located within the Radiation Therapy Department. The treatment machine is housed in a treatment-operating suite with an adjoining scrub area and recovery room. This operating room is modified to comply with all the published standards for a surgical suite: proper air circulation, operating room lights, auxiliary isolated generator, remote patient monitoring devices, operating table, oxygen, vacuum, and anesthetic lines. Similarly, as a radiation treatment facility, the room meets the required radiation therapy standards such as cronal, saggital, and transverse patient motion-detecting laser lights, remote control television monitors, dosimetry cable channels, adequate room shielding to allow 360° gantry rotation for the treatment unit and a conventional radiation treatment table.

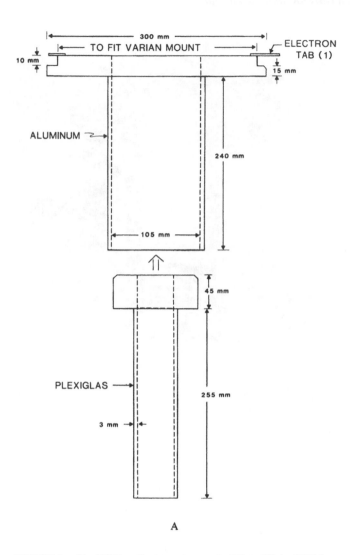

FIGURE 1. The IORT applicator system used at Mayo Clinic. (A) Schematics of the aluminum jacket and the Lucite® applicator; (B) a bevel-end Lucite® applicator inserted in the aluminum jacket; and (C) the complete applicator attached to the linear accelerator. (Courtesy of E. McCullough, Mayo Clinic.)

B. IORT EQUIPMENT

A variety of IORT commercial and noncommercial applicating systems are currently available. Generally, the IORT collimating system consists of a main frame adaptor which attaches to the surface of the accelerator head, a series of single or multisectional applicators which attach to the main frame, and a viewing system for observing the actual treatment area. An example of the IORT system used at Mayo Clinic is shown in Figure 1. A detailed description of the IORT system used at MCO is given in the following section. Other IORT systems are described in separate chapters.

The MCO IORT treatment unit is a Varian® Clinac-18 capable of generating 10-millielectronvolt peak (meVp) photons and 6-, 9-, 12-, 15-, and 18-meV electrons. While both the photon and electron beams are used for conventional external beam treatment, only the electrons are used for IORT.

In the IORT mode, the means by which electrons are produced, the gantry, and the treatment head of the accelerator remain unchanged. Similarly, no modification is made in

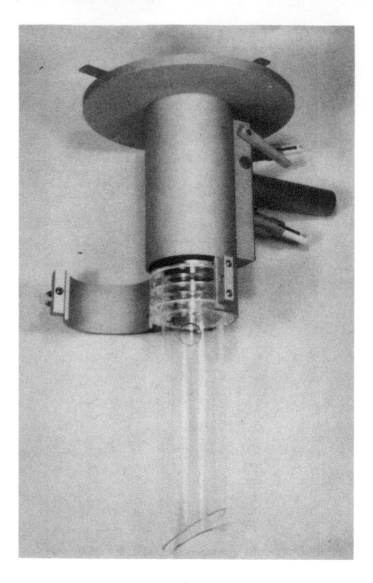

FIGURE 1B.

the upper and lower jaws of the primary photon collimator of the accelerator. Major design modifications, however, exist in the overall configuration of the electron applicator assembly. Figure 2 compares the conventional Varian® Clinac-18 electron applicator for small applicators with the MCO IORT applicator system. Referring to this figure, the three main components of the MCO applicator system are the main attachment, the applicator attachment, and the transparent applicators.

1. Main Attachment

The main attachment of the IORT applicator system is relatively similar to the primary carrier assembly of the Varian® Clinac-18 accelerator. The entire attachment is made of aluminum. The upper portion is circular in cross-section and is essentially a duplicate of the top portion of the Clinac-18 primary carrier assembly. Both systems utilize a set of three short tabs and one long key tab to lock the unit onto the treatment head (Figure 2). The latter tab allows operation of the machine in the electron mode. Both systems contain additional safety screws to secure the attachment to the treatment head housing. The main

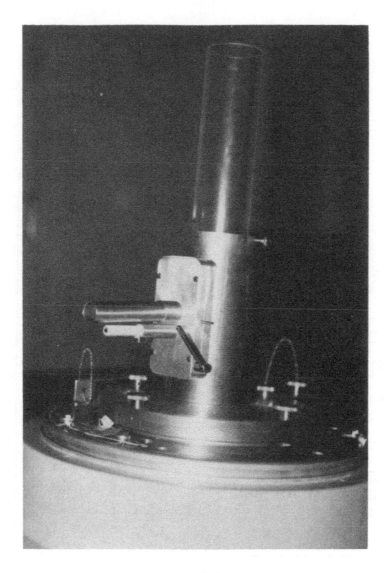

FIGURE 1C.

attachment, however, unlike the Clinac-18 assembly, has a square cross-section. The IORT attachment includes a 90° rigid fiberoptic telescope which allows a "beam's eye view" of the treatment region with minimal optical distortion. The telescope is removable and can be separately sterilized. It is equipped with a variable-intensity light source which allows viewing of the treatment region under any geometrical condition. When documentation of the treatment field is required, a 35-mm camera may be attached to the viewing end of the telescope and photographs of the area taken. Finally, the bottom portion of the main attachment is fitted with a series of precision rails and two pins, one slide-locking, and one manual screw, to allow proper placement of the applicator attachment (Figure 3). The upper portion of the main assembly is draped with a removable thin sheet of clear polyethylene to prevent dirt or dust particles in the accelerator head from falling into the surgical incision.

2. Applicator Attachment

The applicator attachment is made of aluminum. The top plate of the applicator attachment slides into the precision-fitted railings of the main attachment; two pins securely lock

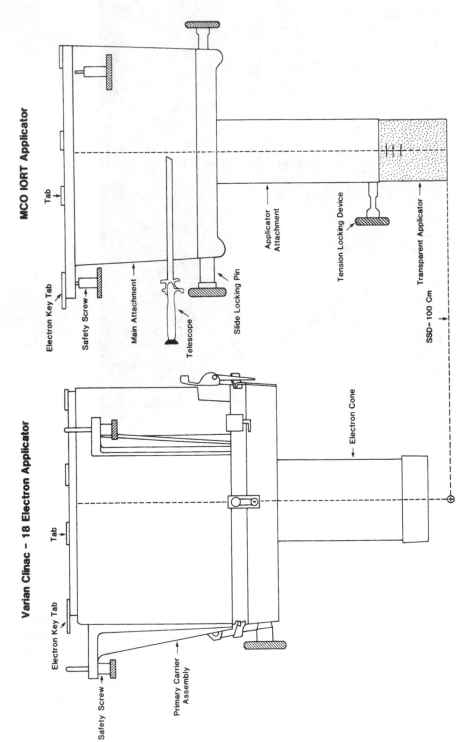

FIGURE 2. The MCO IORT applicator system is compared schematically to a Varian® Clinac-18 applicator for external electron beam therapy.

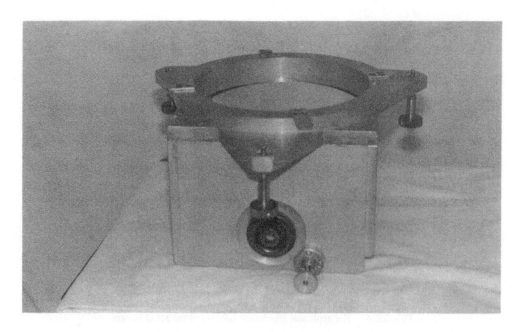

A

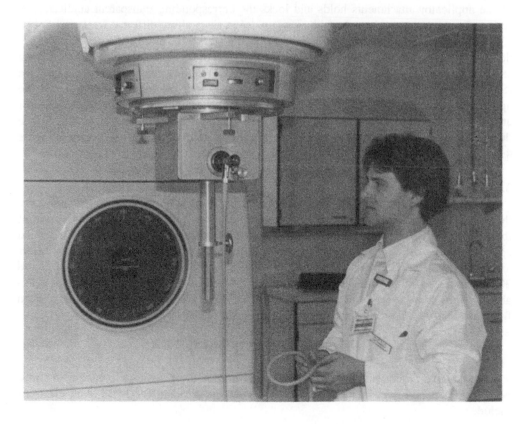

B

FIGURE 3. (A) The main attachment of the MCO IORT system; and (B) the complete applicator system with the fiberoptic telescope in place.

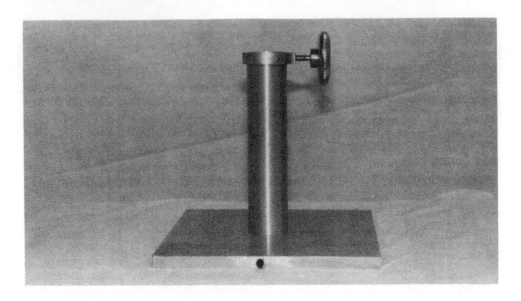

FIGURE 4. The applicator attachment (sleeve) of the MCO system.

the applicator attachment in place. The thickness of the top plate is 0.5 in. The lower sleeve of the applicator attachments holds and locks the corresponding transparent applicator. A series of applicator attachments with varying sleeve sizes allow different treatment fields. The transparent applicator can be locked inside the sleeve by means of a tension locking device. The sleeve is long enough to allow the insertion of transparent applicators to varying lengths. This adjustable length insertion is in turn used to adjust the source surface distance (SSD) at any distance in the clinically useful range. Both the main attachment and the applicator attachment are steam sterilized. Similar to the main attachment, the applicator attachment is anodized (hard coated) to prevent oxidation and discoloration of the surface during the sterilization process. An example of the applicator attachment is shown in Figure 4.

3. Transparent Applicator

The transparent applicators are made of acrylic. Each applicator slides smoothly into the sleeve and then is locked in place. The corresponding SSD is then read on the side of the applicator (Figure 5). The SSD can be set in the range of 97 to 115 cm. The round applicators have a wall thickness of 0.635 cm ($^1/_4$ in.). The inner diameters of the applicators are shown in Table 1. Each size applicator is available in flat end (0° bevel angle), 15, and 30° bevel angles (Figure 5). The transparent applicators are gas sterilized. To ensure availability of the transparent applicators at the time of surgery, multiple applicators have been fabricated for the clinically used diameters and bevel angles.

II. DOSIMETRIC PARAMETERS

Prior to the clinical use of an IORT system, a number of dosimetric parameters must be determined and documented. The necessary dosimetric data for IORT with electrons include

A. Central axis data
    1. Depth of maximum dose (d_m)
    2. Percent depth dose (%DD)

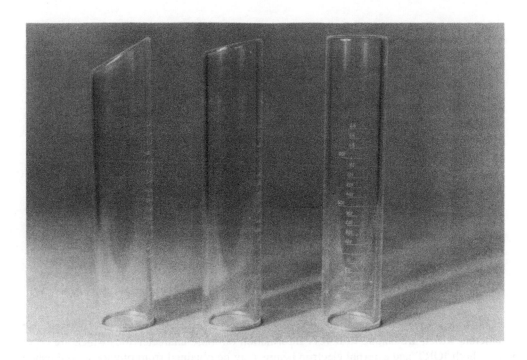

FIGURE 5.   Transparent applicators (flat, 15° bevel end, and 30° bevel end) of the MCO system. The SSD markings are on the side of each applicator.

TABLE 1
Inner Diameters of the Available MCO
Trasparent Circular Applicators

Applicator type	Inner diameter (in.)
Flat; 15° beveled	1
Flat; 15° beveled	$1^1/_4$
Flat; 15° beveled	$1^1/_2$
Flat; 15° beveled	$1^3/_4$
Flat; 15° beveled; 30° beveled	2
Flat; 15° beveled; 30° beveled	$2^1/_4$
Flat; 15° beveled; 30° beveled	$2^1/_2$
Flat; 15° beveled; 30° beveled	$2^3/_4$
Flat; 15° beveled; 30° beveled	3
Flat; 15° beveled; 30° beveled	$3^1/_4$
Flat; 15° beveled; 30° beveled	$3^1/_2$
Flat; 15° beveled; 30° beveled	$3^3/_4$
Flat; 15° beveled; 30° beveled	4

    3. Surface dose
    4. Bremmsstrahlung X-ray contamination
B. Applicator parameters
    1. Output factors
    2. Source-surface distance correction factors
    3. Photon collimator setting
C. Dose distribution data
    1. Isodose curve

TABLE 2
Average Values of the Depth of Maximum Dose (d_m)[a]
and the Variations in d_m and the Surface Energies for
Flat Applicators

Nominal electron beam energy (meV)	Surface energy (meV)	Depth of maximum dose, d_m (cm)
6	5.61	0.6 ± 0.1
9	8.42	1.0 ± 0.1
12	11.15	1.2 ± 0.1
15	13.72	1.6 ± 0.15
18	17.13	1.6 ± 0.1

[a]   Given as a function of nominal electron beam energy.

2. Beam flatness
3. Penumbra

D.   Shielding Data

The following sections are intended to illustrate those features of electron beam dose parameters which are unique to IORT. Information on those characteristics which are common to both IORT and external electron beams may be obtained from previously published data.

A. CENTRAL AXIS DATA
1. Depth of Maximum Dose

The depth of maximum dose, d_m, is an essential factor in IORT since in many institutions the dose is prescribed at this depth. Additionally, other critical dosimetric parameters, including the output factors and %DD values, require the determination of d_m. The depth of d_m, while a function of bevel angle, SSD, and applicator shape and size, can be assigned a single value for each energy. This is because for a given energy d_m varies minimally over the range of applicator variables. Table 2 presents the average values of, d_m as a function of electron beam energy for a Varian® Clinac-18. Also shown is the range over which the value of d_m varies with the applicator size, shape, and bevel angles. For comparison, both the nominal and the surface energy values are given.

2. Percent Depth Dose

Accurate determination of the percent depth dose (%DD) over the clinically used range of energies is particularly important in IORT with electrons because of the frequent use of extended SSD and bevel-ended applicators. A well-organized and comprehensive set of %DD data must be available to the radiation oncologist immediately before irradiation.

Figures 6 and 7 present the %DD curves for flat-end and 15° bevel-end circular applicators of 1 in. diameter. The SSD is 100 cm and the nominal electron beam energies are 6, 9, 12, 15, and 18 meV.

A particular concern when measuring the %DD values for beveled applicators is the choice of the central axis. As shown in Figure 8, three geometrical configurations are possible for defining the central axis:

1.   In the first configuration, the central axis of the beam and the main axis of the tumor volume are congruent. In this situation, an air gap is created on the central axis. The air gap, being geometrically related to the applicator diameter and bevel angle, increases as the latter two parameters increase. While simple in concept, this configuration

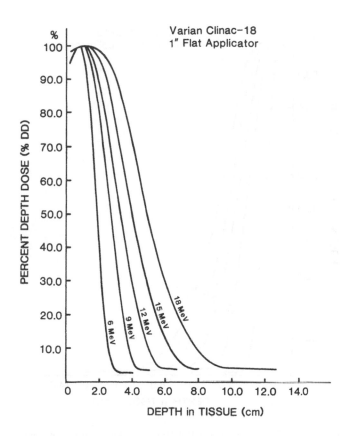

FIGURE 6.   Percent depth dose (%DD) is plotted as a function of depth in tissue for 1-in. flat cylindrical applicator at 6-, 9-, 12-, 15-, and 18-meV electron beam energies. The SSD is 100 cm, and the unit is a Varian® Clinac-18 linear accelerator.

suffers from lack of correspondence to the actual clinical setup. As such, its use is not recommended.

2. In the second configuration, the main axis of the tumor, perpendicular to the surface, is chosen for specifying the beam parameters. In this case, the beam central axis does not coincide with the axis on which data are taken. Because of this noncoincidence, the isodose distribution is not symmetric with respect to the central axis as illustrated in Figure 9. Furthermore, the %DD data underestimate the actual penetration of the electron beams. Figure 10 illustrates this phenomenon. The %DD values along the main axis of the tumor (perpendicular to the surface) and along the beam axis are compared for a 15-meV nominal electron beam using a $3^1/_2$-in.-diameter circular applicator. The bevel angle is 30°. As shown in this figure, the depth of penetration along the central axis is underestimated by a factor of approximately 15%. Another drawback of this configuration is the dependence of SSD on bevel angle and applicator diameter. This dependence arises because the SSD is defined as the distance from the source to the bevel end on the long side of the applicator. As such, the SSD on the central axis is reduced by a factor of $^1/_2$R tan Θ, where R is the diameter of the beveled applicator and Θ is the bevel angle. The major advantage of this configuration is the simplicity with which dosimetry data can be generated. In particular, when data are taken in a water phantom, the detector is simply moved perpendicular to the surface of the water with the gantry rotated by the appropriate bevel angle.

3. The third choice for defining the central axis is a configuration whereby the bevel end is parallel to the surface of the tumor and the central axis of the beam is used for dose

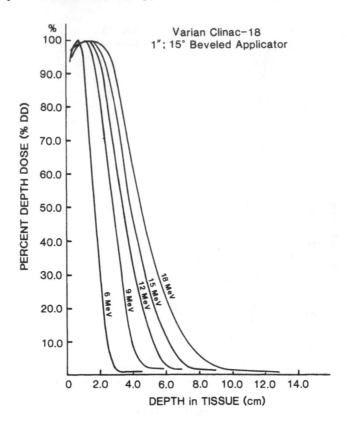

FIGURE 7.   Percent depth dose (%DD) is plotted as a function of depth in tissue for 6-, 9-, 12-, 15-, and 18-meV electrons. The applicator has a diameter of 1 in. and bevel angle of 15°. The SSD is 100 cm, and the applicator was set parallel to the surface of the phantom. The axis of the measurement was perpendicular to the phantom surface.

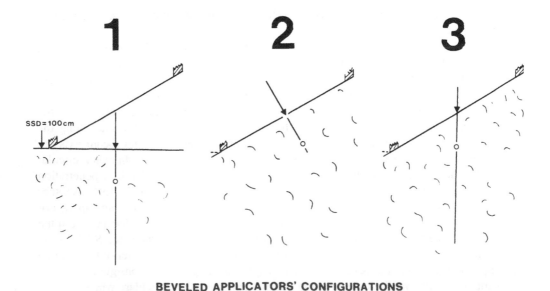

BEVELED APPLICATORS' CONFIGURATIONS

FIGURE 8.   The three possible configurations are shown for bevel end applicators.

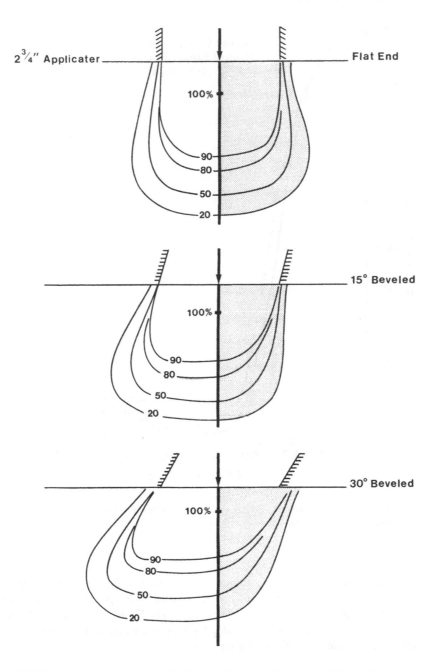

FIGURE 9. The dose distribution for 15-meV electrons. The diameter of the applicators is $2^{1}/_{4}$ in. The data are shown for flat, 15, and 30° bevel end applicators. As shown in this figure, the dose distributions are not symmetric with respect to the central axis if the axis is chosen to be that of configuration 2 (shown in Figure 8).

measurements (Figure 8). Although this configuration creates difficulties in the actual dosimetry, particularly when data are measured in water, it is, nevertheless, recommended for clinical use for a number of reasons. First, the isodose distribution is symmetric with respect to the central axis (Figure 11). Second, the %DD data represent the actual penetration of the beam. Finally, the physical configuration corresponds to the treatment setup. As with the second configuration, however, the current choice results in a central axis SSD which varies with variation in applicator diameter and bevel angle.

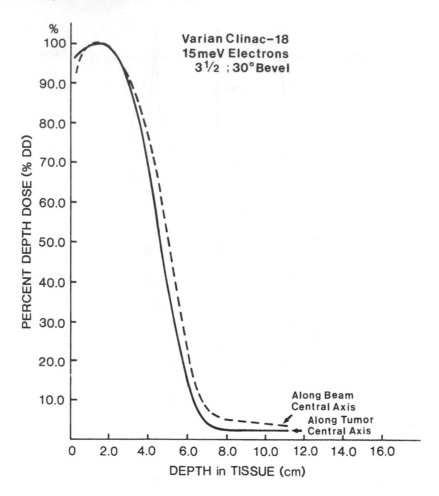

FIGURE 10.   Percent depth dose (%DD) values along the beam axis (configuration 3) are compared with the data along the tumor main axis (configuration 2). The beam consists of 15-meV electrons generated by a Varian® Clinac-18 linear accelerator. The applicator has a diameter of $3^1/_2$ in. and a 30° bevel end.

To simplify generation of %DD values, it is recommended that the %DD data be measured along the main axis of the tumor, perpendicular to the phantom surface, and then the data be geometrically related to %DD on the beam axis. Figure 12 illustrates this method. For a given %DD value, the corresponding depth on the main axis of the tumor, d, is related to the depth on the beam axis, d′, by the equation

$$d' = d(\cos\theta)^{-1} \qquad (1)$$

where Θ is the bevel angle. As shown in Figure 12, good agreement is obtained between the calculated and the measured values once the %DD data are corrected for the depth and SSD variations.

3. Surface Dose

Generally, IORT with electrons involves irradiation of a target volume which extends to the surface. To ensure full coverage of the surface region, it is necessary to accurately determine the surface dose at all beam energies. It is also recommended that the variation of the surface dose with the applicator size, bevel angle, and photon collimator setting be determined.

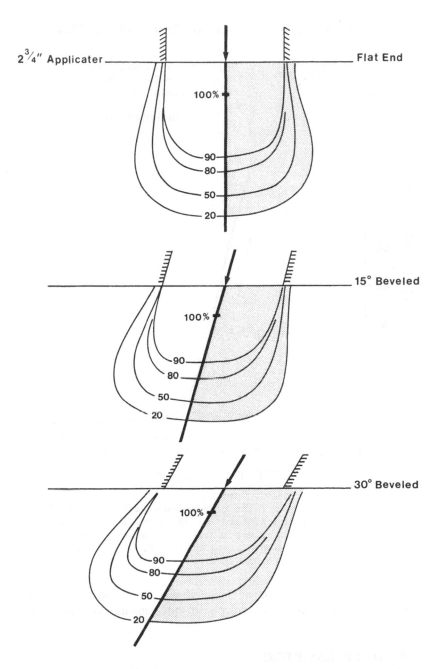

FIGURE 11. Dose distributions for flat, 15, and 30° beveled applicators of $2^3/_4$ in. diameter are plotted. The dose distribution is symmetric with respect to the central axis if configuration 3 (shown in Figure 8) is chosen.

4. Bremsstrahlung X-Ray Contamination

In electron beam IORT, the tumor volume usually overlies a critical organ such as the spinal cord. It is therefore necessary to fully consider the effect of bremsstrahlung X-rays beyond the range of electrons. The bremsstrahlung X-ray contamination is relatively constant beyond the practical range of the electrons. Its contribution is usually in the range of 2 to 10% of the maximum dose, and its magnitude increases with increasing applicator size and beam energy. For the MCO IORT system using a Varian® Clinac-18, the bremsstrahlung X-ray contamination is in the range of 2 to 4%, regardless of the applicator shape or size.

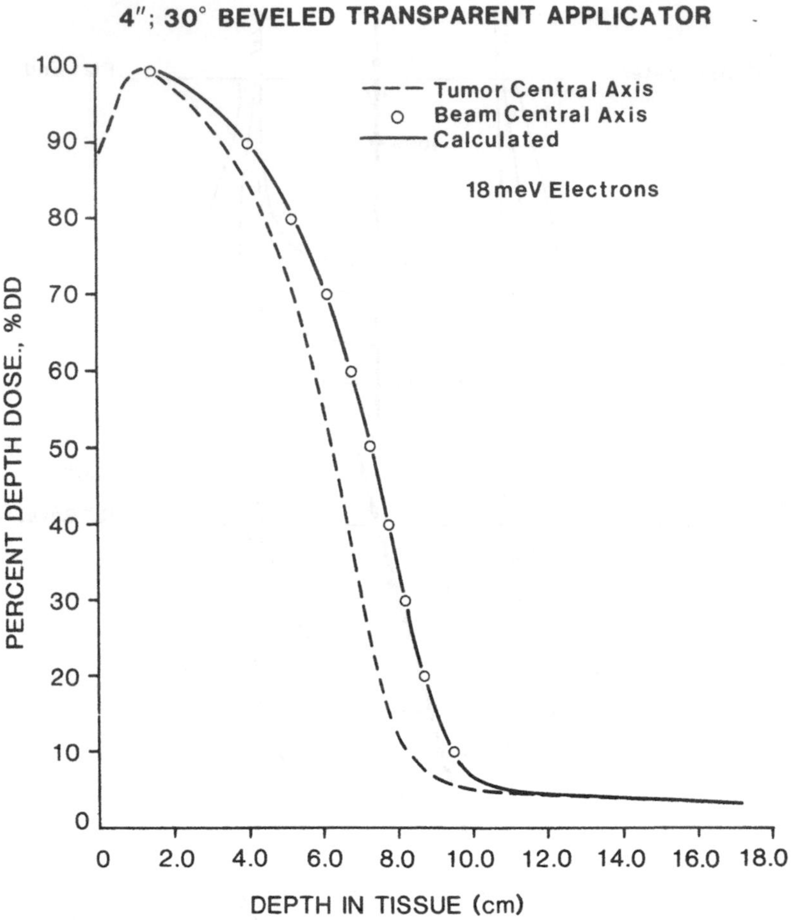

4″; 30° BEVELED TRANSPARENT APPLICATOR

FIGURE 12.   Percent depth dose (%DD) values are plotted as a function of depth in water for a 4-in.-diameter applicator with 30° bevel end. The data measured on the main axis of the tumor (configuration 2) and shown by a dashed line are converted to the data on the central axis of the beam (configuration 3) using Equation 1. The measured data on the beam central axis (○) agree with the calculated values (—).

Generally, the magnitude of this contamination is also a function of the primary photon collimating system. As the photon jaws are opened, the bremsstrahlung X-ray contamination decreases.

B. APPLICATOR PARAMETERS
1. Output Factors

One of the most important dosimetric parameters in IORT is the output factor; namely, the dose at d_m per monitor unit. The output factor is generally a function of photon collimator setting, electron beam energy, SSD, and applicator shape, size, and bevel angle. Consequently, dependence of the output factor on each of the above parameters must be determined.

2. Source-Surface Distance Correction

In general, the inverse-square law does not apply to electron beams. An example of the nonapplicability of the inverse-square law to MCO IORT applicators is shown in Figure 13, where the distance correction factor (DCF) is plotted as a function of SSD for $1^1/_4$-, 2-, and 4-in.-diameter flat-end applicators. The electron beam energy is 12 meV. In this figure, the

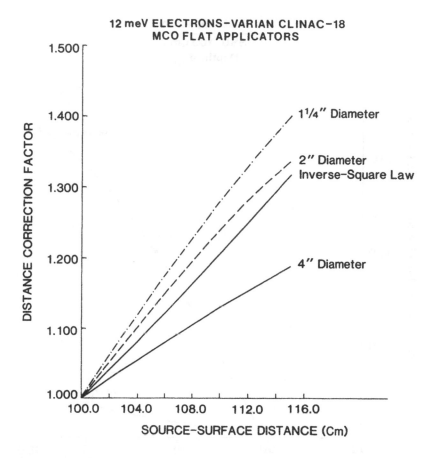

FIGURE 13. The DCF is plotted as a function of SSD for 12-meV electrons generated by a Varian® Clinac-18. The applicators were $1^1/_4$, 2, and 4 in. in diameter. Measurements were made at the depth of maximum dose d_m = 1.3 cm.

DCF is defined as the factor necessary to correct the beam output for the change in SSD. The parameter DCF is given by:

$$D(d_m, SSD, W) = DCF(SSD, W) \cdot D(d_m, S, W) \qquad (2)$$

where d_m = depth of maximum dose, W = applicator size, SSD = source-surface distance, and $D(d_m, S, W)$ = output of the accelerator at SSD and applicator size W. As shown in Figure 13, the inverse-square law does not apply to the MCO IORT system.

Variation of the DCF with the bevel angle of the applicator is exemplified in Figure 14, where the DCF is plotted for 2-in.-diameter applicators with flat-ends and 15 and 30° bevel angles. The beam energy is 12 meV and the depth of measurement is 1.3 cm.

Frequently, empirical relations can be formulated to accurately correct the output for variation in SSD. Studies must be undertaken to assess the degree of change of the DCF with applicator size and shape, bevel angle, energy, and even the photon collimator setting before such empirical relations are used clinically.

3. Photon Collimator Setting

The primary photon collimator setting may have a significant effect on the applicator properties, such as the output and the radiation leakage outside the field. Because of the effect of the photon collimator setting on various dose parameters, it is necessary to ensure that before the radiation beam is turned on, the photon collimator is set appropriately. Because

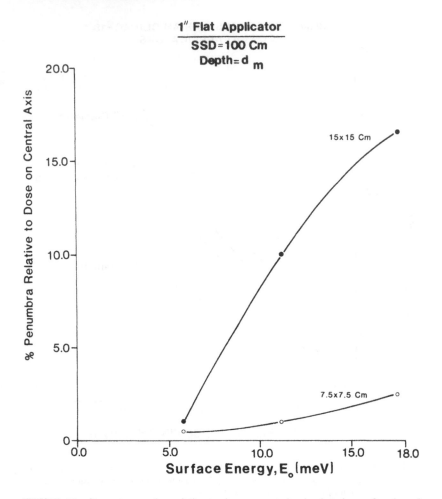

FIGURE 14.   Percent penumbra relative to dose on central axis plotted as a function of energy for photon collimator settings of 7.5 × 7.5 and 15 × 15 cm. The applicator is flat with a 1-in. diameter, and SSD is 100 cm.

of the multidisciplinary nature of IORT, involving radiation oncology, surgery, and anesthesiology staff, and the speed required for setting up the various machine parameters immediately before treatment, many centers use a single photon collimator setting, regardless of the applicator chosen. The most commonly adopted setting for this purpose is 15 × 15 cm.

Figure 15 presents an example of the radiation leakage outside the useful beam when the photon collimator is set at 15 × 15 cm as opposed to 7.5 × 7.5 cm. The percent penumbra relative to the dose on the central axis is plotted as a function of electron beam surface energy for a flat-end applicator with a 1-in. diameter. Measurements were made at the appropriate depths of maximum dose. As shown in this figure, the radiation leakage outside the applicator can be greatly affected by the photon collimator setting. Furthermore, as expected, the radiation leakage is enhanced as the electron beam energy is increased.

Figure 15 presents the beam profiles for a 1-in.-diameter applicator with a 15° bevel angle using photon collimator settings of 15 × 15 and 7.5 × 7.5 cm. The beam energy is 18 meV and the SSD 100 cm. The profiles are measured at 1.6 cm in depth. As indicated by this figure, the leakage is drastically reduced by closing the photon collimator. The dose profile inside the applicator, however, is not substantially affected by the photon collimator setting.

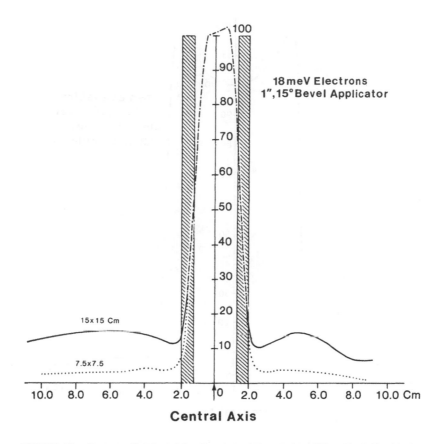

FIGURE 15. Beam profiles for a 1-in.-diameter applicator with 15° bevel end showing the effect of photon collimator setting on the leakage outside and inside the applicator. The beam energy is 18 meV, and SSD is 100 cm.

Such studies are of particular importance in cases where the tumor is adjacent to a critical organ or when the adjoining tissues have been previously exposed to high levels of radiation dose.

C. DOSE DISTRIBUTION DATA

1. Isodose Curves

It is imperative that the isodose curves for all applicators be measured at the clinically used energies. Since the bevel angle of the applicators distorts the shape of the isodose distribution (Figures 9 and 10), the data must be produced not only for flat-end applicators, but also the beveled applicators.

2. Beam Flatness

In general, IORT applicators do not produce a uniform dose across the radiation field. This nonuniformity is caused by radiation scattered from the walls of the applicators. Consequently, regions of high dose are commonly associated with IORT. Figure 16 presents the beam profile for a 3.5-in.-diameter applicator with a 30° bevel end. The data were taken at the d_m along the nonbevel axis of the applicator. As indicated in this example, regions of high dose (horns) are present near the sides of the applicator. The beam profile in Figure 16 shows that for this particular applicator there is as much as 18% nonuniformity across the field when 18 meV electrons are used.

The effect of electron energy on the beam nonuniformity is shown in Figure 17 for a $3^1/_2$-in. flat-end applicator. The percent horn relative to the central axis is plotted as a

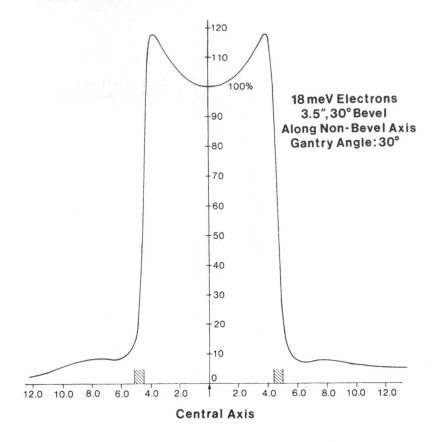

FIGURE 16.   Beam profile is plotted for a 3.5-in. applicator with 30° bevel end; the beam energy is 18 meV.

function of surface energy. Measurements were made at the respective depths of maximum dose. As shown in this figure, the bean nonuniformity increases as electron energy is increased.

Considering the above, it is necessary to measure the variation of dose across the radiation field so that the prescribed dose can be based on full information about the characteristics of the beam in three dimensions.

3. Penumbra

Penumbra for an IORT applicator is the undesired dose outside the radiation field. Penumbra is generally caused by the scattered radiation resulting from interactions inside the radiation field as well as radiation leakage radiation through the sleeve and baseplate of the applicator attachment. The latter depends primarily on the photon collimator setting and the beam energy. The penumbra is particularly important for beveled applicators. Figure 18 presents the relative penumbra outside the useful beam for a $1^{1}/_{2}$-in. applicator with a 15° bevel end. The relative penumbra is the ratio of the highest dose outside the applicator to the dose on the central axis at the same depth. In this figure, the percent penumbra is plotted as a function of electron beam surface energy for the short (S) and the long (L) sides for the beveled applicator. The photon collimator setting is 15×15 cm. All measurements were done at d_m. As shown by this example, the penumbra is much higher at the short side of the applicator than at the long side. Furthermore, the difference in penumbra between the two sides increases with increasing energy. As energy increases, a higher number of unattenuated and unscattered radiation reach the measuring point.

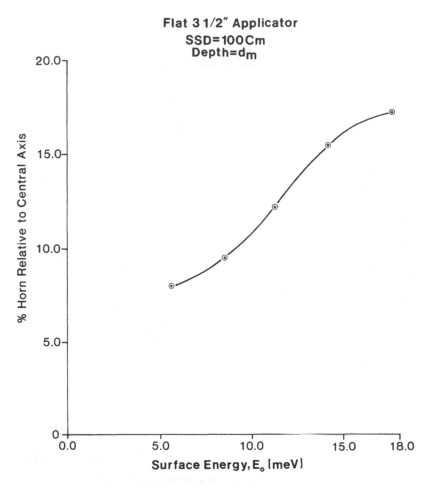

Flat 3 1/2" Applicator
SSD=100Cm
Depth=d_m

FIGURE 17. Percent horn relative to the dose on the central axis is plotted as a function of energy for a flat, $3^1/_2$-in.-diameter applicator.

IV. SHIELDING DATA

Because of irregularities in the shape of the tumor volume and the presence of adjacent critical organs, it is often necessary to partially block the electron beam within the IORT field. Measurements must be made to determine the required thickness of shielding material. Commonly, lead is chosen for this purpose. Table 3 shows the required thickness of lead for electron beam IORT to reduce the dose in the blocked area to less than 10% of the unblocked dose.

It must be mentioned that these data are for illustration only and must not be used for clinical purposes before verification for each individual machine.

V. TREATMENT PLANNING

In IORT treatment planning, two factors are essential: (1) precision in dose calculation; and (2) minimization of the calculation time. Precision in dose calculation is particularly important because the entire dose is delivered in a single fraction. Consequently, any resulting calculation error not only is magnified, but also, unlike conventional external beam therapy, cannot be corrected for subsequent treatments. Minimization of the calculation time, on the other hand, is crucial because the patient is anesthetized for the duration of IORT.

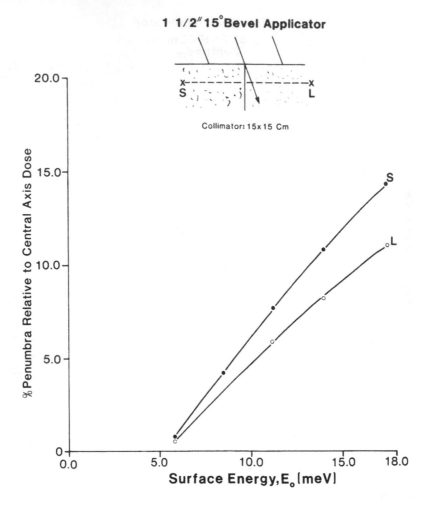

FIGURE 18. Percent penumbra outside the useful beam as a function of electron beam surface energy. Data is generated for a $1^1/_2$-in.-diameter applicator with 15° bevel angle. Letters S and L refer to the percent penumbras along the short and long sides of the applicator, respectively.

TABLE 3

**Lead Shielding Requirements in IORT to
Reduce the Dose to the Blocked Region to
Less than 10% of the Unblocked Field**

Nominal beam energy (meV)	Required number of lead layers	
	$^1/_{32}$ in. thick	$^1/_{16}$ in. thick
6	3	2
9	5	3
12	6	3
15	8	4
18	9	5

Additionally, the patient remains alone in the treatment room during the period between placement of the applicator and completion of the irradiation process. Furthermore, calculation time is delayed because the needed dosimetry and patient data, including the beam energy, SSD, and the applicator size and bevel angle, are not available until immediately prior to irradiation.

At the present time, pretreatment planning and dose calculation are not available for IORT. Accordingly, it is required that all of the necessary information be on hand immediately before radiation treatment. The minimum data necessary are the output factors, %DD data, dose distributions, SSD correction factors, penumbra and field nonuniformity data, and the number of lead layers needed for organ shielding. All of the above data must be in a well-organized and easily accessible form to avoid any unnecessary delay in dose delivery.

VI. VERIFICATION AND DOCUMENTATION

Because the entire radiation dose is given in a single fraction, every effort must be made to ensure the accuracy of dose delivery. It is highly recommended that all of the factors used in calculating the monitor unit setting be checked by an independent but knowledgeable second person. Other methods of patient dose verifications, such as thermoluminescent dosimetry, may also be used to measure the surface dose and in turn relate this value to the dose at d_m. If thermoluminescent dosimetry is used, it is critical that the dosimeters have high precision. Furthermore, it is recommended that more than one dosimeter be used to obtain a lower uncertainty in the final measured dose value.

To verify the region of treatment, a ''beam's eye view'' of the radiation field can be obtained by the use of a right angle telescope. A permanent photographic record of the treatment area can be obtained if the applicator system is equipped with a photographic camera (see Section II.B.1).

It is required to document and initial a number of dosimetric factors at the time of irradiation. Easily accessible forms are used to document the gantry and collimator angles, the shape and size of the applicator, the SSD and the applicable SSD factor, the output factor, surface dose, depths of 80 or 90%, bremsstrahlung contamination, dose to critical organs, bevel angle, photon collimator setting, prescribed dose, the monitor unit setting, and the thickness and type of the shielding material.

VII. CONCLUSION

IORT is a multidisciplinary technique which is rapidly emerging as a standard means of cancer treatment. In order to take full advantage of this modality, it is imperative that the special dosimetric properties and physical characteristics associated with this technique be studied, and all of the necessary treatment planning factors be measured prior to its use.

ACKNOWLEDGMENTS

The author wishes to acknowledge Dr. E. McCullough for providing the figures on the Mayo Clinic IORT system and Mrs. Karen Lehnert and Ms. Lori Donahue for typing this manuscript.

REFERENCES

1. **Abe, M., Fukada, M., and Yamono, K.,** Intraoperative irradiation in abdominal and cerebral tumours, *Acta Radiol. Ther. Phys. Biol.,* 10, 408, 1971.
2. **Bagne, F. R., Dobelbower, R. R., Milligan, A. J., Bronn, D. G.,** Treatment of cancer of the pancreas by intraoperative electron beam therapy: physical and biological aspects, *Int. J. Radiat. Oncol. Biol. Phys.,* 16, 231, 1989.
3. **Bagne, F. R., Samsami, N., and Dobelbower, R. R.,** Radiation contamination and leakage assessment of intraoperative electron applicators, *J. Med. Phys. ,* 15, 530, 1988.
4. **Biggs, P. J.,** The effect of beam angulation on central axis percent depth dose for meV electrons, *Phys. Med. Biol.,* 29, 1089, 1984.
5. **Biggs, P. J., Epp, E. R., Ling, C. C., Novack, D. H., and Michaels, H. B.,** Dosimetry, field shaping and other considerations for intraoperative radiation therapy, *Int. J. Radiat. Oncol. Biol. Phys.,* 7, 875, 1981.
6. **Biggs, P. J. and McCullough, E. C.,** Physical aspects of intraoperative electron beam radiation, in *Intraoperative and External Beam Irradiation,* Gunderson, L. L. and Tepper, J. E., Eds., Yearbook Medical Publishers, Chicago, 1983.
7. **Fraass, B. A., Harrington, F. S., Kinsella, T. J., and Sindelar, W. F.,** Television system for verification and documentation of treatment fields during intraoperative radiation therapy, *Int. J. Radiat. Oncol. Biol. Phys.,* 9, 1409, 1983.
8. **Goldson, A. L.,** Past, present and future prospects of intraoperative radiotherapy, *Semin. Oncol.,* 8, 59, 1981.
9. **Holmes, T. W. and McCullough, E. C.,** Acceptance testing and quality assurance of automated scanning film densitometers used in the dosimetry of electron and photon therapy beams, *Med. Phys.,* 10, 698, 1983.
10. **McCullough, E. C. and Anderson, J. A.,** The dosimetric properties of an applicator system for intraoperative electron beam therapy utilizing a Clinac 18 accelerator, *Med. Phys.,* 9, 261, 1982.
11. **Pillar, D. G., Gillin, M.T., Kline, R. W., and Grimm, D. F.,** A linear accelerator monitor unit totalizer, *Med. Phys.,* 10, 895, 1983.
12. **Rich, T. A., Cady, B., McDermott, W. V., Kase, K. R., Chaffey, J. T., and Helman, S.,** Orthovoltage intraoperative radiotherapy: a new look at an old idea, *Int. J. Radiat. Oncol. Biol. Phys.,* 10, 1957, 1984.

Chapter 6

PHYSICAL ASPECTS OF INTRAOPERATIVE RADIATION THERAPY

Takehiro Nishidai

TABLE OF CONTENTS

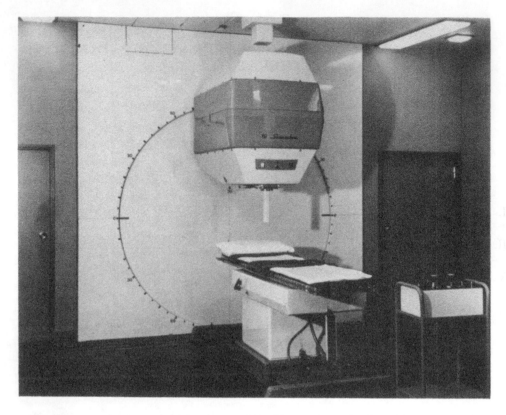

FIGURE 1.   A 32-meV medical betatron with which IORT is performed at Kyoto University Hospital.

I. INTRODUCTION

Megavoltage electron beams are most commonly used for intraoperative radiation therapy (IORT) because they permit delivery of a tumor-sterilizing dose to the target volume with reasonable dose homogeneity and sharp limitation of the volume of tissue included in the high dose range.[1] A fully equipped operating room may be equipped with low-energy X-ray machines (orthovoltage or superficial) for delivering an IORT boost dose in combination with external beam irradiation. In this chapter, the physical aspects of IORT using electron beams will be described, based on our experience at Kyoto University Hospital.

II. MACHINES

At Kyoto University Hospital, IORT is performed with electron beams generated by a BT-32 betatron made by Shimadzu Corporation, Japan (Figure 1). This betatron can produce a wide range of electron energies, beginning with 4 meV and increasing by increments of 2 up to 32 meV. A betatron is suitable for IORT, since electrons are continuously accelerated in the head of the device by the magnetic field, and an optimal energy of electrons is selected easily. However, the efficiency of electron acceleration in a betatron is relatively low, because only a few percent of the electrons injected by the gun are accelerated in an equilibrium circle with a radius within the doughnut.

On the other hand, medical linear accelerators can produce highly intense electron beams. As the dose rate obtained by a linear accelerator is much higher than that obtained by a

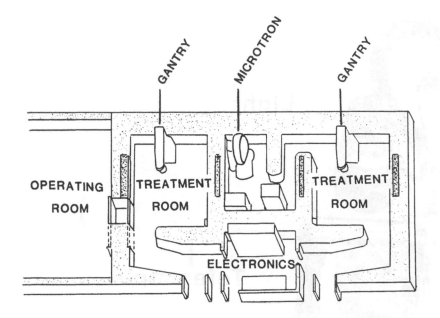

FIGURE 2. Diagram of treatment room for IORT with a microtron at the National Cancer Center Hospital in Tokyo.

betatron, a linear accelerator is used for IORT in many institutions. The possibility of energy selection with a linear accelerator is, however, relatively low as compared with a betatron.

A medical microtron has recently been developed as a new electron accelerator for radiation therapy. Better isodose distributions for electron therapy can be obtained with the microtron than with either the linear accelerator or betatron. Accelerated electron beams from a microtron are characterized by high intensity, excellent energy quality, and various energy steps.[3] An ideal facility for IORT with a microtron was implemented at the National Cancer Center Hospital (NCCH) in Tokyo, where the operating room was installed adjacent to the radiation treatment room (Figure 2).[4] Part of the thick wall of the treatment room can be moved so a patient can be transported from the operating room into the treatment room without passing through an unsterile area.

III. APPLICATOR SYSTEMS

An applicator is used to limit the size of flattened electron beams and to protect tissues outside the target volume from radiation. For IORT, applicators of various sizes and shapes must be provided to adequately cover the lesions to be irradiated. For example, a pentagonally shaped treatment applicator is used for IORT in gastric cancer, and an elliptical applicator for prostatic cancer.[5,6] The applicators for IORT should have sufficient lengths to permit deep insertion into body cavities. In the case of IORT for large lesions, two or more applicators may be used side by side for adequate coverage.

Acrylic or stainless steel applicators are sterilized or covered with a thin sheet of sterile plastic when they are used. The applicators usually slide or dock into a tube attached to the accelerator head. The face plate of the accelerator from which the electrons emerge or the treatment applicator should be covered with a sterilized sheet to prevent the possibility of any particles of dirt or dust from the machine falling into the surgical wound.

A retractable mirror-telescope-light system is desirable to observe the radiation field and to put the applicator into position. A pentagonally shaped treatment applicator with this mirror-telescope-light system is shown in Figure 3. A mirror coupled to a TV camera system

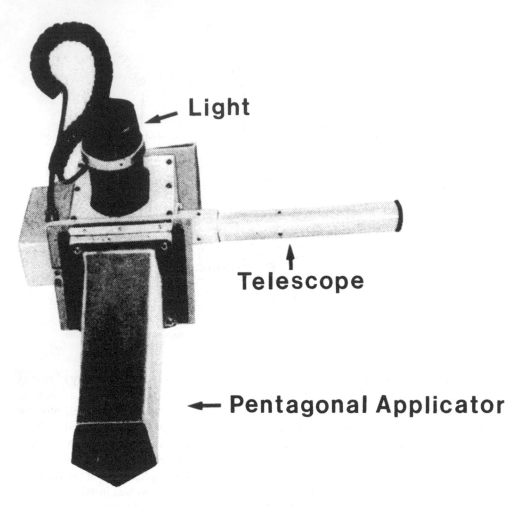

FIGURE 3.   A pentagonally shaped treatment applicator with a mirror-telescope-light system for IORT of gastric cancer.

such as that used at the National Cancer Institute (NCI) in the U.S. is useful to display the field of view on a television monitor during irradiation.

IV. ELECTRON ENERGY

The optimal electron energy for IORT must be chosen according to the thickness of the target volume. Electrons exiting the head of a medical accelerator generally have a very narrow energy spectrum and may be characterized by a single energy value, E_a, the "accelerator energy". However, the electron energy is changed by energy losses in layers of matter traversed by electrons such as the exit window, scattering foil, monitor chamber, and air. These expand the narrow spectrum and shift the effective energy to a lower energy region, as shown in Figure 4. The expanded energy spectrum of electrons at the treatment surface is characterized by the energy value corresponding to its peak, called the "most probable energy", $E_{p,0}$, and by the "mean energy", $\overline{E}_0$.[8] In clinical use of electrons, $E_{p,0}$ is usually used as the treatment energy, and $\overline{E}_0$ is used in calculating the absorbed dose, as shown in the next section. These energies must be measured for each individual accelerator and treatment applicator. A simpler method for energy determination uses the relationship between the energy and range parameters of electron penetration. In an International Com-

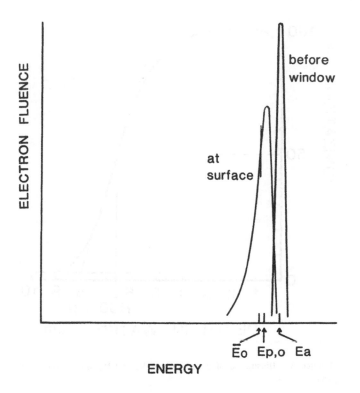

FIGURE 4. Illustration of energy parameters of electron beams. The narrow spectrum of accelerator energy, E_a, is expanded and shifted after the beam traverses an exit window, scattering foil, monitor chamber, and air layer. The expanded energy spectrum of electrons at the treatment surface is characterized by $E_{p,0}$ and E_0 (see text).

mission on Radiation Units and Measurements (ICRU) report (No. 35),[8] the following formulae are recommended for determining $E_{p,0}$:

$$E_{p,0} = C_1 R_p + C_2 \qquad 3 \text{ meV} \leq E_{p,0} \leq 25 \text{ meV} \qquad (1)$$

or, a modified equation

$$E_{p,0} = C_3 + C_4 R_p + C_5 (R_p)^2 \qquad 1 \text{ meV} \leq E_{p,0} \leq 50 \text{ meV} \qquad (2)$$

where R_p is the practical range of electrons, and constants are recommended in water as follows:

$$C_1 = 1.95 \text{ meV cm}^{-1}$$

$$C_2 = 0.48 \text{ meV}$$

$$C_3 = 0.22 \text{ meV}$$

$$C_4 = 1.98 \text{ meV cm}^{-1}$$

$$C_5 = 0.0025 \text{ meV cm}^{-2}$$

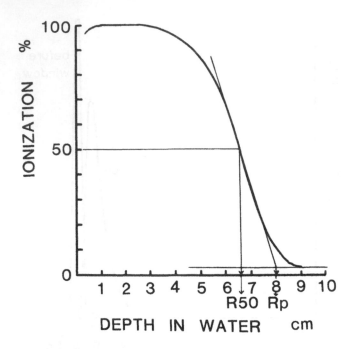

FIGURE 5.   Illustration of definitions of R_p and R_{50} on an ionization curve.

Ionization chambers are used for the determination of R_p. Ionization values are plotted as a function of depth in water as shown in Figure 5. The term R_p is defined as the depth at which the extrapolation line of the straight descending part of the curve meets the extrapolation line of the background due to bremsstrahlung. For example, since R_p is 8.0 cm in Figure 5, $E_{p,o} = 1.95 \times 8.0 + 0.48 = 16.0$ meV from Formula 1.

On the other hand, E_0 is obtained from the half-value depth, R_{50}, in water, as follows:[8]

$$E_0 = C_6 R_{50} \qquad 5 \text{ meV} \leq E_0 \leq 35 \text{ meV} \qquad (3)$$

where $C_6 = 2.33$ meV cm^{-1}. As shown in Figure 5, R_{50} is defined as the depth at which ionization is decreased to 50% of its maximum value. If R_{50} is 6.6 cm, $\bar{E}_0$ is 15.3 meV from Formula 3.

V. DOSIMETRY

ICRU Report No. 29[9] recommends that the whole target volume should be included by an isodose curve of at least 80% of the peak absorbed dose. In IORT, the absorbed dose percentage should be as high as possible throughout the whole target volume, preferably in excess of 90%.[10]

Each radiotherapy department must generate its own data on absorbed doses and dose distributions for each electron beam used for IORT, because the absorbed doses and the dose distributions depend on several factors, such as the quality of the initial electron beams, and the energy degradation in window, foils, transmission chamber, applicator, etc. A practical method of electron dosimetry for IORT with the use of phantoms is described below.

A. TREATMENT DOSE

The absorbed dose at the reference point is a water phantom which is usually used as

TABLE 1
The Reference Depth in a Water
Phantom Recommended in ICRU
Report No. 35.[8]

Energy	Depth of reference plane[a]
$1 \leqslant E_0 < 5$ meV	R_{100}
$5 \leqslant E_0 < 10$ meV	R_{100} or 10 mm[b]
$10 \leqslant E_0 < 20$ meV	R_{100} or 20 mm[b]
$20 \leqslant E_0 < 50$ meV	R_{100} or 30 mm[b]

[a] Here, R_{100} is the depth of maximum depth dose.
[b] The greater depth should always be chosen.

the treatment dose for IORT with electron beams. The reference point is the intersection between the reference plane and the reference axis, where the reference axis (or beam axis) is defined as the line passing through the center of the radiation field.[8] The depth of the reference plane ("the reference depth") in a water phantom is recommended by ICRU Report No. 35,[8] shown in Table 1. For example, an IORT dose is measured at 1.0 cm depth from the phantom surface or at the depth of maximum dose, R_{100}, when electron energies used are between 5 and 10 meV, while 2.0 cm or R_{100} is recommended for 19- to 20-meV electron energies. Ionization chambers are usually used for dose measurement. The ionization chamber is the only device which can be calibrated by the National Standard Laboratory.

The absorbed dose to water, D_w (P_{eff}), at the measuring point in a water phantom, is given by

$$D_w(P_{eff}) = N_D M_E S_{w,air} P_{w,air} \qquad (4)$$

where M_E is the meter reading of an ionization chamber when electrons are irradiated, N_D is the calibration factor giving the absorbed dose to air in the cavity of the chamber calibrated by the national standard with photon beams (cobalt-60 γ-rays or 2-meV X-rays), and $S_{w,air}$ is the water to air stopping power ratio. $S_{w,air}$ values are given in ICRU Report No. 35[8] for different depths in water for incident electron energy $\overline{E}_0$. $P_{w,air}$ is the perturbation correction factor for the ionization chamber. The values of $P_{w,air}$ are also given in the same report. For example, when 16-meV electrons are irradiated in a water phantom and the meter reading of a thimble ionization chamber which has an N_D value of 8.721×10^{-3} J/kg is 400 at the 2.0-cm depth, the absorbed dose at this point is calculated as follows: since $\overline{E}_0$ was calculated at 15.3 meV from Formula 3, the $S_{w,air}$ value at this depth obtained from the table in ICRU Report 35 is 1.006.[8] $P_{w,air}$ for this chamber and for the electron energy at this depth is 0.992, where the inner radius and the cavity length of this thimble ionization chamber are 2.5 and 15 mm, respectively. Therefore, D_w (2 cm) = $8.721 \times 10^{-3} \times 400 \times 1.006 \times 0.992$ = 3.48 Gy from Formula 4. In practical cases, the absorbed dose, D_w, must be corrected by factors such as ion recombination, effective point of measurement in the chamber, and temperature and pressure.[8]

Water is recommended as the standard medium for absorbed dose measurements because the absorbed dose distributions in water and human soft tissue are very similar. However, slabs of solid materials are more easily handled. When a material other than water is used, it is recommended that the solid phantom data be converted into "in-water data".[8] An example of the treatment dose determination in a water equivalent material, Mix D_p, is shown in Figure 6. For practical purposes, a given dose per unit of the monitor chamber

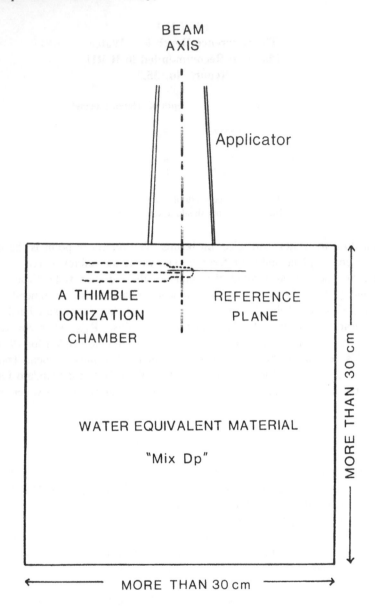

FIGURE 6.   Diagram of standard water equivalent phantom "Mix D_p" for the treatment dose determination with a thimble chamber (see text).

must be determined, where the linearity relationship must be checked over the whole monitor range.

Treatment doses are measured with the beam perpendicular to the surface of the phantom prior to each IORT, as shown in Figure 6. However, the treatment surface of a patient may be curved and there may be an air gap in the actual treatment. Corrections must be made for oblique incidence using the inverse-square law. The dose at depth d along the beam axis, $D'(d)$, can be approximated by correcting the dose value $D(d)$ for a beam of perpendicular incidence as follows:

$$D'(d) = \frac{SSD + d^2}{SSD + d + z} D(d) \qquad (5)$$

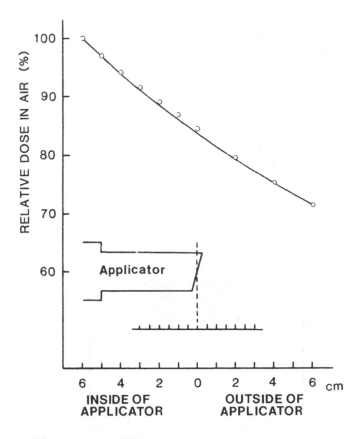

FIGURE 7. Dose variations of 6- or 8-meV electrons as a function of source to surface distance for the pentagonally shaped treatment applicator. Open circles represent thimble chamber measurement values. Solid curve is calculated by the inverse square law.

where z is the length of air gap and SSD is the normal source to surface distance. Figure 7 shows an example of the correction with the inverse-square law along the beam axis in the pentagonally shaped applicator previously described. In this figure, the open circles represent measurement values with a thimble ionization chamber, and the solid curve is calculated by Formula 5. Calculated values fit well to measurement values.

B. PERCENT DEPTH DOSE

Percent depth dose curves are measured on the reference axis. Since the tumor may extend to the surface of surgically exposed tissues and since critical organs may be directly below the tumor, a high surface dose and fast fall-off of dose with depth are required in IORT. Dose measurements in the build-up region are especially important. Examples of percent depth dose curves for 6- and 8-meV electron beams measured with a thimble ionization chamber and a thermoluminescent dosimeter (TLD) are shown in Figures 8 and 9. The percent depth doses measured with the thimble ionization chamber are in good agreement with those obtained by TLD, with an accuracy of $\pm 3\%$. Figure 10 shows various depth dose curves of electrons produced by a BT-32 Shimadzu betatron. For electron beam energies up to 20 meV generated by betatrons or linear accelerators, the radiation dose beyond the peak depth usually falls off rapidly. With further increase in electron energy, the fall-off curves become less steep.

C. SURFACE DOSE

As mentioned above, surface doses and percent depth doses in the build-up region are

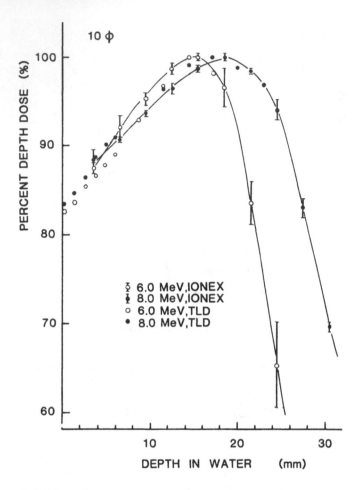

FIGURE 8. Percent depth dose curves for 6- and 8-meV electrons, measured with a thimble ionization chamber and TLD. Applicator size is 10 cm diameter.

particularly important in IORT. An example of the relationship between relative surface doses and electron energies is shown in Figure 11; surface doses measured by TLD and Fricke dosimeter are indicated. The relative surface doses increase with increasing electron energy and field size. For electrons with energy of up to 10 meV, relative surface doses are lower than 90%. For such energies and applicators, bolus is needed to ensure a 90% surface dose. A water equivalent material with a thickness of 5 mm should suffice (see Figures 8 and 9).

D. BEAM PROFILE

Field width, flatness, and symmetry can be determined from the beam profile in the reference plane. The beam profile is important for deciding whether a given applicator provides adequate tumor coverage. Beam profile varies considerably with applicator size and the distance between the reference plane and the end of the applicator, because the applicators function as a source of scattered electrons which may improve flattening of the beam near the surface of the treatment region. The beam profile can conveniently be obtained with film dosimetry. An example of electron beam profiles of 12-meV electrons measured at 2.0 cm depth in a Mix D_p phantom with film dosimetry is shown in Figure 12. Most of

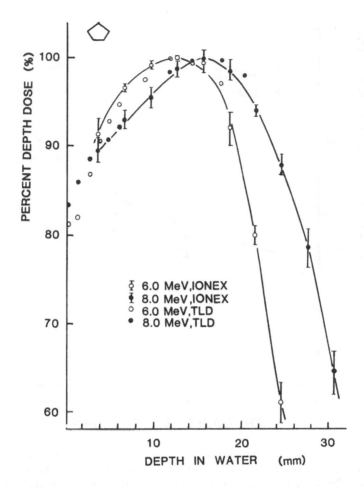

FIGURE 9.   Percent depth dose curves for 6- and 8-meV electrons, measured with a thimble ionization chamber and TLD. A pentagonal treatment applicator is used.

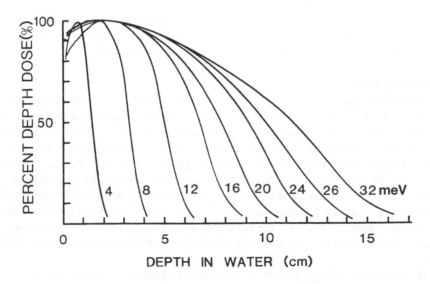

FIGURE 10.   Percent depth dose curves for electrons of various energies (BT-32, Shimadzu Corporation).

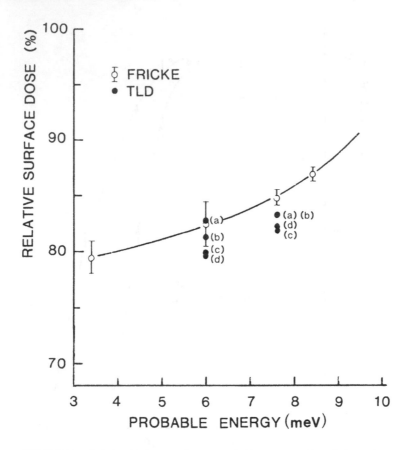

FIGURE 11.   Relationship between the most probable energy and the relative surface dose measured with Fricke dosimeter or TLD at 0.5 mm depth in water. Applicators of (a) 10 cm, (b) pentagon, (c) 8 cm, and (d) 6 cm were measured with TLD, and 10 cm with Fricke dosimeter.

the studies to date, including our own, indicate that a flatness requirement of ±5% and a symmetry requirement of ±2% are usually met.[10-12]

As mentioned above, the field width for IORT is usually defined as the distance between the 90% isodose lines in the reference plane. The penumbra of the field is defined as the average distance separating the 80 and 20% isodose lines ($P_{80/20}$).[8]

E. ISODOSE CURVES

Each radiotherapy department must have its own isodose charts constructed from measurements in a water equivalent phantom for every treatment applicator and each electron energy. These isodose curves can be obtained by films, TLD, diodes, or ionization chambers. Whatever system is used, the aim is to determine distributions of the absorbed dose in water. Raw data from measurements by chambers, or optical density distributions measured by films, cannot be used as isodose curves because the energy spectrum of electrons varies with depth, and therefore the amount of energy imparted to tissue varies with depth (i.e., $S_{w,air}$ and $P_{w,air}$ in Formula 4 change with depth in water). Isodose curves for 8-meV electrons in a water equivalent phantom for the pentagonally shaped treatment applicators are shown in Figure 13. Isodose curves for obliquely incident electron beams tend to be parallel to the surface.

In the treatment of large tumors, two or more treatment applicators may be used side by side in order to increase the irradiated area. In such a case, proper matching of these

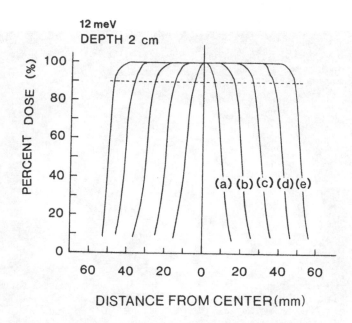

FIGURE 12.   Beam profiles measured with film dosimetry. The electron energy is 12 meV. Applicators (a) 2, (b) 4, (c) 6, (d) 8, and (e) 10 cm in diameter were used.

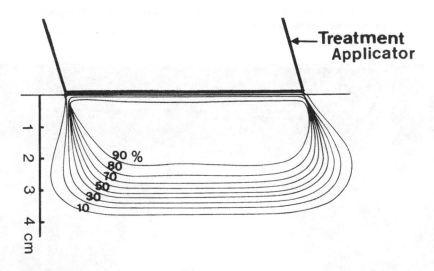

FIGURE 13.   Isodose curves for 8-meV electrons in a water equivalent phantom, Mix D_p, for the pentagonal treament applicator inclined 15°.

electron fields is critical. For IORT, the first field edge is marked by surgical clips in the tissue on the inside edge of the applicator, and the second field edge is then placed adjacent to those clips. Our dosimetric data show some "hot spots" that have not posed any problems clinically for IORT. The same method of field matching in IORT is used at the NCI.[7]

VI. TREATMENT PLANNING WITH A COMPUTER

The dose distribution in a patient differs from that in water phantoms described in the previous section, since the elemental composition, density, and shape of the irradiated tissues

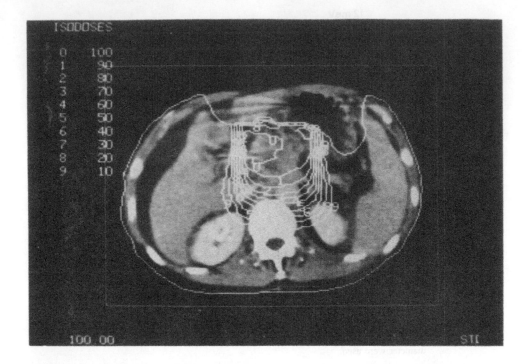

FIGURE 14. Isodose curves for 20-meV electrons through a 7-cm applicator for IORT of pancreatic carcinoma. A pencil-beam algorithm is used for the correction.

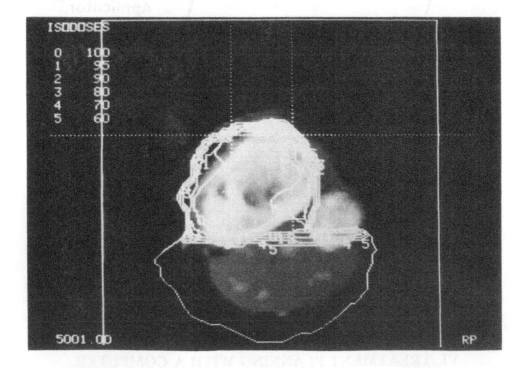

FIGURE 15. Isodose curves for 26-meV electrons with parallel opposing 10 × 10-cm fields for IORT of soft tissue sarcoma. A pencil-beam algorithm is used for the corrections.

differ from that of a water phantom. It is practically impossible to measure the dose distribution in a patient using dosimeters. However, recent developments in electron beam treatment planning with computers have improved the accuracy of determination of dose distribution in a patient. Furthermore, more sophisticated corrections for patient contour, inhomogeneities, etc., can be performed using CT images. Computer programs for electron dose planning are rapidly developing. A number of published algorithms are available for implementation in computerized electron beam treatment planning systems. At present, there is a problem in three-dimensional correction for inhomogeneities, especially in lung tissue, using the published algorithms for electron beam treatment planning. However, since the tissue to be treated by IORT is considered to be almost homogeneous, a computer for electron beam treatment planning with the present algorithms can be used to make corrections for patient contour for IORT.

Examples of the calculated isodose curves using CT images are shown in Figures 14 and 15, where pancreatic carcinoma is treated with a 20-meV electron beam from one portal and soft tissue sarcoma is treated with 26-meV electrons through parallel opposing electron fields. Treatment planning with CT images is especially useful for deciding the treatment volume in IORT.

VII. SUMMARY

Physical aspects of IORT using electron beams have been described:

1. An accelerator for IORT should have the capacity to generate electrons with high intensity, excellent energy quality, and various energy steps, because electron beams from the accelerator must permit delivery of a single sterilizing dose to the target volume with a sharp limitation of the total volume of tissues included in the high dose range without affecting normal structures.
2. Many types of applicators, including special-shaped ones, must be provided for IORT, where they must be adequate in covering the whole lesion(s) to be irradiated. A retractable mirror-telescope-light system and a mirror coupled to a TV camera system are desirable to observe the radiation field and to place the applicator in position.
3. The most probable energy, $E_{p,0}$, is used as the treatment energy. On the other hand, the mean energy, $\bar{E}_0$, is used in calculating absorbed doses. These energies at the treatment surface are measured for each accelerator and treatment applicator.
4. Each radiotherapy department must have its own dosimetric data on electron beams used (i.e., percent depth dose, surface dose, beam profile, and isodose curves in a water phantom) for every treatment applicator.
5. The treatment dose at the reference depth must be measured in a water phantom before IORT is started. The entire IORT target-volume should be within the 90% isodose line.
6. Practical determination of electron dose distributions in a patient can be improved by computer treatment planning using CT images.

REFERENCES

1. **Abe, M.,** Intraoperative radiotherapy — past, present and future, *Int. J. Radiat. Oncol. Biol. Phys.,* 10, 1987, 1984.
2. **Rich, T. A., Cady, B., McDermott, W. V., Kase, K. R., Chaffey, J. T., and Hellman, S.,** Orthovoltage intraoperative radiotherapy: a new look at an old idea, *Int. J. Radiat. Oncol. Biol. Phys.,* 10, 1957, 1984.

3. **Brahme, A. and Svensson, H.,** Radiation beam characteristics of a 22 meV microtron, *Acta Radiol. Oncol.,* 18, 243, 1979.

4. **Egawa, S., Tsukiyama, I., Ono, R., Yanagawa, S., Watai, K., Akiyama, Y., Matsumoto, K., Sakudo, M., Kakehi, M., Kitawgawa, T., and Koyama, Y.,** Clinical experience with the 22 meV microtron at the National Cancer Center Hospital, *Jpn. J. Clin. Oncol.,* 14, 613, 1984.

5. **Abe, M. and Takahashi, M.,** Intraoperative radiotherapy; the Japanese experience, *Int. J. Radiat. Oncol. Biol. Phys.,* 7, 863, 1981.

6. **Takahashi, M., Okada, K., Shibamoto, Y., Abe, M., and Yoshida, O.,** Intraoperative radiotherapy in the definitive treatment of localized carcinoma of the prostate, *Int. J. Radiat. Oncol. Biol. Phys.,* 11, 147, 1985.

7. **Fraass, B. A., Miller, R. W., Kinsella, T. J., Sindelar, W. F., Harrington, F. S., Yeakel, K., Van de Geign, J., and Glalstein, E.,** Intraoperative radiation therapy at the National Cancer Institutes: technical innovations and dosimetry, *Int. J. Radiat. Oncol. Biol. Phys.,* 11, 1299, 1985.

8. Radiation Dosimetry: Electrons with Initial Energies Between 1 and 50 meV, ICRU Rep. 35, International Commission on Radiation Units and Measurements, Washington, D.C., 1984.

9. Dose Specification for Reporting External Beam Therapy with Photons and Electrons, ICRU Rep. 29, International Commission on Radiation Units and Measurements, Washington, D.C., 1978.

10. **Gunderson, L. L., Tepper, J. E., Biggs, P. J., Goldson, A., Martin, J. K., McCullough, E. C., Rich, T. A., Shipley, W. U., Sindelar, W. F., and Wood, W. C.,** Intraoperative ± External beam irradiation, in *Current Problems in Cancer,* Vol. 7, Yearbook Medical, Chicago, 1983.

11. **Biggs, P. J., Epp, E. R., Ling, C. C., Novack, D. H., and Michaels, H. B.,** Dosimetry, field shaping and other considerations for intraoperative electron therapy, *Int. J. Radiat. Oncol. Biol. Phys.,* 7, 875, 1981.

12. **McCullough, E. C. and Anderson, J. A.,** The dosimetric properties of an applicator system for intraoperative electron-beam therapy utilizing a Clinac 18 accelerator, *Med. Phys.,* 9, 261, 1982.

Chapter 7

ANESTHESIOLOGIC CONSIDERATIONS FOR INTRAOPERATIVE RADIATION THERAPY

Paul E. Hodel and John T. Martin

TABLE OF CONTENTS

I. INTRODUCTION

The concept of intraoperative radiation therapy (IORT) involves the combination of two dissimilar treatment modalities in a potentially hazardous fashion. An anesthetized patient experiencing an ongoing and unfinished surgical procedure is transported to a high-energy radiation source where the anesthetic must be safely continued while all attendant personnel are away from the immediate vicinity of the patient during tissue irradiation. Compounding the problem is the fact that patients who have recognizable cancer are often at an increased risk of complication for any type of anesthesia.

II. MANAGEMENT ALTERNATIVES

Where space is limited, particularly in older institutions, it may be necessary to perform the surgical portion of intraoperative radiation therapy in surgery, then to transport the anesthetized patient a perilous distance through halls, elevators, and public spaces to reach and return from the distant radiation facility. There is real potential for mishap with this alternative, despite careful surveillance by knowledgeable participants. Monitors and intravascular lines may dislodge or become damaged; the inevitable jostling during transport can upset a patient's vital signs sufficiently to require interventions that are impossible en route; accidents can occur in public areas; unacceptable public spectacles may be created; the surgical wound may disrupt or become contaminated; etc. The hazards of the return trip to the operating room are compounded by the additional duration of anesthesia plus whatever stresses may have been added by the physiologic trespass of irradiation. Unless the absence of a suitable alternative forces its use, this method would not seem to serve the patient's best interest.

When space can be allocated, either in designing new construction or in the renovation of an existing structure, a surgical site can be constructed in the department of radiation therapy in close proximity to the high-energy treatment machine. After the induction of anesthesia, the tissue target can be exposed surgically, the operating table repositioned under the treatment beam, irradiation of the patient accomplished, and the table returned to the original operative position for closure of the wound. Anesthesia is then terminated and the protective reflexes of the awakened patient offer him increasingly adequate support during the move to the recovery unit. We have constructed such a facility because of our concerns about controlling the hazards of extensive patient movement. It is an effective and acceptable patient-care solution, despite the valid criticism that accomplishing anesthesia and surgery at the linear accelerator site interferes with the primary mission of the machine.

III. FACILITIES TO SUPPORT ANESTHESIA

To be accomplished, IORT requires some form of anesthesia. If either regional or general anesthesia is used, a method must be found to allow anesthesia personnel to depart the treatment area during the brief but usually repetitious intervals in which the high-energy beam is activated. Competent remote analog, digital, and visual electronic monitoring becomes an obvious necessity. Equally evident is the need for members of the anesthesia team to have almost instant physical access to the patient at the irradiation site should the monitors indicate either equipment malfunction or unacceptable changes in vital signs.

A. HOLDING AREA

Immediately outside the accelerator room, in the radiation therapy suite of the Medical College of Ohio Hospital, an area has been created to receive a patient on a stretcher. Adequate lighting, telephone, and record-keeping facilities are present, as are piping outlets

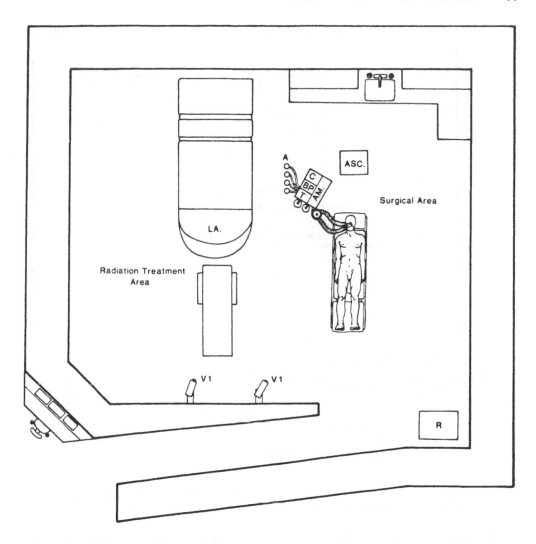

FIGURE 1.   IORT surgical area. (A) Anesthesia hose drops (ceiling mounted); (AM) anesthesia machine; (ASC) anesthesia supply cart; (BP) automated noninvasive blood pressure monitor; (C) carbon dioxide monitor; (LA) linear accelerator; (R) standardized resuscitation cart; (S) speaker for stethescope microphone; (T) Tektronix® (or equivalent) multifunction monitor (deriving signals from patient); (To) secondary (outside) Tektronix® monitor; (V1) video cameras; and (V2) video displays.

for oxygen and vacuum. Portable anesthesia supply carts are available to permit installation of intravascular lines. Sensors for physiologic monitors can be applied. While unexpected effects of prior medication can be dealt with here, the patient holding area is not intended to be an anesthetizing location.

B. THE SURGICAL AREA

Our linear accelerator room was structurally converted into an operating room by changing lighting, air handling, electrical circuitry, ceiling surface, and piped anesthesia services to comply with existing local hospital construction codes. Air handling was improved to provide 25 exchanges per hour without recirculation. Electrical circuits from two separate sources were brought in, each with a sufficient number of grounded double deluxe outlets to exceed anticipated demands for service. Surgical lights were hung from the ceiling and are augmented as needed with fiberoptic headlights worn by members of the operating team. Background lighting was enhanced by additional fluorescent ceiling fixtures.

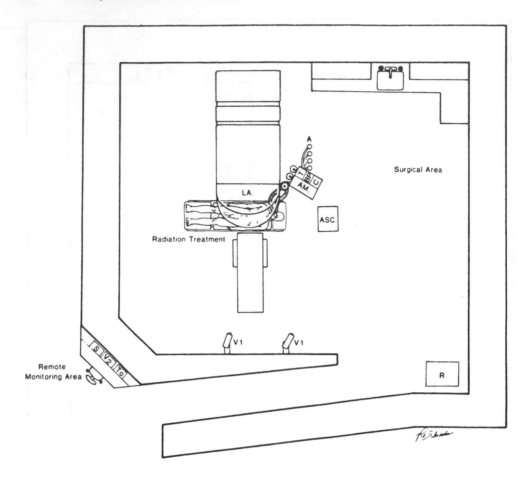

FIGURE 2.   Remote monitoring of the IORT/surgical area. (S) Speaker for stethoscope microphone; (To) secondary (outside) Tektronix® monitor; (V2) video displays; other abbreviations as in Figure 1.

A fixed position on the ceiling was located from which anesthesia service hoses could drop vertically to the anesthesia machine whether during the operative procedure or while irradiation is in progress (Figure 1, Item A). Oxygen, nitrous oxide, compressed air, and dual vacuum lines (one always available for aspiration of the patient's airway, and the other used for scavenging of waste anesthetic gases) were extended to the room from the central piping source of the hospital. Surgical vacuum is derived from separate wall outlets away from the anesthesia area. Preacceptance testing of the piping systems was carried out under the joint supervision of management personnel from the departments of anesthesiology and respiratory care. Because of the optimally short distance required for patient movement in this configuration of equipment, the anesthesia machine needs to be rotated only 90° around the point of the hose drop and moved several feet toward or away from the accelerator.

Adjacent to the 18-meV linear accelerator (Figure 1, Item LA) is an area large enough for an operating table, a stretcher for patient transfer, surgical back tables, the anesthesia machine (Figure 1, Item AM), a departmentally standardized anesthesia supply cart (Waterloo® or Craftsman®) (Figure 1, Item ASC), a floor-standing thermal unit, and the appropriate i.v. poles. Storage cabinets and a double sink were previously present on the back wall of the room. Surgical scrub sinks and a clothing change area are located elsewhere in the radiation therapy department to allow for multipurpose use.

Standard alarms, an anaerometer, an oximeter, a mechanical respirator with visible bellows, and a gas-scavenging attachment are all on the anesthesia machine. Its shelves contain (1) a portable Tektronix® ECG, temperature and dual pressure monitor with paper and oscilloscopic displays (Figure 1, Item T); (2) an automated, noninvasive blood pressure monitor (Figure 1, Item BP); and (3) an infrared carbon dioxide monitor (Figure 1, Item C) with its sensor interposed between the endotracheal tube and the Y-piece of the breathing circuit. Pressure transducers for intravascular catheters (arterial, central venous, or pulmonary artery as needed) are affixed either to the operating table or to a floor-standing i.v. pole. Supplementing the contents of the anesthesia supply cart are materials for resuscitation and defibrillation; these are always present on a mobile cabinet cart that is standard for all areas of our hospital (Figure 1, Item R).

C. THE REMOTE MONITORING AREA

Outside the treatment room, as a permanent installation immediately above the control console of the linear accelerator, is a Tektronix® unit (Figure 2, Item To) that is functionally identical to the one on the anesthesia machine (Figure 1, Item T). The outside unit is connected to its counterpart within the treatment enclosure by a cable that runs through a contorted channel ("maze") in the protective wall of the room. The biologic signals from the patient are received by the room unit, displayed, and immediately relayed to a simultaneous read-out at the functionally similar secondary unit in the remote monitoring area. Both oscilloscopic and paper displays are available from the outside unit with the signal gains of each being identical to those of the unit attached to the patient in order to permit accurate comparison and surveillance.

Also present at the remote monitoring site is a loudspeaker (Figure 2, Item S) which is connected by cable through the maze to a microphone in the esophageal stethoscope tubing just outside the mouth of the patient; the anesthesiologist can then continuously hear both heart and breath sounds during treatment. Consequently, apnea from a disconnected breathing circuit would at once become audibly evident before resultant changes appeared in other physiologic parameters of the paralyzed, ventilated patient.

Two wall-mounted television cameras (Figure 2, Item V1) in the treatment room have their monitors and controls at the remote linear accelerator console (Figure 2, Item V2) so that the patient can be viewed constantly by team members from a protected location during irradiation. One camera can be aimed and zoomed toward the front of the anesthesia machine to show flowmeters, respirator bellows, pulse oximeter, and the digital displays of the carbon dioxide monitor. The other offers a wider view of the treatment area and lets the anesthesia personnel identify patient movement or other problems. Should access to the patient be needed in an emergency, opening the door of the accelerator room shuts down the linear accelerator and instantly renders the area safe for attendants. Less than 10s is needed for a person at the remote monitoring station to reach the patient.

D. RECOVERY FACILITIES

At the conclusion of IORT, the operating table and anesthesia equipment are returned to their original orientation in the accelerator room, and the surgical wound is closed. Anesthesia is terminated in the usual manner. Disposition of the patient is decided upon according to his general physical condition as well as his progress in eliminating the anesthetic agents and adjuvants. A recovery room exists in the radiation therapy suite; however, the high cost of its use in terms of equipment and personnel has deterred us from using it. We prefer, as soon as the patient's cardiorespiratory status permits, to move the patient with supplemental oxygen and any necessary ventilatory support to the main Post Anesthesia Recovery Unit in the surgical area or, if appropriate, directly to the patient's bed in an intensive care unit.

IV. ANESTHETIC CONSIDERATIONS

A. TYPE OF ANESTHESIA

During the intraoperative radiation procedure, considerable time may be spent in positioning the patient so that the applicator of the linear accelerator can reach a peculiarly situated tumor bed. This is specifically true for transanal applicators. In the process, the maneuvers and comments involved may be uncomfortable and inelegant enough to constitute major emotional trauma for anxious, awake patients. A time-limited regional anesthetic, despite the most meticulous preliminary planning between anesthesiologist and surgeon, may have insufficient duration to accommodate unexpected alterations in the surgical program. Major regional anesthetic techniques usually incorporate supplementary sedation. We question the advisability of leaving a sedated patient unattended during the period of irradiation lest he move in such a way as to adversely affect the positioning of the body part being irradiated. Therefore, we consider regional anesthesia to be indicated only in those rare instances in which an unusually self-composed and cooperative patient can be expected to tolerate the immobility and solitude required during the period of irradiation. Combined regional and general anesthetic techniques may occasionally offer an advantage.

Any general anesthetic agent, technique, or precaution that is applicable to the cancer patient in the main surgical suite is also applicable when the patient is anesthetized for IORT in the facility described herein. Despite a location, remote from normal departmental traffic patterns, the careful planning of supplies and equipment, plus a minimal requirement to stress an anesthetized individual by extensive movement, allows the conduct of anesthesia to be familiar, predictable, and safe.

1. Practical Problems and Solutions

a. Transportation of the Anesthetized Patient

As is obvious from previous comments, we do not advocate extensive movement of an anesthetized patient. However, for a variety of reasons, our arrangements may not be applicable elsewhere, and we do not wish to imply that our opinions should serve as standards of practice to which others must adhere. Where anesthesia and transport must be combined, attention to the following hazards will benefit the patient.

1. Movement, whether from table to cart or while the cart traverses bumpy terrain, can easily stress the brittle autoregulation of anesthetized vasculature sufficiently to produce vasomotor decompensation and perfusion instability. Monitoring is needed en route to detect a sudden requirement for protective interventions with vasoactive drugs.
2. A volatile agent, sloshed within a vaporizer during jerky movement of an anesthesia machine, can, in some anesthetic machines, enter the delivery line in liquid form and produce a potentially lethal concentration in the breathing circuit.
3. When an anesthesia machine is towed along behind the patient's cart, uneven movement may stretch the breathing circuit and cause either disconnection or extubation. The resultant chaotic events for the anesthesia team and patient alike have to be experienced to be appreciated.
4. Travel through public spaces and in elevators creates the potential for equipment damage, physical injury to the patient, and contamination of the surgical wound. Significant invasion of privacy can occur, and the entire process often creates a very poor public image.

B. THERMAL CONTROL DURING ANESTHESIA

An environmental problem of consequence to the poikilothermic anesthetized patient in the accelerator unit is the low room temperature that must be maintained in order for the radiation therapy equipment to function properly. Inadvertent hypothermia is a significant problem with small or frail patients unless extraneous heat is provided. Careful humidified warming of the breathing circuit will usually maintain normothermia adequately. Accurate core or surface monitoring of the patient's body temperature is a necessity, as is the presence of a thermometer in the heated respiratory circuit.

Although a channeled mattress that circulates water with which to regulate the body temperature of the patient is generally useful, it may not always be an acceptable addition to the operating table. Diagnostic roentgenography is sometimes needed during the surgical exposure of the tumor and the water channels of the mattress can introduce shadows from different penetration densities that may complicate interpretation of the film. Fortunately, this problem can be eliminated almost completely by draining the water from the mattress before exposing the film. We prefer to have a heating/cooling machine present and its mattress routinely in place as an additional heat source with which to combat hypothermia. It can also serve as a cooling surface if hyperpyrexia is either feared or recognized.

C. CONCURRENT THERAPY

Infrequently, we find that the patient who is scheduled for IORT is also receiving antineoplastic drugs. The potential influences of the presence, side effects, or residual consequences of the various chemotherapeutic agents now available are significant issues for the anesthesiologist as well as the radiation therapist. For a detailed discussion of some of these issues, the reader is referred to an excellent review by Selvin.[1]

D. CONTROL OF ANESTHESIA

Although equipment for remote monitoring of the patient is readily available, the means with which to regulate the anesthesia machine from a distance do not exist. Stimuli during surgery and the positioning of the applicator require significant and titratable concentrations of anesthesia. After placement of the applicator, stimuli lessen as treatment is imminent and all personnel move away from the patient and the anesthesia machine to the shelter of the remote monitoring site. Simultaneously, the diminished stimuli usually permit a decreased concentration of the anesthetic. Without the opportunity to titrate anesthetic doses while away from the machine, the anesthesiologist must estimate the needs of the patient, leave the room during the treatment, and follow the results at the monitoring station. Any variation from acceptable vital signs during the treatment requires that the irradiation be temporarily suspended while anesthesia personnel return to the patient to make the necessary adjustments.

E. LOGISTICS

Because the radiation therapy area is remote from the surgical suite, the anesthesiology and nursing teams must carefully plan their supply and equipment requirements as well as the logistics of resupply during a procedure. Competent arrangements are not difficult to develop and the quality of support should be the same as that enjoyed in the main operating theater. A messenger system can deliver samples for rapid laboratory testing, supply transfusion therapy products, and can acquire unanticipated material.

REFERENCES

1. **Selvin, B. L.,** Cancer chemotherapy: implications for the anesthesiologist, *Anesth. Analg. (Cleveland)*, 60, 425, 1981.

Chapter 8

NURSING AND TECHNOLOGICAL CONSIDERATIONS IN INTRAOPERATIVE RADIATION THERAPY

D. Ann Hollon

TABLE OF CONTENTS

I. INTRODUCTION

Although oncology nursing as an art and science is relatively modern, nursing in actual practice (the spirit of nursing) has existed since the beginning of time. The impulse to serve is the basis on which the spirit of nursing has been fostered through the ages. As the needs of humanity have changed during the process of civilization, nursing has developed broader interest and functions. Now nursing means many things — to nourish, to protect, to prevent illness, to avoid injury, to educate, to sustain, to give.

The concept of intraoperative radiation therapy (IORT) is not new. Intraoperative X-ray treatment was used in Germany in 1915 and in the U.S. and Great Britain during the 1940s. Although technical problems prevented it from being widely applied, these early experiences demonstrated its potential.[1] Now there is renewed interest in IORT because of improved technology and a better understanding of the limitations of surgery and radiation for specific types of cancers.[2] Most importantly, this encourages surgeons and radiotherapists to expand collaborative investigations. This procedure also presents nurses with a challenge and many new responsibilities.

IORT demands very close interdisciplinary cooperation and teamwork. The team must work in cooperation and harmony, bringing to the patient all the knowledge and skill available in combating the cancer. Every member of an IORT group must work together so that the corps of workers may function not as individuals, but as one unit having one common interest — the welfare of the patient.

The responsibilities of everyone associated with the IORT procedure should be outlined clearly. This eliminates confusion and allows for the maximum in safety for the patient and staff.

IORT is not for all tumors, certain eligibility criteria must be met for consideration. The protocol should include, but not necessarily be limited to, the following: (1) biopsy-proven cancer, (2) unresectable tumor or high likelihood of local recurrence, (3) tumor size compatible with inclusion in the high-dose intraoperative boost volume, and (4) no contraindications to surgical exploration.

IORT is a treatment technique designed for certain cancer patients. Both surgery and radiation have significantly improved survival rates, but each has its limitations.[3] Despite aggressive therapy, local failure continues to be a major problem in the treatment of malignant disease, especially in advanced tumors of the abdomen and brain. Limitations in the surgical approach may possibly spread microscopic disease beyond the operative site. External radiation alone may be inadequate, because the dose that can safely be delivered to the tumor is restricted by the limited radiation tolerance of normal surrounding tissues. IORT can theoretically overcome these limitations by directly irradiating the tumor site with a high dose of radiation.

II. TECHNIQUES OF TREATMENT

The surgical procedure involves excising portions of the tumor that can be removed safely. Then, radiosensitive structures, such as the liver, intestines, and other organs, are temporarily moved out of the path of the radiation beam. After the tumor is exposed, the exact extent of the disease is determined. Particular attention is directed to the size of the primary lesion and presence or absence of metastatic disease in adjacent tissues. Biopsy and frozen-section examinations confirm the diagnosis and identify the tumor type.

In most instances the IORT will be given. Exceptions occur when lesions can be surgically removed with clean margins or when the ratio of probable therapeutic benefits to complications is too low.

When using the Medical College of Ohio IORT device, the radiation oncologist and the surgeon select an acrylic applicator of appropriate diameter. The applicator is attached to an aluminum sleeve which slides onto the main assembly attachment. It is connected to the treatment head of the linear accelerator in much the same fashion as a conventional electron beam apparatus. The clear Lucite® applicator with $^1/_4$-in.-thick walls not only serves to identify the area of the electron beam, but it also helps to retract tissue from the path of the radiation beam. The patient is moved so that the incision is directly under the treatment machine. The operating table is moved up to the desired height and the applicator is brought down. This is a delicate maneuver which demands total cooperation of everyone involved. When the radiation oncologist and the surgeon judge the applicator to be in a satisfactory position, a fiberoptic right-angle periscope is inserted through the main assembly attachment. This allows for direct visual placement of the applicator into the body and directly on the tumor as "seen" by the therapy machine.

If the IORT dose is to be delivered by means of an orthovoltage unit, the radiation oncologist and surgeon select an appropriate size treatment cone made of lead-lined brass. The cone is attached to the treatment head of the machine and stabilized in the patient allowing for tumor coverage plus a 1- to 2-cm margin.

Once the radiation oncologist and the surgeon are satisfied with the IORT applicator placement, the entire team leaves the room, closely observing the patient's vital signs via remote monitors, TV, and/or direct visualization through a leaded-glass viewing window. The patient is maintained under anesthesia with automatic equipment.

Should the need arise for immediate access to the patient, the radiation power source shuts off automatically when the door is opened. This occurs because the doors are equipped with safety switches interfaced with the treatment machines. Neither the linear accelerator nor the orthovoltage unit can generate radiation without electrical power. The treatment can also be interrupted or stopped by depressing the beam "off" button on the console of the linear accelerator or by turning the timer switch off on the orthovoltage unit.

III. DOSAGE-TIME FACTORS

The average dose given during an IORT procedure ranges from 10 to 40 Gy. A single dose of 20 Gy may not be biologically equivalent to a total dose of 40 to 60 Gy delivered at the usual 1.8 to 2.0 Gy per fraction over 4 to 6 weeks time. The dose delivered is dependent upon the bulk and histology of the residual tumor. The energy of the electron beam or the orthovoltage kilovolt peak (kVp) is selected on the basis of the thickness of the residual tumor (from 6 to 18 meV or from 15 to 300 kVp). The time required to deliver the dose is dependent upon the prescribed dose, the area to be covered, the thickness of the tumor, and the target tumor distance (TTD). The time will vary between 5 and 15 min for the electron beam and 15 to 25 min for orthovoltage X-ray.

IV. TREATMENT ROOM

In some institutions, the anesthetized patient is transported to the radiation therapy department after initial surgical exposure of the tumor. After the tumor is exposed, the patient's incision is temporarily closed with stay sutures and covered with sterile drapes. The patient is then transferred with the surgical team and all life support systems to the radiation therapy department. After IORT is given, the patient is returned to the operating room if additional surgery is required, or he may remain in the radiation therapy department for routine wound closure.

Another approach is to have the IORT machine in the operating room, so patients do not have to be transported while anesthetized. This approach can be used when orthovoltage

TABLE 1
Intraoperative Radiation Therapy: Operating Practices[a]

Procedure/parameters	Timing and frequency	Responsible individual(s)
Calibrate linear accelerator or orthovoltage machine	Always: morning of procedure	R.T.(T.)[b]
Monitor system (intercom, TV, Textronix® slave)	Always: evening preceding procedure	R.T.(T.)
Room "surgically cleaned"	Always: evening preceding procedure	Housekeeping
Ordering case cart	Always: evening preceding procedure	R.N.[c] O.R.[d]
Check anesthesia machines, equipment	Always: evening preceding or morning of procedure	Anesthesiologist
Removing unneeded equipment from room	Evening preceding procedure	R.T.(T.)
Place operative equipment in room	Always: evening preceding procedure	R.T.(T.) R.N. radiation therapy
Patient consent signed, witnessed	Always: evening preceding procedure	Radiation oncologist
Proper identification of patient	Always: morning of procedure	R.T.(T.), R.N. O.R.
Patient to recovery room	Immediately after procedure	Anesthesiologist
Removal of instruments case carts to central supply room	Always: immediately after procedure	R.N. O.R.
Removal of linen	Always: immediately after procedure	R.N. O.R.
Removal of operative equipment from linear accelerator room	Always: immediately after procedure	R.T.(T.)
Removal of anesthesia equipment	Always: immediately after procedure	Anesthesiologist
Cleaning of linear accelerator room	Always: immediately after procedure	Housekeeping

[a] For IORT procedures, all operating room protocols will be followed. The above protocols are followed when the IORT facilities are located in the radiation therapy department. There would be slight modification on the above protocol if IORT were done in the operating room or if the patient is transported to the radiation therapy department after the initial surgical exposure.

[b] R.T.(T.) — radiation therapy technologist.

[c] R.N. — Registered Nurse.

[d] O.R. — operating room personnel.

is employed. The orthovoltage unit is much smaller and less complex than the linear accelerator. The linear accelerator is a large, costly, and complex unit, not convenient or cost effective for installation in an operating room in ordinary clinical circumstances.

Still another approach is to administer IORT in a combined operating room and radiation treatment room. The patient does not need to be transported, and the linear accelerator can be used for outpatient radiation treatments at other times. If the latter approach is used, strict cleaning procedures are adhered to, and the room is dedicated solely to surgery on days that an IORT patient is scheduled (Table 1). When this approach is used, patients who normally would receive treatment from this machine are treated with another linear accelerator. To be able to achieve this, the radiation therapy department must have more than one treatment machine and the beam shaping blocks must be interchangeable between treatment machines.

V. ELECTRONS VS. X-RAYS

The approximate cost of an orthovoltage X-ray unit is $^1/_{10}$ to $^1/_{20}$ the cost of an electron beam treatment machine. Orthovoltage X-rays have poorer penetration and deliver a higher dose to the bone. There is also more secondary scatter of radiation with conventional X-rays. These disadvantages can be minimized by treating small tumors (less than 5 cm thick) and by carefully shielding bone where possible. A high dose to bone could be associated with latent radiation effect, and patients treated in this fashion should be followed carefully for these effects.

The general rationale for using IORT is to improve the therapeutic ratio of local control vs. complications. Most major advances in radiation therapy for the treatment of cancer have been premised on the difference in radiation dose distribution between tumor and normal tissue. For most tumors, the likelihood of achieving local tumor control improves as larger radiation doses are delivered to the tumor mass. However, in many clinical situations, the dose that can safely be delivered to the tumor is restricted by the limited radiation tolerance of normal surrounding tissues. Hopefully, the higher IORT dose may mean improved cure rates and better palliation for some cancers.

VI. THE NURSE'S ROLE

The IORT procedure, as stated previously, presents the nursing staff with a challenge and many new responsibilities. The nurse is not only involved with patient care before, during, and after the procedure, she/he is also involved in the physical planning and delivery of this multidisciplinary treatment regimen.

Planning for the individual patient, the perioperative nurse carries out a thorough and sensitive preoperative assessment, identifying the patient's learning, emotional, and physical needs. Any and all nursing personnel must be involved in patient assessments if continuity of care is to be established. A postoperative nursing assessment should be done to establish the effectiveness of the plan and to assess if any additional nursing measures are needed for optimal care.

The physical, emotional, and psychological needs of the patient must be identified and met. There are three stresses facing the patient simultaneously: (1) the diagnosis of cancer, (2) the surgery, and (3) the radiation. It is of utmost importance for the nurse to evaluate a patient's emotional status and anxiety level.

For some patients, a diagnosis of cancer seems a death sentence, regardless of the extent of disease and even when a cure may be anticipated. They may have a perceived misconception about radiation. Anxieties are often heightened when the patient must cope with the thoughts of cancer, radiation, and surgery at the same time. Time must be allowed for questions and answers. Nursing personnel must give special attention to verbal as well as nonverbal communication of anxieties. The nurse must be attuned to unshown fears and unasked questions.

A patient's emotional reaction to his or her illness and treatment management may reflect one or more of the following: (1) basic personality and level of emotional stability, (2) attitude toward the underlying disease, and (3) relationship of the patient to professional staff members, family, and friends with whom he/she has discussed his illness. Mental comfort for the patient may be provided by allaying fears and worry. The patient may find many things to fear in his immediate situation. He may be afraid that the IORT procedure will endanger his life. He may be fearful of the anesthetic agent, dreading the experience of going to sleep, and the thought of dying may produce real terror.

When evaluating a patient's emotional status, anxieties, and learning needs, it is important to remember that more damage can occur from misinterpretation and misunderstanding than has ever been reported in a medical literature review of the side effects of IORT.[4] This fact reinforces the need for patient education.

Teaching is a tool available to the nurse and is invaluable in lowering an IORT patient's anxiety level. Some patients may be relieved to know that their treatment regimen will be shortened by having both the radiation and surgery at the same time. The IORT dose of radiation may eliminate or decrease the need for repeated trips to the outpatient radiation therapy center.

In evaluating the patient's physical condition, the evaluation should center on the overall condition of the patient, the patient's past and present illnesses, his medical and surgical history, a review of body systems, and identification of any allergies or physical limitations. If the patient is afraid of pain and physical discomfort, which may follow the IORT, he may be greatly reassured that pain and discomfort can be controlled by medications. If the treatment plan involves pre- or postoperative external beam irradiation, nursing care plans must be made to maintain skin integrity and promote wound healing.

VII. FACTORS TO TEACH THE PATIENT

- Both surgery and irradiation have significantly improved patient survival rates.
- The patient is under constant observation during the IORT dose delivery.
- Repeated trips to an outpatient radiation therapy center may be eliminated or decreased by having radiation and surgery at the same time.
- Pain and discomfort can be controlled by medications.
- Assure mental comfort by allaying fears and worries.
- Include family members and loved ones in pre- and post-IORT planning.

VIII. EDUCATION AND PERSONNEL

Just as IORT is not for every patient, it is not a procedure that can be handled routinely. Extensive planning and in-service education is essential in preparing personnel for this procedure. In-service training sessions should be held with all personnel involved in the IORT procedure. These in-service training sessions allow everyone the time to ask questions and express their concerns. Valuable input is obtained which proves to be a very important part of preplanning.

IORT by both orthovoltage X-ray and electron beams are under continuing investigation as a means of improving palliation and increasing cure rates. There will be a continuation of assessments of the acute and potential latent effects of IORT.

Much remains to be done in evaluating what part IORT plays in the management of certain malignancies. It is hoped that this innovative procedure will improve survival and the quality of life for certain cancer patients.

REFERENCES

1. **Bane, C. L. and Rich, R. A.,** Intraoperative radiation therapy, *AORN J.,* 37, 1983.
2. **Abe, M. and Takahashi, M.,** Intraoperative radiotherapy — the Japanese experience, *Int. J. Radiat. Oncol. Biol. Phys.,* 7, 863, 1981.
3. **Goldson, A. L.,** Past, present, and prospects of intraoperative radiotherapy, *Semin. Oncol.,* 8, 59, 1981.
4. **Bane, C. L. and Shurkus, L.,** Caring for intraoperative radiation patients, *J. Am. O.R. Nurse,* 37, 841, 1983.

Chapter 9

THE DEVELOPMENT OF AN INTRAOPERATIVE RADIATION THERAPY PROGRAM — THE GRONINGEN IORT PROJECT

H. J. Hoekstra, D. M. Mehta, J. Oldhoff, J. Vermeij, and M. Crommelin

TABLE OF CONTENTS

I. INTRODUCTION

Surgery is no longer the sole major method of cancer treatment. Combined therapies utilizing surgery, chemotherapy, and radiation therapy have improved the 5-year survival rates of patients with a variety of malignancies. The disadvantages of these combined therapies are reflected in increased morbidity. Improvements in technical equipment and in methods of radiation therapy have decreased the radiation-induced morbidity. Still, the delivery of tumoricidal doses of radiation for various malignancies with external beam techniques can be accomplished by significant short- and long-term toxicity to normal tissues.

In the early part of this century, gastrointestinal malignancies were treated with ortho-voltage radiation during surgery.[1-3] The limitations of equipment and surgical and anesthetic techniques hampered the further use of this combined therapy of surgery and radiation. Our interest in intraoperative radiation therapy (IORT) came when several Japanese and American centers demonstrated that megavoltage radiation could be safely and effectively given to areas within the abdomen.[4-9]

IORT, single high-dose electron beam irradiation during a surgical procedure, is still an experimental treatment. The technique has potential advantages over current conventional fractionated external beam irradiation by limiting the exposure of normal tissues to irradiation and therefore limiting radiation toxicity. IORT is used in combination with macroscopic tumor resection in gastric cancers, colorectal carcinomas, pancreatic cancers, retroperitoneal sarcomas, and pelvic tumors, as well as in unresected pancreatic cancers, biliary tract cancers, and bladder cancers.[6,9] There are differing opinions about the optimum use of IORT. At the National Cancer Institute (NCI), Howard University, and Kyoto University, single high-dose (>20 Gy) electron beam irradiation is delivered to the tumor bed and potential areas of locoregional spread following gross surgical resection. The Mayo Clinic, The Medical College of Ohio (MCO), Massachusetts General Hospital (MGH), and the Joint Center for Radiation Therapy (JCRT) combine conventional fractionated external beam irradiation (45 to 50 Gy) with an IORT boost (15 to 20 Gy) of high-energy electrons (Mayo, MCO, and MGH) or 300-kV X-rays (JCRT).[6] The optimum use of IORT is still unknown. It is believed that IORT has its greatest value in a combination of macroscopic surgical resection with or without conventional fractionated external beam radiation therapy.

Although at present IORT must be considered experimental, preliminary reports suggest that IORT has advantages over current conventional radiation therapy.[4-10] Therefore, in 1983, the Division of Surgical Oncology and the Department of Radiotherapy of the University Hospital Groningen, Netherlands, initiated a program for IORT at their new hospital. This chapter describes the development of the Groningen IORT project.

II. THE IORT GROUP

Intraoperative delivery of radiation is not a simple procedure. It requires active participation of surgeons, radiation oncologists, anesthetists, physicists, operating room nurses, and radiation technologists. For the evaluation of the IORT treatment, the support of a radiobiologist and pathologist is imperative. Table 1 summarizes the participants in the IORT group. The objective of the IORT group was to develop an IORT program for IORT facilities at the Groningen University Hospital, based on existing clinical experiences. It was necessary to (1) analyze the IORT literature, (2) investigate the technical IORT requirements, (3) study the radiobiological effects of varying doses of IORT, (4) acquire logistic experience with IORT, and (5) identify potential patient populations for IORT treatment.

III. THE IORT PROGRAM

More than one hundred articles and abstracts about IORT have been published; the

TABLE 1
Participants in IORT Group

Surgery	Intraoperative radiation	Treatment evaluation
Surgeon	Radiation therapist	Surgeon
Anesthetist	Physicist	Radiation therapist
O.R. nurse	Radiation technologist	Pathologist
Radiation therapist	Surgeon	Radiobiologist
		Physicist

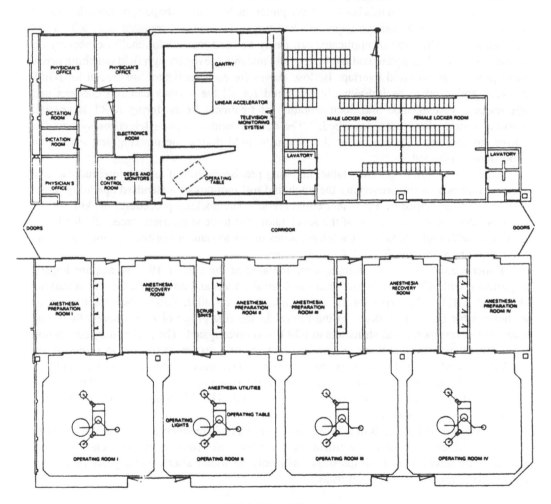

FIGURE 1.   Floor plan of operating rooms with dedicated IORT facilities.

majority during the last 5 years. Over 1500 patients have been treated with IORT, most with resectable or unresectable abdominal or pelvic malignancies that sometimes required extensive surgical resections. In general, the IORT experience is limited to a few centers in Japan and the U.S. Most of these institutions have IORT facilities in the department of radiation therapy. For a more efficient IORT program, we decided to construct a dedicated IORT facility within the general operating suites of the new hospital (Figure 1). With this situation, the opportunity exists to treat patients with IORT at any time, only requiring transfer over a short distance from the operating room to the room which contains the radiation equipment. If necessary, more than one IORT procedure can be performed on the same day. The dedicated IORT room is a standard operating room with a 20-meV linear accelerator. The whole procedure of surgery and irradiation can be performed in the IORT room. A linear accelerator with electron energies up to 20 meV was selected, as opposed to orthovoltage equipment. Although orthovoltage equipment is less expensive, it is not recommended for IORT because of its poor depth-dose characteristics, wide-angle setting, absorbed dose enhancement in bone, and the low exposure rate causing longer treatment times.

Applicator systems are not widely available commercially. A number of applicator systems, circular and rectanglar, different sizes and bevels, are described in the periodic literature and elsewhere in this book.[11-14] We prefer the horseshoe-shape applicator developed at NCI.[14] The horseshoe-shape applicator has one square and one rounded side, with a 15° beveled angle. This type of applicator can easily be used intra-abdominally, especially on sloping surfaces. The square end facilitates field matching, even though field matching needs extra precautions to avoid overlap. Isodose curves for each applicator are crucial for IORT delivery and need to be individually measured for all the various electron energies and applicators. Visualization and documentation of treatment fields during IORT is crucial. Various systems have been described.[15] The development of a color television system that allows continuous visualization of the treatment field during the docking and irradiation procedure is planned.

A dedicated IORT operating table, allowing precise control of lateral, longitudinal, and vertical motions, while preserving the pitch and roll motions of a standard operating table, was recently described by Fraas and co-workers.[14] The docking procedure, docking of the electron applicators to the head of the accelerator, has to be simplified, especially for IORT treatment with multiple fields. Therefore, adjustments to standard operating tables allowing the necessary versatility for IORT are necessary.

Experiments with large animals were initiated at the end of 1983 to acquire logistic experience with IORT and to study radiobiological effects and dosimetric aspects of varying doses of IORT. The experiments were carried out on adult female beagles to provide guidelines for the clinical doses in the future. In the first group of experiments, the tissue tolerance of retroperitoneal structures to IORT was investigated. The preliminary conclusion from our investigation is that the primary dose-limiting organs in the retroperitoneum are the kidneys and ureter. Doses in excess of 30 Gy induce irreversible damage to the kidneys and ureter. In the second group of experiments, the effect of varying doses of IORT to the bronchial stump after pneumectomy was investigated. The follow-up is too short to draw any definitive conclusions.

As mentioned before, IORT is still an experimental treatment, and it is important to determine which methods of treatment are the most cost effective and convenient for the patient. The answers to these questions will only be found after several years of various prospective, randomized clinical trials.

IV. SUMMARY

IORT requires considerable expenditure of effort by surgical, radiotherapeutic, and anesthetic staffs. It is still an experimental treatment with potential advantages over current conventional radiation therapy. At the moment it is unknown if this ''new'' cancer treatment justifies dedicated IORT facilities. Prospective, randomized clinical trials utilizing IORT are necessary to investigate the effect of IORT.

ACKNOWLEDGMENTS

Thanks are due to the many individuals who have made it possible to undertake the

IORT project at Groningen. Experimental studies were supported by the Jan Kornelis de Crockstichting and the Groningen Pediatric Oncology Foundation.

REFERENCES

1. **Beck, C.**, An external roentgen treatment of internal structures (eventration treatment), *N.Y. Med. J.*, 89, 621, 1909.
2. **Eloesser, L.**, The treatment of some abdominal cancers by irradiation through the open abdomen combined with cautery excision, *Ann. Surg.*, 106, 645, 1937.
3. **Barth, G. and Menel, F.**, Intraoperative Kontakttherapie in den grossen Körperhölen, *Strahlentherapie*, 109, 386, 1959.
4. **Abe, M., Takahashi, M., Yabumoto, E., Adachi, H., Yoshi, M., and Morik, K.**, Clinical experience with intraoperative radiotherapy of locally advanced cancers, *Cancer*, 45, 40, 1980.
5. **Goldson, A. L.**, Past present and prospects of intraoperative radiotherapy (IORT), *Semin. Oncol.*, 8, 59, 1981.
6. **Gunderson, L. L., Tepper, J. E., Biggs, P. J., Goldson, A.L., Martin, J. K., McCullough, E. C., Rich, T. A., Shipley, W. U., Sindelar, W. F., and Wood, W. C.**, Intraoperative ± external beam irradiation, *Curr. Probl. Cancer*, 7, 11, 1983.
7. **Tepper, J. E. and Sindelar, W. F.**, Summary of the workshop on intraoperative radiation therapy, Meeting report, *Cancer Treat. Rep.*, 65, 911, 1981.
8. **Sindelar, W. F., Kinsella, T. J., Tepper, J. E., Travis, E. L., Rosenberg, S. A., and Glatstein, E.**, Experimental and clinical studies with intraoperative radiotherapy, *Surg. Gynecol. Obstet.*, 157, 205, 1983.
9. **Kinsella, T. J. and Sindelar, W. F.** Intraoperative radiotherapy, in *Cancer Principles and Practice of Oncology*, 2nd ed., DeVita, V. T., Hellman, S., and Rosenberg, S. A., Eds., Lippincott, Philadelphia, 1985.
10. **Tepper, J. E., Wood, W. C., Cohen, A. M., Shipley, W. U., Orlow, E., Hedberg, S. E., Warshaw, A. L., Nardi, G. L., and Biggs, P. J.**, Intraoperative radiation therapy, in *Important Advances in Oncology 1985*, DeVita, V. T., Hellman, S., and Rosenberg, S. A., Eds., Lippincott, Philadelphia, 1984, 226.
11. **Biggs, P. J., Epp, E.R., Ling, C. C., Novack, D. H., and Michaels, H. B.**, Dosimetry, field shaping and other considerations for intraoperative electron therapy, *Int. J. Radiat. Oncol. Biol. Phys.*, 7, 875, 1981.
12. **McCullough, E. C. and Anderson, J. A.**, Dosimetric properties of an applicator system for intraoperative electron beam therapy utilizing a Clinac-18 accelerator, *Med. Phys.*, 9, 261, 1982.
13. **Mondalek, P. M.**, A clinical telescoping intraoperative electron radiation therapy device, *Int. J. Radiat. Oncol. Biol. Phys.*, 10, (Suppl. 2), 181, 1984.
14. **Fraass, B. A., Miller, R. W., Kinsella, T. J., Sindelar, W. F., Harrington, F. S., Yeakel, K., Van der Geijn, J., and Glatstein, E.**, Intraoperative radiotherapy at the National Cancer Institute: technical innovations and dosimetry, *Int. J. Radiat. Oncol. Biol. Phys.*, 11, 1299, 1985.
15. **Fraass, B. A., Harrington, F. S., Kinsella, T. J., and Sindelar, W. F.**, Television system for verification and documentation of treatment fields during intraoperative radiation therapy, *Int. J. Radiat. Oncol. Biol. Phys.*, 9, 1409, 1983.

Chapter 10

THE ROLE OF ORTHOVOLTAGE EQUIPMENT FOR INTRAOPERATIVE RADIATION THERAPY

Tyvin A. Rich, Richard W. Piontek, and Kenneth R. Kase

TABLE OF CONTENTS

I. INTRODUCTION

Equipment selection based on machine energy has played a major role in past and present applications of intraoperative radiation therapy (IORT). Before high-energy electrons from betatrons or linear accelerators became available, orthovoltage X-ray units with increasing kilovoltage potential (50 to 250 kilovolt peaks [kVp]) were used. In this chapter, we discuss the development of early orthovoltage equipment and the role of modern equipment in contemporary radiotherapeutic practice.

A. HISTORIC BACKGROUND

In the earliest IORT studies, low-kilovoltage machines ("deep ray", <100 kVp) were used to treat surgically exposed, deeply seated tumors in a treatment called "eventration".[1] First reported in 1909, it was based on the concept that an improved therapeutic ratio could be achieved by bringing the tumor to the abdominal surface during surgery.[2] Equipment limitations prevented the widespread use of this type of IORT, and interest in IORT waxed and waned over the next decades until technologic advancement rekindled clinical interest.

In Germany in the 1920s, contact therapy X-ray machines were used to simulate the dose distribution obtained with radium, but at lower cost and greater intraoperative convenience. The introduction of these low-energy machines, which were portable and electrically safe, allowed large single doses of X-rays to be given intraoperatively to selected patients who had small unresected or residual cancer after surgical debulking. Chaoul described the results of 60-kVp contact therapy (2 mA, 0.2 mm Cu, 5 cm target-to-skin distance) for 11 patients with incompletely resected gynecologic and bladder cancers.[3] Surface doses of 7600 to 11,400 roentgens (R) were used for 11 patients, of whom 3 survived longer than 3 years and were considered cured. Palliation without reported complications was achieved for many patients who had gross residual or unresected disease. Other investigators found contact therapy useful for palliation in patients with head and neck, gynecologic, and rectal cancers.[4,5] A novel application of contact therapy was reported for superficial bladder and stomach cancers.[6,7] The short X-ray penetration was particularly suited to the treatment of early cancers in hollow viscera. From a radiobiologic point of view, these investigators also realized the advantage of fractionating the IORT dosage. By temporary surgical exposure of the urinary bladder for several weeks, multiple daily X-ray doses could be delivered to superficial bladder cancers, thus providing the possibility for a high therapeutic ratio. This practice is not unlike the "radiosurgery" done today for small rectal cancers by repeated applications of intracavitary 50-kVp X-rays.[8]

The introduction of higher energy orthovoltage equipment (90 to 150 kVp) led to further studies of IORT for patients with more extensive cancers in the neck, thorax, abdomen, and pelvis.[9,10] The most successful approach combined the use of multiple doses of X-rays to temporarily exposed cancers in surgical neck wounds. This technique was most suitable for patients who had partially resected disease because the radiotherapy dose could be delivered uniformly to these patients' tumor area; when the "subcutaneous" therapy was completed, the skin flaps could be sutured in place. Among patients treated for 48 head and neck primary cancers by Barth with 3000 to 15,800 r, using IORT plus external beam X-rays (<2000 R), some patients were disease-free 3 to 4 years later, and many experienced remarkable palliation.[4] All patients had had advanced disease, so that any prolonged survival was considered a major success. Barth concluded that IORT to the head and neck was useful for patients with advanced cancers, but he cautioned on its use for those with extensive tumors that involved major osseous or vascular structures. Watson advocated a similar approach to treating axillary and groin regions.[11]

For unresectable tumors, Eloesser, at Stanford University, in 1937 advised a slightly different intraoperative treatment — the use of 250-kVp X-rays in single doses.[12] IORT doses ranging from 2900 to 4500 R were combined with fractionated doses of external beam irradiation ranging up to the tolerance of the surrounding normal tissues. To increase the therapeutic ratio further by decreasing dose inhomogeneity, Fairchild and Shorter used dual coaxial 250-kVp units for IORT of patients with unresectable gastric cancer.[13] administering 500 to 1300 R plus external beam irradiation. Of 32 patients, 2 lived beyond 2 years without complications.

The introduction of megavoltage irradiation reduced interest in IORT because it raised the expectation that deep-seated tumors could be controlled by external beam techniques alone. The initial experience with orthovoltage IORT had, however, uncovered many features that are now recognized as important to successful IORT. Acute morbidity of IORT was low, and high single doses to localized areas in the pelvis, abdomen, thorax, and head and neck regions could be combined with external beam irradiation. The most favorable IORT results were achieved in patients with minimal gross or only microscopic residual disease after surgical resection. Rapport between radiation therapists and surgeons was enhanced and required a continuing multidisciplinary effort.

II. THE NEW ENGLAND DEACONESS HOSPITAL EXPERIENCE

As interest in electron beam IORT reawakened at many institutions in Japan and the U.S., investigators at the Joint Center for Radiation Therapy in Boston decided in 1979 that the ideal location for a dedicated IORT machine was the operating room. This circumvented the high expense of a linear accelerator for electron beam IORT by using orthovoltage X-rays, which cost 10 to 20 times less. Placing the machine in the operating room, the radiotherapists believed, would eliminate problems of moving anesthetized patients and avoid some scheduling disruptions in the radiotherapy department. Since orthovoltage therapy units are relatively inexpensive and widely available, any demonstrated benefit of this therapeutic modality could potentially have a large impact on the intraoperative management of many patients. The machines are very reliable, easy to maintain, and maneuverable.

The Phillips® RT 305 X-ray machine, a heavily filtered orthovoltage X-ray unit operating at 300 kVp and a current of 10 mA, was permanently installed in an operating room at the New England Deaconess Hospital. The machine is suspended from ceiling tracks by a counterbalanced, telescopic suspension arm permitting free motion in all directions. The relatively light weight (320 kg) and small size of the unit allows great flexibility of use and convenient storage. Controls for the electromagnetic locks are placed for easy intraoperative handling for positioning and docking to the intraoperative applicator. Figure 1 shows the IORT machine in the treatment position. The X-ray tube is designed for sort focus-to-skin distances (FSD) using a rod-anode configuration. The 300-kVp radiation is filtered by 3.2 mm copper (Cu) in addition to the inherent filtration that produces a beam of a half-value layer (HVL) of 3.8 mm Cu (160 kVp effective), and an energy spectrum that has been described.[14] Figure 2 shows the room layout.

IORT treatment applicators are designed for use at either 25 or 30 cm FSD, which, in our experience, has been adequate to clear the tube shield above the patient's surface. The applicator system consists of two parts: a removable docking device attaches directly to the X-ray tube housing; and a family of detachable, cylindrical brass applicators attach to the docking device. A sterile plastic bag covers the head of the unit during the treatment and is secured by being sandwiched between the tube housing and the sterilized applicator docking assembly. The applicator system, located outside the bag, is sterilized by autoclaving. Treatment applicators are circular in cross-section, with internal diameters ranging from 6.1 to 9.9 cm.

The radiation dose rate at the tissue surface varies from 1.10 to 1.65 Gy/min depending on the FSD, field size, and bevel angle of the applicator tip (15 or 30°). Examples of the

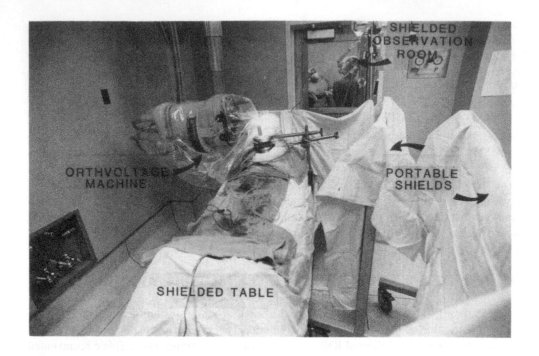

A

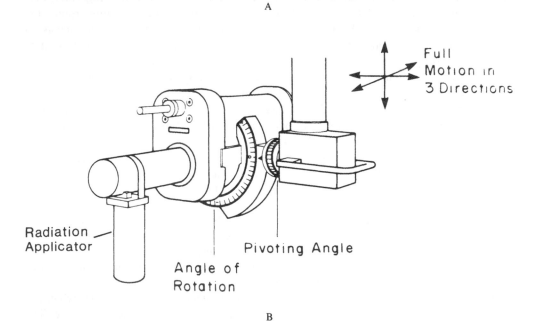

B

FIGURE 1.   (A) The orthovoltage machine is shown docked to the treatment applicator which has been positioned for treatment of a pancreatic cancer. Also shown are the shielded observation room and portable shields. (B) A schematic diagram of the Phillips® RT 305 orthovoltage machine used for IORT at New England Deaconess Hospital.

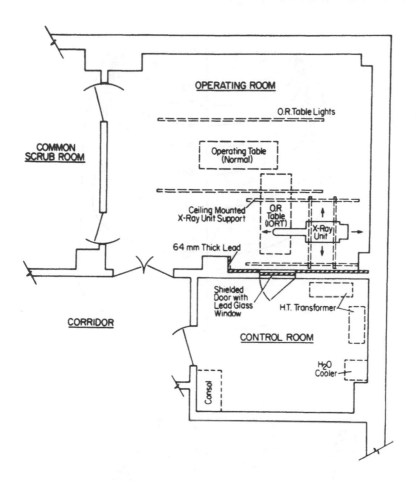

FIGURE 2.   Floor plan of IORT facility.

isodose distributions for a straight and beveled-tip applicator are shown in Figures 3A and 3B, respectively. For this illustration, the internal diameter of the applicator was 9.9 cm. Beam profiles measured perpendicularly to the central axis of the applicators indicated less than 5% lateral dose inhomogeneity throughout the field. Measurements outside the applicator at the tissue surface showed that the radiation dose immediately outside the applicator was approximately 15% of the central axis dose. Approximately 90% of the radiation dose outside the field defined by the applicator is caused by backscattered radiation from tissue within the beam. The details of the construction of the applicators and docking mechanism, as well as the radiation dosimetry, have been described elsewhere.[15]

The room chosen for IORT, an outside corner of the hospital on the third floor above ground, was ideal because of minimum radiation shielding requirements. The cost of retrofitting an operating room for IORT, including shielding, was low ($25,000) because major renovations were already being done to all the operating suites. The design of the IORT facility (Figure 2) shows the wall and door which are shielded with 6.4-mm-thick lead to the height of 2.14 m above the floor, separating the control room from the operating room (OR). The walls and door separating the common scrub room from the OR contain no shielding. Two 1.2 × 0.9-m portable shields with 6.4-mm-thick lead serve to shield the scrub room and corridor door during treatment. After the patient is prepared for IORT, the shields are positioned as close to the table as possible and parallel to the patient's longitudinal axis. Four removable sections of 12.7-mm-thick lead encased in stainless steel were placed in the operating room table to shield the room located directly below the OR from the direct

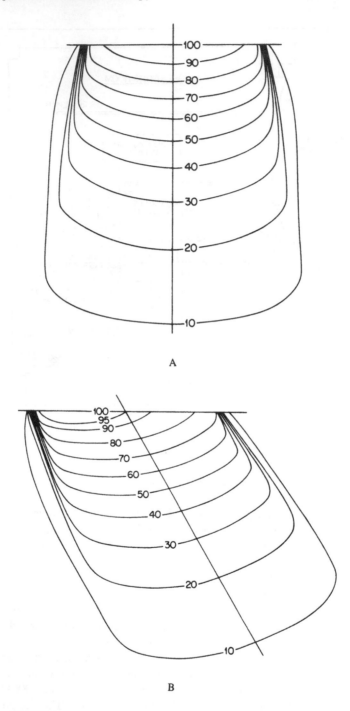

FIGURE 3. (A) Isodose curves for the 30-cm FSD straight-tipped intra-operative applicator. (B) Isodose curves for a 30 cm FSD intraoperative applicator with a 15° beveled tip. Internal diameter of applicator, with both straight and beveled tips, is 9.9 cm.

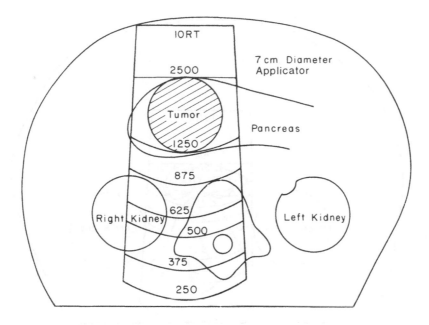

FIGURE 4.   Isodose distribution for an unresectable carcinoma of the head of the pancreas.

beam. The concrete ceiling (20 g· cm^{-2}) is adequate shielding for the room above. Shielding calculations were based on a beam time of 2.5 h/week, with design criteria for the weekly permissible exposure outside the OR being 5 mrem/week. These were easily met by the arrangements described.

By locating the IORT machine in the OR, the capability of direct, remote anesthetic monitoring of the patient during treatment was provided by placing shielding access ports in the wall through which the anesthetists can monitor the patient directly while maintaining visual contact through the leaded-glass window. The control room is also a suitable place for the surgeon and radiotherapist to wait while maintaining sterility until the end of the IORT procedure. After IORT is completed, the machine is undocked, the applicators are removed, and the surgeon and nurses regown and complete the procedure with the operating table in the usual position.

Another consideration regarding the orthovoltage IORT machine is the relative biologic effect (RBE) of 300-kVp X-rays compared with that of higher energy radiations.[16] The RBE of orthovoltage X-rays, about 1.15 that of super- or megavoltage radiations, results from denser ionization along the radiation path.[17] The RBE difference between orthovoltage and megavoltage electrons will be undetectable, however, because of the large dose inhomogeneity and the probable variation in biologic response which exceeds the RBE difference. The magnitude of the dose inhomogeneity is proportional to target depth and may vary from 10 to 15% to well over 100%, depending on the clinical situation. Examples of this dose inhomogeneity are shown in Figures 4 and 5. In clinical situations in which IORT is directed at a tumor bed after gross disease has been removed, dose inhomogeneity is reduced (10 to 20%), and the dose distribution across the target is quite similar to that of electrons (Figure 5).

A relative disadvantage of orthovoltage X-ray compared with megavoltage electron beam irradiation is the potential for radiation-induced bone injury because of the preferential energy absorption in bone caused by the photoelectric process. For low-energy X-rays (<80 kVp), the absorption in bone may exceed four times the absorption in soft tissues.[18] In the past, treatment with orthovoltage radiation beams occasionally resulted in radiation bone necrosis of the femoral heads,[19] ribs,[20] and mandible,[21] but this preferential damage may be related

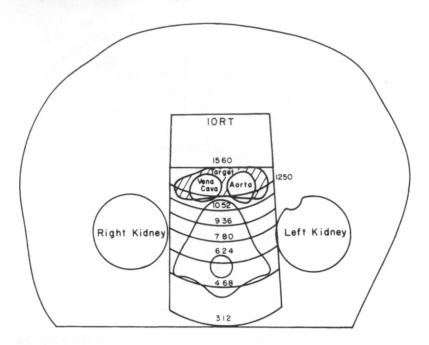

FIGURE 5. Isodose distribution for a resected tumor volume in the retroperitoneal area. The isodose distribution shows approximately 20% inhomogeneity across the target volume.

to the fact that these anatomic components are served by single-nutrient arteries. In IORT, bones likely to be irradiated are the vertebrae, sacrum, and portions of the other pelvic bones, which are supplied by either posterior vessels or multiple perforating blood vessels. Other important variables in radiation injury to adult bone include pattern of application and volume of radiation, patient's age, antecedent trauma, and pre- or postirradiation conditions that predispose to injury.[22]

Use of a heavily filtered radiation beam spectrum is one method of minimizing bone injury. The effects of radiation on adult bone are believed to be a consequence of injury to the cellular (osteocytic and osteoblastic) and vascular components residing in small cavities (5 to 50 micra) surrounded by material of high effective atomic number. For IORT, the problem of avoiding bone injury requires special consideration of the influence of cavity size and radiation beam spectral degradation with increasing depth in tissue. The dose to cells in small cavities may be 1.4 to 2 times the dose to the surrounding tissues. For comparison, the dose to large cavities (>250 micra) show the differences to be insignificant (Figure 6). Large doses of orthovoltage IORT carry a potential for increased bone damage, but the possibility of severe complications will be minimized if the following precautions are taken. Doses used for the boost technique should be only about 25% of the total dose to the target volume. Multiple large fractions should not be used nor should patients with evidence of bone involvement or periosteal infiltration by tumor, which results in nutrient arterial compromise, be candidates for IORT. In some clinical situations, it is possible to shield the anterior vertebral edge with lead, thereby reducing the bone dose by 70%. Furthermore, the exit dose across the bone will fall off rapidly and only a small volume of bone will be treated. There is some radiobiologic evidence that osteocytes may be relatively hypoxic, which may afford some radioprotection.[21]

III. RESULTS OF IORT AT THE NEW ENGLAND DEACONESS HOSPITAL

Between January 1981 and May 1984, 44 patients were treated with IORT: 16 males and 28 females whose ages ranged from 9 to 83 years. The majority (85%) had unresectable

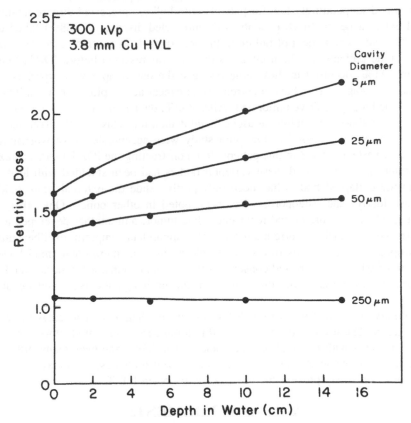

FIGURE 6. Demonstration of the magnitude of bone absorption with orthovoltage X-rays as a function of depth and cavity size.

disease, and 11 patients had all tumor resected before IORT. Biopsy examinations were done for all patients with unresectable disease and for all but one patient whose tumors were resected. The one patient without biopsy-proven disease had suspected residual cancer in the porta hepatis, and, at the time of IORT, biopsy was considered too hazardous.

Tumor sites treated with IORT consisted of pancreatic (19), biliary (6), colorectal (1), retroperitoneal lymphoma (1), and recurrent Wilm's tumors (2). In 14 patients, only IORT was used because of previous X-ray therapy or because they had unresectable symptomatic cancers of the pancreas with metastatic disease (5 patients). The other 30 patients were treated with combinations of external beam radiation therapy, consisting of 45 to 50 Gy given in fractions of 1.8 to 2 Gy/d, 5 d/week, and an IORT boost. The IORT dose was 12.5 Gy (tumor minimum) for the first 30 patients, and increased to 17.5 Gy for the next 14 patients.

The primary goal of this pilot study was to assess the feasibility of performing IORT in the operating room. We found that the approach caused little disruption in the operating room and radiotherapy department. We encountered no major technical problems and were able to provide maximum patient safety regarding infection control and anesthetic monitoring during the IORT procedure. An unquantifiable factor that made the program a success was greatly improved interdisciplinary management, partly as a result of the full interaction of surgeons, radiotherapists, and medical oncologists before IORT.

The results of treatment from our pilot study have been analyzed, and preliminary data have been reported in detail elsewhere.[23] There were, however, several important aspects of orthovoltage IORT that we noted with this small group of patients. Complete local tumor regression was disappointingly low for patients with bulky, unresected disease treated with IORT and external beam. In 18 patients with unresected disease, 16 (88%) failed overall and 14 (78%) had a component of failure in the area treated. In contrast, a better result was achieved in nine patients in whom all gross disease was resected before IORT. Only one local failure (11%) occurred in these nine patients; the one relapse was experienced by a patient who was diagnosed to have recurrent rectal cancer at reexploration when IORT was delivered to the biopsy-positive tumor bed. After IORT, the patient had recurrence of cancer in the pelvis and abdomen (malignant ascites) and distant metastases in the liver and lungs.

The complications assessed in this pilot study were acceptable. Most worrisome was the collapse of vertebrae L1-3 in one patient. In reconstructing the IORT fields and external beam treatment plan, we found these vertebral bodies had been shielded with lead during IORT, and the collapsed bodies had been only partly inside the external beam field. The patient was elderly, and osteoporosis had been noted in other bones. One other patient developed an obstructed ureter and recurrent pelvic tumor, and another developed a pelvic abscess also associated with recurrent tumor. Three patients had symptoms of either cutaneous nerve neuropathy, porta hepatis fibrosis and mild ascites, or intermittent small bowel obstruction, all of which were treated conservatively. Complications, after more than 3 years, have not been fully assessed in this pilot study, and all surviving patients are under continuing observation.

In summary, the modern era of IORT offers many challenges and areas for exciting clinical research. The use of orthovoltage IORT in our series was satisfactory, particularly for selected patients with minimal residual cancer. The IORT approach using orthovoltage may be appealing to some clincians at institutions in which the case load may be small and technical constraints may prevent the use of electron beam IORT.

ACKNOWLEDGMENTS

This work was supported in part by grants CA06294 and CA16672 from the National Cancer Institute, U.S. Department of Health and Human Services, Washington, D.C.

REFERENCES

1. **Finsterer, H.,** Zur Therapie inoperable Magen- und Darmkarzinome mit Freilegung und nachfelgender Rontgenbestrahlung, *Strahlentherapie,* 6, 205, 1915.
2. **Beck, C.,** External roentgen treatment of internal structures eventration treatment, *N.Y. Med. J.,* 89, 621, 1909.
3. **Chaoul, H.,** Weiterer Beitrag zur Rontgennahbestrahlung des Karzinoms, *Strahlentherapie,* 50, 446, 1934.
4. **Barth, G.,** Experience and results with short distance irradiation of surgically exposed tumors, *Strahlentherapie,* 91, 481, 1953.
5. **Drescher, H.,** Uber intraabdominale Nahbestrahlungen, *Strahlentherapie,* 78, 503, 1948.
6. **Levine, S. C., Pack, G. T., and Gallo, J. S.,** Intravesical roentgen therapy of cancer of the urinary bladder, *JAMA,* 112, 1314, 1939.
7. **Fuchs, G. and Uberall, R.,** Die intraoperative Rontgentherapie des Blasenkarzinoms, *Strahlentherapie,* 135, 280, 1966.
8. **Papillon, J.,** Conservative treatment by irradiation — an alternative to radical surgery, in *Rectal and Anal Cancers,* Springer-Verlag, New York, 1982, 63.
9. **Barth, G. and Wachsmann, F.,** Zur Methode der Nahbestrahlung operativ freigelegter Tumoren, *Strahlentherapie,* 77, 585, 1948.
10. **Barth, G. and Meinel, F.,** Intraoperative contact therapy in the large body cavities, *Strahlentherapie,* 109, 386, 1959.

11. **Watson, T. A.,** Subcutaneous X-ray therapy, *Br. J. Radiol.,* 13, 113, 1943.
12. **Eloesser,L.,** The treatment of some abdominal cancers by irradiation through the open abdomen combined with cautery excision, *Ann. Surg.,* 106, 645, 1937.
13. **Fairchild, G. C. and Shorter, A.,** Irradiation of gastric cancer, *Br. J. Radiol.,* 20, 511, 1947.
14. **Chen, T. S., Kase, K. R., and Bjarngard, B. E.,** Photon energy spectra of a heavily filtered 30 Kv X-ray unit, *Acta Radiol. Oncol.,* 19, 411, 1980.
15. **Piontek, R. W. and Kase, K. R.,** Design and dosimetric properties of an intraoperative radiation therapy system using a Phillips RT-305 X-ray unit, *Int. J. Radiat. Oncol. Biol. Phys.,* in press.
16. **Johns, H. E. and Cuningham, J. R., Eds.,** *The Physics of Radiology,* 3rd ed., Charles C Thomas, Springfield, IL, 1971, 679.
17. **Sinclair, W. K.,** The relative biologic effectiveness of 22 meVp X-rays Cobalt 60 gamma rays and 220 kVp X-rays, Parts I to VII, *Radiat. Res.,* 16, 336, 1962.
18. **Wilson, W.,** Dosage of high voltage radiation within bone and its possible significance for radiation therapy, *Br. J. Radiol.,* 23, 92, 1950.
19. **Smithers, D. W. and Rhys-Lewis, R. D. S.,** Bone destruction in cases of carcinoma of the uterus, *Br. J. Radiol.,* 18, 359, 1945.
20. **Gratzek, F. R., Holmstrom, E. G., and Rigler, L. G.,** Post-irradiation bone changes, *Am. J. Roentgenol.,* 53, 62, 1945.
21. **Gowgiel, J. M.,** Experimental radio-osteonecrosis of the jaws, *J. Dent. Res.,* 39, 176, 1960.
22. **Parker, R. G. and Berry, H. C.,** Late effects of therapeutic irradiation on the skeleton and bone marrow, *Cancer,* 37, 1162, 1976.
23. **Rich, T. A., Cady, B., McDermott, W. V., Kase, K. R., Chaffey, J. T., and Hellman, S.,** Orthovoltage intraoperative radiotherapy: a new look at an old idea, *Int. J. Radiat. Oncol. Biol. Phys.,* 10, 1957, 1984.

Chapter 11

THE USE OF SUPERFICIAL X-RAY EQUIPMENT FOR INTRAOPERATIVE RADIATION THERAPY

R. M. Krishnamsetty, M. Khalil, and J. I. Pearce

TABLE OF CONTENTS

I. INTRODUCTION

The use of low-energy machines for intraoperative irradiation is not a new idea.[1] Its use was started back in the 1930s, but interest in this technique decreased with the introduction of megavoltage machines. The interest in intraoperative radiation therapy (IORT) was renewed again by Abe and co-workers in the 1960s, but with the use of more sophisticated machinery.[2] In this chapter we will review the experience at Roswell Park Memorial Institute (RPMI) in the use of superficial X-ray equipment for IORT. At RPMI we understand the advantages of the high output and rapid fall-off of electron beams, but due to the impracticality of their use at our institution without major renovations, we considered it would be helpful to perform a phase I study using superficial X-ray equipment. The main advantages of the use of superficial X-ray equipment[3] are (1) low cost, which is about one tenth of that equipment capable of generating electron beams, (2) minimal shielding requirements in the operating room, (3) machine mobility for cleaning and treatment purposes, and (4) ease of maintenance. The disadvantages of those machines are (1) low dose rate, resulting in longer treatment times, (2) inhomogeneous dose distributions, (3) high exit doses compared to those of electron beams of comparable penetration, and (4) increased bone absorption, especially in the energy range of our machine. The bone absorption in the superficial energy range is approximately four times that of soft tissue.

II. EQUIPMENT DESCRIPTION

IORT is delivered using a Picker Zephyr® 120-kV X-ray machine permanently installed in an operating room at RPMI. The X-ray tube support structure has been modified to provide a compact unit with good mobility to facilitate easy alignment to the treatment cone that has been positioned over the tumor volume. A compromise was necessary between the addition of filtration for improved penetration and the maintenance of an acceptable dose rate. An added filter of 1.5 mm of aluminum results in a 3.5-mm Al half-value layer (HVL) and surface dose rates at 31 cm focus-to-skin distance (FSD) of 77 to 88 cGy/min. Typical treatment times range from 15 to 30 min depending on the prescribed dose, cone selection, and treatment gap. A variety of treatment cones are available from 6×6 to 20 cm diameter.

III. BEAM CHARACTERISTICS

The depth dose characteristics of the beam are such that typically 85 and 70% of the surface dose are present at 1 and 2 cm depth in tissue, respectively. The presence of bone, however, poses a significant problem[4] at these X-ray energies with as much as four times the absorption in bone as compared to that in soft tissue. The possibility of bone damage and the shielding effects of overlying bone must be evaluated in treatments with these low-energy X-rays. In addition, the presence of large blood vessels can result in a 20 to 30% reduction in dose to the underlying tissue.

IV. RADIATION SAFETY

The operating room was modified to provide adequate radiation protection for the personnel involved in the procedure. This included the addition of shielding materials to the doors and some wall surfaces, provision of leaded-glass viewing windows, warning lights, and interlocks on all access doors.

V. PATIENT SAFETY

The anesthesiologist can observe the patient and the anesthesia equipment through a

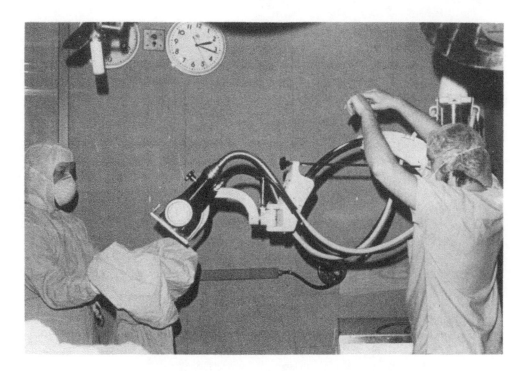

FIGURE 1. The X-ray head is "docked" to the cone and locked in place over the operating room table.

leaded-glass window, and the door interlock will instantaneously terminate treatment if the anesthesiologist enters the room. The head of the machine is draped with special sterile sheets above the treatment cone to completely isolate the X-ray tube from the sterile field. Because of the use of oil cooling in conjunction with a remote heat exchanger, the X-ray tube housing can be draped totally without risk of overheating.

VI. TECHNIQUE OF IORT

At the time of surgery, every attempt is made to resect the tumor completely. The radiation therapist is present during surgery to evaluate the initial tumor size and location. After surgery is completed, all sensitive structures are moved out of the radiation field. The appropriate cone size is selected to cover the area of the primary tumor with a 1- or 2-cm margin, if possible. Lead rubber shields are used to shield sensitive structures within the cone. The X-ray unit is moved over to the operating room table and the X-ray head is "docked" to the cone and locked in place using a special clamping system (Figure 1). A hole located near the top of each cone allows for viewing of the treatment field by means of an endoscopic device (Figure 2). This provides for confirmation of the cone position prior to the initiation of treatment and at intervals during treatment when required (e.g., for suction of fluids that accumulate in the field). All personnel are outside the room during the treatment itself. The radiation dose is usually 15 Gy surface dose. At the completion of the exposure, the X-ray head is undocked, the unit moved back away from the table, and the cone removed.

VII. EXPERIENCE WITH SUPERFICIAL X-RAY MACHINES

As mentioned previously, the exit dose and the high bone absorption are major limitations. This was most obvious in advanced gynecological tumors adherent to the pelvic walls and in gastric and pancreatic tumors where the tumor thickness usually is more than

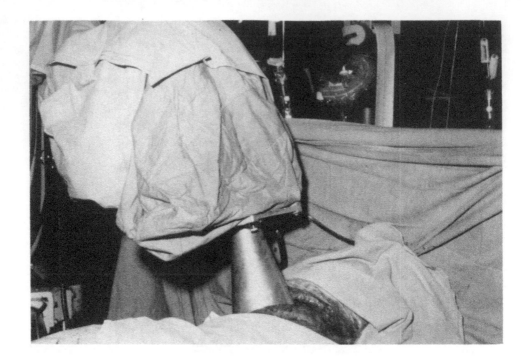

FIGURE 2.   A hole located near the top of each cone allows the viewing of the treatment field by means of an endoscopic device.

2 cm. The use of this machine was intended only to deliver a single boost dose to be supplemented with external beam irradiation. Because of the referral pattern to the institution, the majority of patients we have treated had advanced disease, and some of these had been already irradiated to the tolerance of the normal tissues.

Between October 1981 and August 1985, we treated a total of 55 patients with IORT. In the first 3 years (October 1981 to September 1984), we treated 27 patients. During the last year, 28 patients were admitted for IORT due to an increased interest in the field. We are presently reporting the results of the first 27 patients.

Eighteen patients with various types of soft tissue sarcomas were treated. Eight patients received external beam irradiation following the IORT. Five of these had local control of disease with a median survival time of 23 months. Of the remaining three patients, two had disease recurrence outside the field and one had progression of lung metastases present at the time of the IORT. Two of the ten patients who did not have external beam irradiation had local control of disease.

There were seven patients with advanced carcinoma of the lung who received IORT following resection. None of them had external beam irradiation. One of those patients expired 39 d following surgery because of severe infection. One patient had local recurrence of cancer in the irradiated field associated with brain metastases. Five patients did have local control of disease without evidence of distant metastasis with survival time ranging from 2 to 19 months following IORT. Two patients with advanced malignant melanoma were treated. One of them did not have external beam irradiation and expired 2 months following the procedure. There was no evidence of tumor in the treatment field at autopsy. The second patient had 45 Gy external beam irradiation in addition to the IORT; this patient is alive 14 months following IORT with no evidence of disease.

Three patients received treatment to two or more adjacent fields. There were no complications related to overlapping fields.

We observed two complications of IORT. One patient died of severe infection and a second patient developed enteritis that responded to conservative therapy. The emphasis must be made that most of these cases were very advanced or locally recurrent tumors.

VIII. FUTURE CONSIDERATIONS

The use of IORT is in its early days. There is a lack of well-planned, prospective randomized studies. The results from several institutions are encouraging. The use of the electron beam with the advantages it offers (dose homogeneity, less differential absorption between bone and soft tissues, and the rapid fall-off of dose with depth) is attractive. We are now in the process of converting our 35-meV linear accelerator room into an operating suite. This will enable us to randomize patients with no residual or minimal residual disease (less than 1 cm in thickness) between the use of electrons and superficial X-rays.

We think that more radiobiological studies on the effect of single, large radiation doses are needed. This will become clearer with longer follow-up periods.

REFERENCES

1. **Finsterer, H.,** Zur Therapie Inoperable Magen- und DarmKarzinome mit Freilegung und nachfolgender Rontgenbestrahlung, *Strahlentherapie*, 6, 205, 1915.
2. **Abe, M., Fukada, M., Yamano, K., et al.,** Intraoperative irradiation in abdominal and cerebral tumors, *Acta Radiol.*, 10, 408, 1971.
3. **Gunderson, L. L., Tepper, J. E., Biggs, P. J., Goldson, A., Martin, J. K., McCullough, E. C., Rich, T. A., Shipley, W. U., Sindelar, W. F., and Wood, W. C.,** Intraoperative external beam irradiation, in *Current Problems in Cancer*, Year Book Medical, Chicago, 1983, 40.
4. **Rich, T. A., Cody, B., McDermott, W. V., Kase, K. R., Chaffey, J. T., and Hellman, S.,** Orthovoltage intraoperative radiotherapy: a new look at an old idea, *Int. J. Radiat. Oncol. Biol. Phys.*, 10, 1957, 1984.

Chapter 12

GENERAL SURGICAL ASPECTS OF INTRAOPERATIVE RADIATION THERAPY

Hollis W. Merrick, III

TABLE OF CONTENTS

I. INTRODUCTION

Intraoperative radiation therapy (IORT) offers the surgeon a logical extension to the effectiveness of operative procedures. Whether the surgery is complete or partial excision, or mere exposure of the tumor, the ability to irradiate the tumor has potentially significant advantages. As with external beam radiation therapy, IORT would seem to be most effective in treating microscopic residual disease. However, even in instances where the tumor cannot be completely excised, the ability to precisely define intraoperatively the limits of the gross tumor and the areas of potential spread is important in allowing direct treatment of these areas.

This modality (IORT) allows direct appositional treatment excluding all or part of the adjacent normal tissue. This can be accomplished by surgical mobilization or shielding of the electron beam with Lucite® or metal. The use of appropriately sized Lucite® treatment applicators permits the tumor to be encompassed and prevents electron beam scatter to adjacent tissue.

External beam irradiation can be used postoperatively as an additive boost to IORT. Conversely, patients who have failed standard external beam therapy are candidates for additional therapy with exploration, tumor excision or debulking, and IORT. This last advantage offers some hope of palliation to patients who have otherwise failed all the conventional treatments.

II. TISSUE TOLERANCE

From the surgical perspective, it is essential for the surgeon to be aware of the tissues which may potentially be damaged by IORT. Different organs and tissues have different maximum tolerated doses of radiation which can be administered without clinical complications. While the tolerance to external beam irradiation is well documented, less is known about intraoperatively administered single-dose treatments. Table 1 outlines the tolerances of single-dose treatments administered intraoperatively to experimental animals. Of special note is the particular sensitivity of the small bowel and colon to radiation injury. During treatments a major concern is to mobilize the intestine out of the beam path and prevent its irradiation. In addition, it is important to note the sensitivity of the kidney, ureter, and bile duct. In radiating the lower abdominal cavity, it would be important to mobilize the ureters and retract them laterally, and it may also be beneficial to shield the kidney or bile ducts during treatment.

Table 2 outlines the radiotolerance of anastomoses after certain surgical manipulations. The healing of any anastomosis will be significantly retarded by a full dose of radiation. In planning an IORT procedure, it would be wise to delay these aspects of the procedure until the radiation is administered. For example, in a patient with gastric carcinoma, irradiation can follow resection of the gastric tumor and the gastrojejunostomy can be performed subsequent to the irradiation.

III. REPORTED CLINICAL PROBLEMS

Some problems secondary to IORT have been reported. Generally speaking, doses in the range of 10 to 30 Gy are delivered in various treatment situations. Duodenal hemorrhage has been reported as a late complication in patients following irradiation of the head of the pancreas for carcinoma.[1] This is probably due to ulceration of the margin of duodenum that is included in the radiation field. Great care should be taken in carrying out this procedure to exclude all duodenum to prevent this complication. Peripheral neuropathies may result from direct radiation damage to nerve or nerve roots.[1] Such neuropathies have been noted

TABLE 1
Collected Animal Studies Attempting to Define Radiation Tolerance of Various Normal Tissues and Organs to Intraoperative Single-Dose Irradiation[1]

Organ or tissue	Animal	Maximum dose without clinical complication (Gy)	Comments and findings
Aorta	Dog	50	Patency and structural integrity preserved; dose-related subintimal and medial fibrosis at doses $\geq$ 30 Gy
Vena cava	Dog	50	Patency and structural integrity preserved; dose-related fibrosis at doses $\geq$ 30 Gy
Small bowel	Dog	<20	Dose-related mucosal atrophy, mucosal ulceration, muscularis fibrosis, and luminal stenosis at doses $\geq$ 2000 rad; functional small-bowel segments obstruct or perforate at doses $\geq$ 3000 Gy, but defunctionalized bypassed segments maintain structural integrity
Colon	Dog	<20	Dose-related mucosal atrophy, mucosal ulceration, muscularis fibrosis, and luminal stenosis at doses $\geq$ 20 Gy; obstruction can develop at doses $\geq$ 20 Gy, perforation expected at doses $\geq$ 40 Gy
Liver	Rabbit	30	Parenchymal atrophy, fibrosis necrosis at doses $\geq$ 30 Gy
Bile duct	Dog	20	Dose-related fibrosis and stenosis at doses $\geq$ 20 Gy, can lead to biliary cirrhosis
Kidney	Dog	<20	Dose-related fibrosis and stenosis at doses $\geq$ 20 Gy, can lead to biliary cirrhosis
Ureter	Dog	30	Parenchymal atrophy at doses $\geq$ 30 Gy
Bladder	Dog	30	Structural integrity preserved; dose-related contraction and ureterovesical narrowing at doses $\geq$ 30 Gy

TABLE 2
Collected Animal Studies Attempting to Define Radiation Tolerance of Various Surgically Manipulated Tissues and Organs to Intraoperative Single-dose Irradiation[1]

Organ or tissue	Animal studied	Surgical manipulation	Maximum dose without clinical complications (Gy)	Comments and findings
Aorta	Dog	End-to-end anastomosis	20	Dose-related fibrosis and stenosis at doses $\geq$ 20 Gy, sometimes producing occlusion; no clinical signs of arterial insufficiency and no anastomotic disruption to 45 Gy
Small bowel	Dog	Closure of defunctionalized intestinal loop	45	Dose-related fibrosis and stenosis at doses $\geq$ 20 Gy; no suture line disruption to 45 Gy
Bile duct	Dog	End-to-side biliary-enteric anastomosis	<20	Anastomotic disruption at doses $\geq$ 20 Gy
Bladder	Dog	Closure cystotomy	30	Dose-related contraction at doses $\geq$ 30 Gy; no suture line disruption to 45 Gy

following pelvic irradiation, resulting in severe pelvic pain due to local nerve injury. In addition, in the NCI series,[2] sciatic nerve injury has occurred resulting in disabling late neuropathy.

IV. SURGICAL TECHNIQUE

The use of IORT generally implies some measure of transportation while the patient is under general anesthesia. Some institutions have a dedicated operating room which occupies the same room as the linear accelerator. In this case, transportation involves merely draping the patient and moving a short distance. However, at most institutions the patient must be transported a considerable distance from the operating room to the radiation therapy suite. This implies significant hazards as the patient is transported after the initial phase of the surgical procedure, whether it be resection or merely exposure of the tumor. The wound is packed or temporarily closed and multiple layers of drapes are applied over the operative field. The patient is then transported through corridors and down elevators to the radiation therapy suite. Following administration of the treatment, the patient is either closed in the radiation therapy suite or returned to the operating room for closure or additional procedures.

The logistics of IORT are complicated and require careful planning. There must be close cooperation between the surgeon and the radiotherapist. In addition, other services such as anesthesiology, nursing service, radiation therapy, technicians, support services, and even hospital security need to be closely coordinated and well rehearsed.

Despite the significant potential for complications, most centers do not report problems secondary to the transport of the patient. The Massachusetts General Hospital noted 4 wound infections in their series[3] of 35 patients, 3 of which they attributed to problems related to the surgery.

V. SURGICAL PROCEDURE

The surgical procedure requires more planning than for the equivalent procedure performed without IORT. The surgeon must consider additional factors in carrying out surgery when IORT is being administered, regardless of whether the surgery involves complete excision, a palliative procedure, or merely exposure of the tumor.

A. INCISION
The type of incision used must be carefully thought out in advance of the procedure. Generally, a more extensive exposure than usual will be required. This is to allow entry of the treatment applicator into the body cavity in such a manner so as to completely encompass the tumor from the best possible angle. The radiotherapist will be concerned about completely treating the tumor and adjacent regional area, but also will want to adjust the radiation energy, dosage, and angle of the applicator in order to spare normal tissue. The depth of penetration of the electron beam can be accurately controlled by varying the voltage employed. Midline incisions will be adequate for most abdominal procedures; however, some may need to be carried out through a transverse or bilateral subcostal incision. Occasionally, for a high-lying abdominal or low thoracic lesion it may be necessary to perform a thoracoabdominal incision. Lateral chest incisions are usually sufficient, although for a mediastinal lesion, a median sternotomy may be utilized.

B. EXPOSURE
The use of self-retaining retractors is important to facilitate exposure of the radiation fields. The Lucite® collimator of the treatment head will prevent irradiation of the small bowel and other viscera which may be in contact with it. However, it may be difficult to

gain optimal placement of the collimator in certain positions. The two most difficult areas to treat are the upper abdomen and the pelvis. We have found that the upper-hand retractor is particularly useful in elevating the costal margins and allowing full access to the upper abdomen. For mid-abdominal lesions, the Buchwalter retractor has been very useful. Abe[4] has developed a pentagonally shaped applicator for use in the upper abdomen. This retractor fits well along the costal margins and allows excellent application for radiation of upper abdominal and, particularly, gastric carcinomas. Low-lying pelvic lesions can be treated through a perineal incision by positioning the linear accelerator horizontally.

C. SURGICAL PROCEDURE

The type of case for which IORT is most useful is often the patient with the most advanced or difficult to treat tumor. In order to gain the most effectiveness with this adjuvant modality, it is often necessary to combine IORT with major resections of either primary or recurrent disease. This implies a long operation with concomitant blood loss and increased general risks to the patient. This is in addition to the added risk of transportation over a long distance or the performance of the operation in the radiation therapy suite. This setting is remote from the main operating room with all of its ready resources of personnel and equipment. In order to minimize the danger of this situation, careful planning and organization of services available is required.

VI. INSERTION OF THE TREATMENT DEVICE

One of the most difficult aspects of carrying out IORT is the actual placing of the treatment applicator on the tumor. This can be accomplished by either bringing the tumor in contact with the collimator or placing the collimator on the tumor and "docking" it with the treatment applicator. At our institution we bring the patient to the applicator. The operative table is maneuvered underneath the accelerator head, and the gantry of the linear accelerator is angled in what is felt to be the best position to administer the radiation. The operative table is then progressively elevated until the collimator rests on the tumor. The collimator slides in and out within an aluminum steel sleeve so that final, small adjustments can be made at this point. The distance to the tumor is easily determined and this information is used to calculate the amount of energy required to deliver the desired dosage. There are operative tables available which not only pitch and roll, but have lateral and longitudinal movement, and this greatly facilitates the ease of placement of the treatment applicator. The ability to adjust the table along multiple axes permits rapid and accurate alignment of applicator positions within the body cavities.

VII. ADMINISTRATION OF THE IORT

In fitting the applicator to the radiation field, it is important to assure that blood does not accumulate as this interferes with proper dose delivery to the tumor. Blood acts as a tissue and will absorb the electron beam prior to its reaching the targeted tissue. It is therefore important to obtain adequate hemostasis before attempting to initiate treatment. We have emphasized this as important, and hemorrhage has not been a problem. We have found that suctioning of the area under the Lucite® collimator prior to administration of the treatment is usually sufficient.

The IORT treatment unit should have some means of visualizing the operative field. Our IORT unit makes use of a retractable right-angle periscope which also illuminates the field area to be treated. This permits direct visualization after the collimator has been positioned. This allows not only verification that the proper area is being treated, but also that there is no blood present.

TABLE 3
Types of Cancer Treated

Rectum	16
Colon	16
Pancreas	14
Cervix	7
Ovary	6
Breast	4
Brain	4
Stomach	4
Prostate	3
Sarcoma	
Chest	2
Abdomen	2
Pelvis	2
Head and neck	1
Vulva	1
Vagina	1
Uterus	1
Bladder	1
Anus	1
Lung	1
Kidney	1

VIII. MONITORING THE PATIENT

The radiation treatment with a linear accelerator takes only a few minutes to administer. However, during this period, all personnel must be evacuated from the operating room and the patient is thus unattended. We have monitored these patients remotely using a number of devices. The blood pressure and pulse are monitored via a radial artery catheter using a Techtronix® 414 monitor which has a remote unit at the linear accelerator treatment console. In addition, we utilize two controllable TV cameras connected to a TV monitor. Another very useful device is a speaker/amplifier system which amplifies an esophageal stethoscope. This provides reassuring monitoring of heart beats and breath sounds. These devices offer accurate and immediate monitoring of the patient.

The radiation treatment can be interrupted at any time. The linear accelerator can be quickly stopped and the room reentered to deal with any anesthetic or surgical problems. In practice, we commonly reentered the treatment room half-way through the treatment to evaluate the patient's conditions and verify that the radiation field is properly positioned and free of blood.

IX. EXPERIENCE WITH IORT AT THE MEDICAL COLLEGE OF OHIO

Between 1983 and 1985, 93 patients have undergone IORT at the Medical College of Ohio. There were 66 female and 37 male patients, with an average age of 56.7 years.

A wide variety of cancers have been treated, as listed in Table 3. Diagnoses included 32 patients with colorectal cancer, 14 with cancer of the pancreas, 16 with gynecological tumors, 4 with breast tumors, 4 with gastric carcinoma, 3 with carcinoma of the prostate, 1 with carcinoma of the lung, and 4 with brain tumors. The surgical procedures were performed by several different surgeons, including general and thoracic surgeons, gynecologists, urologists, and neurosurgeons. A variety of doses of radiation have been utilized in conjunction with the surgery as outlined in Table 4. However, most of the patients received dosages in the range of 15 to 25 Gy.

TABLE 4
Dosages Used (Gy)

10	4
15	24
20	29
25	29
30	1

TABLE 5
Morbidities

Atelectasis	4
Wound infection	4[a]
Hematuria	2
U.T.I.	2
Deep vein thrombosis	2
Enterocutaneous fistula (short duration)	2
Splenic infarct	1
Septicemia	1
Postoperative ileus	1
Cholangitis	1
U.G.I. bleed	1
Wound dehiscence	1
Abominal abscess	1
Proctitis requiring colostomy	1

[a] Two occurred secondary to postcraniotomy bone flap necrosis.

A wide variety of procedures have been carried out, ranging from curative resection to mere exposure of the tumor. We have carefully examined the postsurgery course of each of these patients for at least 30 days in order to assess the early morbidity and mortality of surgery in combination with IORT. Table 5 outlines the morbidities which have occurred in these 93 patients. The rate of occurrence of these morbidities is comparable to that expected in a similar group of patients undergoing surgery alone for advanced malignant conditions. In addition, we were concerned about the rate of infection as the procedure was performed in an operating room in the radiation therapy suite. Of particular note is the occurrence of only 4 wound infections in this group of 93 patients. Two of these infections were in patients undergoing brain irradiation who developed scalp wound infections secondary to necrosis of the bone flap. The reason for this necrosis is not apparent, but it appears that the circulation of the galea may have been compromised by prior irradiation. One other major problem was the occurrence of proctitis in a patient with sarcoma who had irradiation of three separate fields in the pelvis. The patient developed severe pelvic pain due to proctitis which required colostomy. The pain slowly resolved over a 3-month period.

Two surgical mortalities occurred in this series of patients. The first occurred in a 68-year-old female undergoing irradiation for cancer of the pancreas. She was found to have extensive hepatic metastases at the time of surgery as well as a large pancreatic mass. Postoperatively, the patient developed a splenic infarct with septicemia, from which she succumbed on the ninth postoperative day. It is hypothesized that the pressure of the collimator compressed the splenic vessels posterior to the pancreas onto the vertebral column and resulted in their temporary occlusion. Unfortunately, we were not able to obtain an autopsy to confirm this diagnosis. The second postoperative death also occurred on the ninth postoperative day in a 30-year-old patient with a very extensive malignant histiocytoma in the abdomen and was considered due to natural progression of the disease.

TABLE 6
Reasons for Nontreatment

23 (25%) of 93 Patients Explored
were not Treated with IORT

Abdominal tumor implants	14 (61%)
(peritoneal, omental, bowel)	
Liver metastases	5 (22%)
IORT not indicated	1 (04%)
Abdominal abscess	1 (04%)
No cancer found	2 (09%)

TABLE 7
Pelvic Pain Following Pelvic Irradiation

4 of 11	Gynecological carcinomas
0 of 20	Rectal carcinomas
1 of 4	Transanal irradiation for rectal cancer

TABLE 8
Pancreatic Cancer Patients Undergoing IORT

	No. of patients	Median survival (months)	Pain relief
With metastatic lesion	3	4.0	2
Without metastatic lesion	6	10.5	5

All patients undergoing exploration and IORT had a comprehensive therapeutic evaluation, including CT scan of the appropriate area, prior to surgery. However, 23 of the 93 patients explored (25%) were not treated with IORT. Table 6 outlines the reasons for this. The main reason was the presence of extensive intra-abdominal or hepatic cancer which was not detected prior to surgery and was not amenable to management by IORT. In particular, the presence of peritoneal seeding is difficult to detect and has led to consideration of the use of preexploration laparoscopy.

Analysis of the late posttreatment course of the patients has revealed pelvic or sciatic pain following pelvic irradiation to be a problem (Table 7). Of 11 patients with a gynecological malignancy, 4 have developed sciatic pain, whereas no pain has developed in any of 20 patients with pelvic disease due to rectal cancer. The probable explanation for this is that rectal carcinomas usually require midline irradiation, whereas gynecological malignancies involve lateral pelvic irradiation. One of four patients receiving six courses of transanal irradiation developed low pelvic pain which was completely relieved when she subsequently underwent abdominoperineal resection.

Our follow-up time is too short to have extensive survival data; however, the group undergoing treatment for cancer of the pancreas show some interesting preliminary data (Table 8). Three patients with metastatic disease present at the time of surgery had a median survival of 4.0 months, while those without metastatic spread survived 10.5 months (median). These survivals show minimal improvement over bypass surgery alone. However, seven of the nine patients experienced significant relief of pain.

REFERENCES

1. **Kinsella, T. J. and Sindelar, W. F.,** Intraoperative radiotherapy, in *Cancer: Principles and Practice of Oncology,* 2nd ed., Devita, V. T., Hellman, S., and Rosenberg, S. A., Eds., Lippincott, Philadelphia, 1985.
2. IORT: NCI finds preliminary results are equal to conventional therapy, *Clin. Cancer Lett.,* 9 (1), 1986.
3. **Gunderson, L. L., Shipley, W. W., Suit, H. D., Epp, E. R., Nardi, G., Wood, W., Cohen, A., Nelson, J., Battit, G., Biggs, P. J., Russell, A., Rockett, A., and Clark, D.,** Intraoperative irradiation: a pilot study combining external beam photons with "boost" dose intraoperative electrons, *Cancer,* 49, 2259, 1982.
4. **Abe, M., Takahashi, M., Yabumoto, E., Onoyama, Y., and Torizuka, K.,** Techniques, indications and results of intraoperative radiotherapy of advanced cancers, *Radiology,* 116, 693, 1975.

Chapter 13

NEUROSURGICAL CONSIDERATIONS IN INTRAOPERATIVE RADIATION THERAPY

Samuel H. Greenblatt and Mark Rayport

TABLE OF CONTENTS

I. INTRODUCTION

The main theme of this chapter will be the development and discussion of a *rational protocol* for the use of intraoperative electron beam radiation therapy (IOEBT) in the treatment of primary cerebral malignancies. Since the histological classification and associated terminology of these malignancies is presently in flux, we will use the term *malignant glioma* to include: anaplastic astrocytoma, astrocytomas grades III and IV of Kernohan and Sayre,[4] glioblastoma multiforme, and malignant astrocytoma.

II. THE RADIOBIOLOGICAL BACKGROUND

The radiobiological behavior of all malignant gliomas is fairly well known.[10] When these tumors reach sufficient size to be clearly apparent, they consist of four definable zones (Figure 1). The necrotic central zone may be clinically significant because of mass effect, but it is of limited radiotherapeutic interest because the tissue is dead. The next, the paracentral zone, consists of hypoxic cells that survive large doses of radiation because they are not metabolically active. This zone, which is probably no more than 150 μm thick, is thought to be responsible for most of the inevitable recurrences of malignant gliomas after high-dose, external beam, conventional radiation therapy (CRT). The more superficial zone of growing tumor cells is most sensitive to standard CRT because the cells are dividing actively. There is some evidence that this zone of active growth might be largely sterilized by sufficiently high doses of external beam CRT, but only at the price of radiation necrosis in the surrounding brain.[7] Finally, there is a "peripheral zone of infiltration",[2] the radiobiological behavior of which is less well characterized at present. In computed tomography (CT) scans, the tumor tissue of this zone is actually located in the region of peritumoral edema.

Since the maximum allowable dose of CRT is relatively fixed at around 60 Gy, regardless of the size or configuration of the tumor, surgical removal of tumor mass ("debulking") is important because it decreases the tumor load and thereby enhances the effect of CRT. Thus, we consider "standard" treatment of malignant gliomas to be surgical removal to the greatest extent consistent with a decent quality of life during survival, followed by CRT to the maximum safe dose. An extensive literature on the application of this standard treatment to glioblastoma (grade IV) shows that the median survival time is about 9 months;[6,8] grade III astrocytomas have a median survival of about 10 months. If the presence or absence of micronecrosis is used as a distinguishing criterion, patients whose tumors show micronecrosis have a median survival of 8 months as compared to 28 months for those without micronecrosis.[6]

In the simplest possible terms, the fundamental goal of any tumor therapy is to eradicate the malignancy without damaging the surrounding tissue. IOEBT has the potential to do this within the brain, because the ionizing radiation can be delivered directly and uniformly to the tumor. Autopsies on the IOEBT-treated patients of Abe, et al.[1] have shown that "the irradiated part was completely destroyed and no cancer cells were found in the field." This statement refers to patients who had malignant gliomas. We have had a similar experience with one patient who had metastatic carcinoma in the brain (see Medical College of Ohio [MCO] Case 3 below). Therefore, the modality of IOEBT may have a potential to "cure" intracerebral malignancies, if it can be applied in a sufficient dose and in a configuration that encompasses all viable tumor cells.

III. AN OPTIMAL PROTOCOL FOR IOEBT IN MALIGNANT GLIOMAS

The preceding data about the biological behavior and survival of malignant gliomas

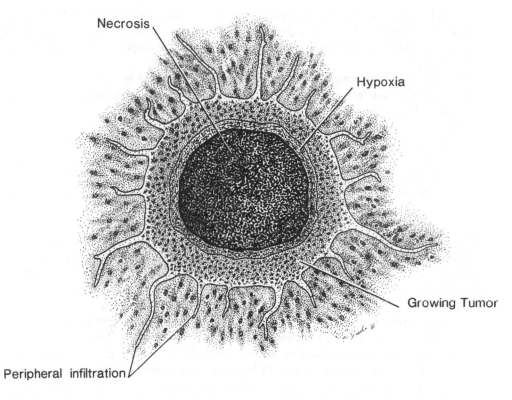

Necrosis

Hypoxia

Growing Tumor

Peripheral infiltration

FIGURE 1. A schematic representation of the four biologically different zones in an untreated malignant astro-cytoma.

constitute the empirical basis of our protocol for the use of IOEBT in cerebral malignancies. In essence, the tumor load should be smallest after the standard modalities of surgery and CRT have been applied. Therefore, we should expect the best results if an extra dose of radiation is given at this point in the course of the patient's disease, when most of the cells in the zone of active growth have been damaged or killed, but the cells in the hypoxic zone are still viable. Moreover, Burger et al.[2] showed that there is little tumor in the peripheral zone of infiltration when glioblastomas are in remission after standard treatment with surgery, radiation therapy, and chemotherapy. Thus, our "optimal" protocol is as follows:

1. For any lesion that is suspected of being a malignant glioma, histological diagnosis is essential and maximum surgical removal of the tumor bulk is highly desirable. Simple biopsy (whether by open or percutaneous technique) is acceptable for lesions in critical brain areas. Standard CRT is then given to full dose (approximately 60 Gy). This requirement for complete "standard" treatment of the tumor has two goals:
   a. Maximum reduction of tumor load and lesion size.
   b. Careful compliance with currently standard treatment so that results can be mean-ingfully compared to survival data in the literature. This point is methodologically critical, because it may be the only way to evaluate the results of IOEBT without randomized surgical studies, which are very difficult to carry out in the circum-stances of patients who have these tumors.
2. An interval of some weeks or, at most, a few months is allowed to elapse before performing or reopening the craniotomy for IOEBT. This time period is important to give the scalp and dura time to heal after CRT and to allow completion of cell death and shrinkage in the tumor. On the other hand, this period should not be allowed to

extend into the time when recurrence is likely, because the efficacy of the "extra" dose of radiation (IOEBT) would then be diminished by its application to a larger cell mass. In addition, the zone of peripheral infiltration enlarges very rapidly during recurrence.[2]

3.   The tumor must be reasonably superficial, i.e., there should be a minimum of intervening brain tissue between the brain surface and the tumor, especially in "eloquent" areas such as motor- and language-related cortex.

4.   The tumor should be well encompassed by the width and depth of the electron beam of the IOEBT equipment being used. The accumulating information about the peripheral zone of infiltration makes this point especially important. We have not yet irradiated significantly beyond the obvious boundaries of the tumor, as defined by CT ring enhancement and/or by surgical observation or biopsy, but it may be important to do so.

Our own experience with the preceding "optimal protocol" is still so small as to be simply anecdotal (see MCO Case 1 below), but there is some support for this approach from the Japanese experience. Terao[9] reported a total of 15 patients who received IOEBT for malignant gliomas (see also Chapter 14). His first four cases were given IOEBT 3 to 4 weeks after initial craniotomy or biopsy, apparently without intervening CRT. When the results of this approach proved to be unsatisfactory, he then did the next 11 patients with malignant gliomas according to a regimen that was very close to our "optimal protocol". The primary difference was in the dose of preliminary CRT, which was only 30 to 40 Gy in Terao's series. Seven of the patients in his series had grade IV astrocytomas and the remainder were grade III. With four patients still alive at the time of his report (two grade IV and two grade III), the mean survival from the time of IOEBT was 20 months and the median was 13 months. One patient with a grade IV astrocytoma was still alive at 54 months, after having two applications of IOEBT. Since the median survival for Terao's patients should have been 9 to 10 months from time of initial surgery, even with full-dose CRT, we believe that his results speak strongly for our rationale.

IV. OTHER PROTOCOL CONSIDERATIONS

Given the many vagaries of human disease, it is obvious that rigid adherence to any protocol is often impossible. Compromises must be made in a variety of individual circumstances. In some situations this is reasonable on the basis of what limited data are available, but in others it is unwise because experience has shown that no good ends are achieved.

A. IOEBT AT INITIAL SURGERY
Although the use of IOEBT at the time of the first surgery obviates many of the biological advantages of prior CRT, it does have the attraction of avoiding a second surgical procedure. Nonetheless, we have not used this approach and we strongly recommend against it. The application of IOEBT to previously unirradiated malignant gliomas has resulted in massive brain swelling in several patients and the associated death of at least one patient.[3] Even when application of IOEBT was done at repeat craniotomy 3 to 4 weeks after surgical diagnosis and bulk removal, the survival data were poor when external beam CRT was not given prior to IOEBT.[9] On the other hand, we have done intracranial pressure monitoring after IOEBT in patients who had large recurrent tumors that had previously been treated with CRT. There were never any sustained periods of intracranial hypertension.

B. RECURRENT MALIGNANT GLIOMAS
The situation of a patient with a recurrent malignant glioma is desperate. Therefore, it may be reasonable to try any therapeutic modality that might hold some glimmer of promise

for these patients, despite our claim that this is not the optimal circumstance for application of IOEBT. The only data in the English language literature about results of IOEBT in recurrent malignant gliomas are from Abe's[1] group in Japan (see also Chapter 14). In 1980, they reported a series of four patients whose recurrent tumors were treated with 20 to 40 Gy of IOEBT. None had had initial IOEBT. All of their patients had had partial resections and CRT, though one glioblastoma patient had only 17.4 Gy of CRT plus chemotherapy after initial surgery. The survival times ranged from 3 to 26 months, but the longest survival time was for a patient who had two applications of IOEBT to his recurrent astrocytoma (? grade III). The lesions in the other patients were glioblastomas in two and fibrosarcoma in one. In the original report, it was not clear whether the stated survival times were measured from the time of original discovery of the tumor or from the time of IOEBT. A more recent review by the same group indicates that all four of these patients died within 12 months of IOEBT,[11] so the stated survival periods were probably from the time of tumor discovery.

A more recent report from Abe's[11] group contains data on seven more patients whose recurrent malignant gliomas were treated with IOEBT. Two had tumors in unresectable areas, and they too survived less than 12 months after IOEBT. The next five patients, however, were treated in the CT era. More importantly, their recurrent tumors were localized in the frontal or occipital lobes. At the time of the report, they were all alive at periods of 4 to 31 months after 25 to 30 Gy of IOEBT had been given following gross removal of their recurrences. All of these important data from the original group of IOEBT investigators in Japan indicate that IOEBT does have the potential to eradicate sufficiently localized tumors, whether primary or recurrent. The difficulty, of course, relates to the problem of "sufficiently localized". Most recurrent malignant gliomas are not well localized, so it still makes sense to apply IOEBT according to our "optimal protocol" whenever possible.

C. REPEAT APPLICATION OF IOEBT

When malignant gliomas recur after treatment with IOEBT, it is reasonable to presume that their radiographic and pathologic features are the same as those of recurrences after standard treatment. Thus, it is likely that the peripheral zone of infiltration is aggressive and widespread.[2] Nonetheless, the foregoing data on the use of IOEBT for recurrent tumors would appear to lend some credibility to its repeated use in this circumstance. We will discuss only three patients who have been subjected to second applications of IOEBT for treatment of malignant gliomas (but see also Chapter 14).

Two patients who had IOEBT in an optimal protocol have had second treatments when their malignant gliomas recurred. Case 1 (Table 1) of Terao[9] was a 29-year-old male who was given an initial external dose of 40 Gy to his right frontotemporal grade IV astrocytoma, followed by 10 Gy of IOEBT. When his tumor recurred approximately 3 years later, he was given another 30 Gy of CRT and 15 Gy of IOEBT. He was still alive at 54 months after initial treatment at the time of Terao's report. The other patient who received a second dose of IOEBT after treatment in an "optimal protocol" was the first patient in our own series.

1. MCO Case 1

This 35-year-old woman had a previous history of ovarian carcinoma. It had been treated with total abdominal hysterectomy and chemotherapy. Approximately 3 years later she complained of headaches. A CT scan showed a mass lesion in the left lateral frontal lobe, with contrast enhancement and surrounding edema. Partial excision was performed, but with care not to extend the tissue removal too close to Broca's area (Figure 2A). The histological diagnosis was anaplastic astrocytoma without micronecrosis (grade III of Kernohan and Sayre[4]) (Figure 3A). Postoperatively she received external beam CRT to a dose of 50 Gy; 11 weeks after the first craniotomy, the patient received 15 Gy of IOEBT. At this second

TABLE 1
Miscellaneous Brain Tumors Treated by IOEBT

Author(s)	Tumor type	Age	Location[a]	CRT dose (Gy)	IOEBT dose (Gy)	Outcome
Abe et al.[1]	Fibrosarcoma	57	R occipito-temporal	?	35	Died — 6 months
Goldson et al.[3]	Mixed oligodendroglioma and astroblastoma	51	L frontoparietal	20 (after IOEBR)	15	Died — 1 month
	Oligodendroglioma	37	R parietal	55 (after IOEBR)	15	Died — 8 months (trauma)
	Juvenile pilocytic astrocytoma	19	L frontal	55 (after IOEBR)	15	Alive — 9 months
	Meningioma	44	L temporal	30 (after IOEBR)	15	Alive — 33 months
	Recurrent meningioma	53	L frontoparietal	40	15	Alive — 42 months
Terao[9]	Rhabdomyosarcoma	3	L middle fossa	None	15	Died — 4 months

[a]   R = right, L = left.

surgical procedure the fluid-filled cavity left by the first procedure was found. There was little necrotic tissue to be removed, but multiple needle biopsies were obtained through the wall of the cyst to guide the configuration of the IOEBT beam.

The patient remained neurologically normal. A CT scan 12 weeks after IOEBT showed only minimal evidence of abnormality (Figure 2B). Because of necrosis and infection in the incision, the craniotomy bone flap had to be removed 10 months after IOEBT. At 14 months after IOEBT, she complained of headaches, anomia, and short-term memory problems. A CT scan showed recurrent tumor with major edema and left-to-right shift. The edema was controlled with steroids, and a second dose of IOEBT was given. At this time, a large block of obviously abnormal but firm tissue was removed. It was entirely well-differentiated fibrillary astrocytoma (grade II of Karnohan and Sayre) (Figure 3B). After this procedure, the patient had some continuing nonfluency of speech and intermittent headaches. She remained at home, but completely able to care for herself. A CT scan without contrast 3 weeks after the second dose of IOEBT showed a low-density area in the region of the lesion, but little edema and no shift.

The patient died abruptly $3^1/_2$ weeks after the second application of IOEBT and 16 months after the original discovery of her tumor. Her husband, an experienced RN, called her from work at 8:00 p.m. and her condition was unremarkable. When he returned home at 11:30 p.m., the house was entirely in order and she had gone to bed. However, she was comotose and the craniotomy site (with no overlying bone flap) was bulging massively. An autopsy was not performed, but the most likely explanation for her sudden terminal ictus was intracerebral hemorrhage.

Despite its recurrence, the histological nature of this tumor improved after the *first* dose of IOEBT. Whether there was higher grade recurrent tissue deeper in the left frontal lobe will never be known, but no suspicious area was observed surgically or by CT. We speculate that there may have been some immunological idiosyncrasy in this person, because she had an earlier, cured malignancy, and part of its treatment had been chemotherapeutic. In any case, her sudden death was a great disappointment. Whether the presumed hemorrhage was directly related to the second application of IOEBT will never be known, but the outcome of the case does call for some caution about this possibility.

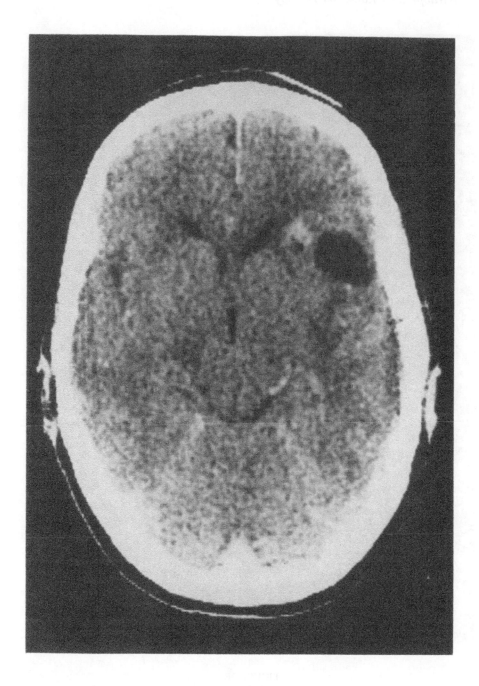

A

FIGURE 2.   Computed tomography (CT) scans of MCO Case 1. (A) 2 months after initial decompressive surgery, i.e., before secondary craniotomy for IOEBT; (B) 2 months after first application of IOEBR, i.e., approximately 3 months after scan in 2A.

Another patient who has been subjected to a second application of IOEBT for malignant glioma is Case 1 (Table 1) of Abe, et al.[1] This patient was a 36-year-old male whose right frontal astrocytoma was initially treated by partial resection and 60 Gy of CRT. The timing of the two doses of IOEBT (20 and 30 Gy, respectively) is not given, but it is clear that the first dose of IOEBT was given when the tumor recurred. The total survival time was 26 months.

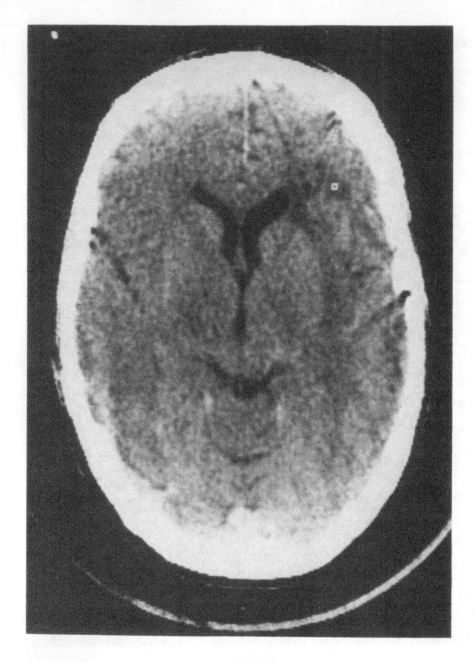

FIGURE 2B.

A total experience of three patients who have been subjected to repeated doses of IOEBT for malignant glioma is little more than anecdotal. Terao[9] has also treated one other case of metastatic tumor with repeated doses of IOEBT to the same right frontotemporal field. He feels that repeated usage of IOEBT is safe because the field of irradiation is narrow. This is probably true as far as it goes, but we suspect that IOEBT will prove to be most effective when the electron beam covers a significant margin beyond the obvious tumor. Thus, we may find ourselves in the usual dilemma of trying to decide whether our goal is tumor eradication or simply palliation for each invididual case.

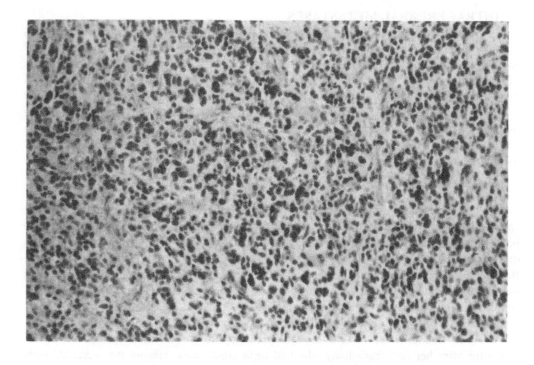

A

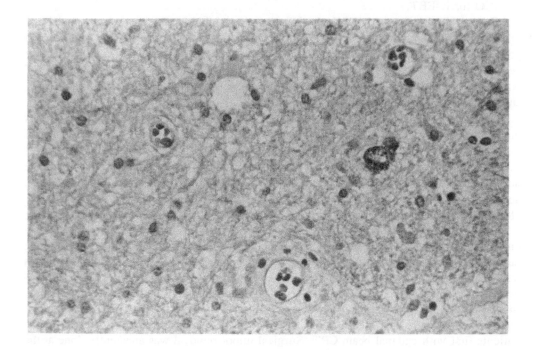

B

FIGURE 3. Photomicrographs of representative areas of tumor in MCO Case 1 (by courtesy of Manuel Velasco, M.D.). (A) Tumor removed at original surgery is anaplastic astrocytoma without micronecrosis. (B) Tumor removed at surgery for second application of IOEBT (after CRT of 50 Gy and IOEBT of 15 Gy) is entirely well-differentiated fibrillary astrocytoma. (Courtesy of Manuel Velasco, M.D.)

D. INTRACEREBRAL METASTASES

The fundamental radiobiology of metastatic tumors in the brain is probably the same as that of primary tumors, with one major exception. Since metastases do not arise from glial or neural elements, they probably do not have peripheral zones of infiltration such as those of gliomas. In theory, at least, it may be more feasible to eradicate any individual metastasis than to eradicate a seemingly focal malignant glioma. But recurrence of metastasis could still arise from the original primary or from other, untreated metastases. Our own experience includes two cases of cerebral metastasis. The first originated from a carcinoma of unknown origin. It serves well to illustrate the potential and the problems in the application of IOEBT to intracerebral metastases.

1. MCO Case 3

This 42-year-old woman presented to another center with right hemiparesis. CT and angiography showed a large tumor in the left parietal lobe. At surgery, it was thought to be a glioblastoma, but histological study revealed poorly differentiated carcinoma. This diagnosis was confirmed by the Armed Forces Institute of Pathology, Washington, D.C. Because a CT of the abdomen suggested a tumor in the ovarian area, a laparotomy was performed, but the only abnormality was a uterine fibroid. Exhaustive search for the primary source was unrevealing.

The patient's neurological condition improved markedly after initial surgery. She received 40 Gy of external beam CRT through opposing ports over a 1-month period. However, 3 months after her first craniotomy, she had some right-sided seizures and increased right hemiparesis. CT showed areas of enhancing tumor around the margins of the postoperative cavity in the left parietal lobe and another mass near the left occipital pole. She was referred to MCO for IOEBT.

Prior to application of IOEBT, the left parieto-occipital craniotomy was reopened and all reachable tumor was removed. We knew that some tumor remained both anterior and posterior to the craniotomy site, although the craniotomy margin was extended another centimeter medially. After 16 days, the craniotomy was again reopened and 20 Gy of IOEBT was delivered to the tissue within the margins of the bone opening; 3 weeks after IOEBT she had recovered some strength in her right arm.

At 7 weeks after IOEBT, the bone flap had to be removed because of *Staphylococcus aureus* infection. The dura was tense. Computed tomography scan showed recurrence of tumor both at the occipital pole, which was inspected, and at the frontal pole, which was not. She died 6 months after discovery of her tumor and 2 months after IOEBT. Complete autopsy did not reveal any primary source of her tumor. However, examination of the brain showed that the tumor that had been directly within the IOEBT beam had been sterilized. Her recurrence had come from tumor which was not encompassed by the field of IOEBT.

Another reported experience with IOEBT for the treatment of cerebral metastatic carcinomas is by Terao.[9] In his series of five patients, four had carcinoma of the lung and one had a breast origin. As mentioned above, one man with metastatic lung carcinoma was treated twice. In addition, a woman with lung carcinoma was apparently treated simultaneously for separate right occipital and right temporal tumors. At the time of his report, four of the five patients were still alive at 4, 7, 8, and 10 months after IOEBT. One patient with lung carcinoma had died at 19 months. In all of these cases, Terao had treated the patients first with external beam CRT. Surgical tumor removal was apparently done at the time of IOEBT. Although these survival times may be encouraging, it is difficult to interpret their significance, because Terao does not indicate the total survival times from the point of the discovery of the brain metastasis. More importantly, the clinical circumstances of patients with cerebral metastases are quite variable. We do not have any reliable, large group survival statistics against which to compare these results.

Finally, we have recently applied IOEBT to one patient with a posterior fossa metastasis.

E. POSTERIOR FOSSA TUMORS

None of the reported series known to us has mentioned anything about the application of IOEBT in the posterior fossa. Since our recent experience appears to be unique, we report it here with admittedly short follow-up.

1. MCO Case 4

This 40-year-old woman developed a malignant cutaneous melanoma over the right shoulder blade in 1981. Wide excision and skin grafting were performed. She was well for about $1^1/_2$ years, when local recurrence was associated with right axillary metastasis. The skin lesion was reexcised; axillary lymph nodes were removed. Postoperatively, the right axilla was treated with radiation therapy. She received immunotherapy elsewhere during the ensuing 27 months. Liver and lung metastases developed. These were controlled with interferon therapy under the supervision of the MCO Division of Hematology/Oncology during the 6 months preceding her admission. At 4 weeks prior to admission, a subcutaneous melanoma nodule was excised from the right inguinal region. About the same time, she began to experience increasingly severe headaches. Neurosurgical consultation 1 week prior to admission revealed that she had incoordination of the left hand (dominant for writing), mild ataxia of gait, and Romberg's sign. A CT scan of the head demonstrated a large (4.5 × 3.5 cm) mass in the left cerebellar hemisphere, compressing and displacing the adjacent fourth ventricle and associated with noncommunicating hydrocephalus of moderate severity. Oral steroid therapy was initiated, and the neurological examination became normal. In February 1986, through a suboccipital craniectomy, near-total excision of the mass was carried out. Postoperative recovery was uneventful. The neuropathologist's report was this: amelanotic melanoma, histologically similar to the previously resected skin neoplasm. The tumor cells had a strong reaction to immunoperoxidase for S-100 protein and a negative reaction for GFA and keratin, supporting the diagnosis of melanotic melanoma (M.E. Velasco, M.D.). After 10 d, the suboccipital craniectomy was reopened and the tumor bed explored. A small amount of residual tumor was removed. She received a 20-Gy dose of IOEBT to the tumor bed, the electron beam being aimed from medial to lateral to exclude the brain stem from the axis of the beam. Her postoperative course was again uneventful. She was discharged home, neurologically intact, on the sixth postoperative day; 3 months later, she was admitted to another hospital with a recurrent cerebellar mass. She expired with extensive metastatic melanoma.

F. OTHER TUMOR TYPES

Aside from the malignant gliomas and metastatic carcinomas, a small miscellany of other brain tumors have been treated with IOEBT. None of these is within our own experience. The reported cases are summarized in Table 1. Although the survivals with malignant tumors have been poor, we feel that it would be justifiable to apply IOEBT to such cases, precisely because their outlooks are so dismal. None of the malignant tumors in Table 1 was treated in a manner similar to our optimal protocol. Doing so might well improve their survivals. With regard to nonmalignant tumors, we have taken a much more cautious attitude, primarily because the long-term effects of IOEBT are not known. Late radionecrosis is a particular concern, though no such problems have been reported to our knowledge. Another concern about the use of IOEBT for nonmalignant tumors is the problem of measuring the influence of this modality on the patient's survival. Since these patients often live for many years, and there are no useful group statistics, it would be very difficult to know whether IOEBT really had any influence on the course of the patient's illnesses.

V. COMPLICATIONS

A. ACUTE BRAIN SWELLING

As mentioned above (in the section on IOEBT at initial surgery), Goldson et al.[3] have observed acute brain swelling after applying IOEBT at the time of initial decompressive surgery and when IOEBT was given immediately after open biopsies. Terao did not mention this problem in his initial group of four patients who were given IOEBT by repeat craniotomy soon after the diagnosis of tumor was confirmed histologically. Abe's reports[1,11] also say nothing about any similar problems, but Abe's patients apparently all had recurrences which had been previously treated with external beam CRT. Matsutani also describes one death due to postoperative brain swelling in his chapter (Chapter 14) of this book. No prior CRT had been given, but it is not clear whether a previous debulking procedure had been done. We conclude that the application of intracranial IOEBT at the time of initial surgery is a dangerous undertaking, with or without tumor decompression.

B. RADIONECROSIS

Since the field of irradiation in IOEBT is largely restricted to tumor, late radionecrosis in normal surrounding brain should not be a major problem. To date, no such complication has been reported. Among the various reported case series discussed in this chapter,[1,3,9,11] the longest survival has been 54 months. There have been several patients who lived into and past their second post-IOEBT years. Goldson et al.[3] do mention that two of their surviving glioma patients have CT density changes that could be consistent with either necrosis or recurrence. However, neither of these patients was symptomatic at the time of the report, so it was very difficult to distinguish between the two possible causes for the CT changes. The number of patients who have survived more than a year after receiving IOEBT for brain tumors is very small. To complicate the issue further, many of these patients have also received external beam CRT. For these reasons we can only recommend an appropriate sense of caution with regard to the possibility of late radionecrosis after IOEBT for cerebral malignancies.

C. INTRACEREBRAL HEMORRHAGE

Two instances of intracerebral hemorrhage have been reported following IOEBT for malignant gliomas, albeit in very different circumstances. Patient 2 in the series of Goldson et al. (1980) "developed an intratumoral hematoma in the immediate postoperative period, necessitating re-exploration and drainage." Those authors attributed the bleeding to both the surgery and the IOEBT, which is probably the only fair statement that can be made. In a much more chronic situation, our first patient (MCO Case 1, described above) apparently died of an intracerebral hemorrhage $3^1/_2$ weeks after a second dose of IOEBT, but no autopsy was done, and this diagnostic conclusion remains unproven.

D. WOUND INFECTIONS AND SCALP NECROSIS

No mention of wound infection or scalp necrosis is found in any of the available literature on IOEBT for cerebral lesions. However, three patients in our small series have required removal of their bone flaps at 2, 3, and 6 months after IOEBT. *Staphylococcus aureus* was cultured from all three wounds. One patient (Case 2) had Gram-negative organisms as well. Without the bone flap, good healing was eventually achieved in all three patients, but one (Case 1) required plastic maneuvers for her scalp closure because of loss of tissue in the wound edge. IOEBT had been given at first or second reopenings of the craniotomies. The patients had received 40 to 50 Gy of external beam CRT, completed at intervals of 1 to 2 months before IOEBT was given. In Case 1 (50 Gy completed $1^1/_2$ months before IOEBT), it appeared that the infection was actually secondary to breakdown of the scalp wound, rather than vice versa. In response to these problems, we have initiated a more vigorous program of preoperative antibiotic prophylaxis. Other considerations would be to use a smaller dose of CRT before IOEBT (with completion later) and/or to increase the interval between CRT and IOEBT.

VI. CONCLUSIONS

Malignant gliomas have been tenaciously recalcitrant to a large variety of seemingly ingenious treatments. In view of the basic biology of these tumors, IOEBT probably will not be the ultimate answer to the problem. However, we do believe that the fundamental logic of our "optimal protocol" is sound. Although the early results surveyed in this chapter are in no way definitive, they do justify continued investigation of this modality in the treatment of these tumors. The most important technical problem is adequate postoperative definition of the zone of peripheral infiltration, as defined pathologically by Burger et al.[2] Clearly, all of this zone must be included in the radiation field if IOEBT is to have any chance of producing long-term remission or cure. Early results of comparing CT scanning to nuclear magnetic resonance (NMR) scanning show that the latter technique gives more definitive results.[5] Thus, the advent of NMR scanning may well improve our ability to plan appropriate use of IOEBT in patients with malignant cerebral gliomas.

ACKNOWLEDGMENTS

Dr. and Mrs. M. Ahito provided an English translation of the paper by Terao.[9]

REFERENCES

1. **Abe, M., Takahashi, M., Yabumoto, E., Adachi, H., Yoshii, M., and Mori, K.,** Clinical experiences with intraoperative radiotherapy of locally advanced cancers, *Cancer,* 45, 40, 1980.
2. **Burger, P. C., Dubois, P. J., Schold, S. C., Jr., Smith, K. R., Jr., Odom, G. L., Crafts, D. C., and Giangaspero, F.,** Computerized tomographic and pathologic studies of the untreated, quiescent, and recurrent glioblastoma multiforme, *J. Neurosurg.,* 58, 159, 1983.
3. **Goldson, A. L., Streeter, O. E., Jr., Ashayeri, E., Collier-Manning, J., Barber, J. B., and Fan, K.-J.,** Intraoperative radiotherapy for intracranial malignancies, *Cancer,* 54, 2807, 1984.
4. **Kernohan, J. W. and Sayre, G. P.,** Tumors of the central nervous system, in *Fascicle 35, Atlas of Tumor Pathology,* Armed Forces Institute of Pathology, Washington, D.C., 1952.
5. **Laster, D. W., Ball, M. R., Moody, D. M., Witcofski, R. L., and Kelly, D. L., Jr.,** Results of nuclear magnetic resonance with cerebral glioma. Comparison with computed tomography, *Surg. Neurol.,* 22, 113, 1984.
6. **Nelson, J. S., Tsukada, Y., Schoenfeld, D., Fulling, K., Lamarche, J., and Peress, N.,** Necrosis as a prognostic criterion in malignant supratentorial, astrocytic gliomas, *Cancer,* 52, 550, 1983.
7. **Salazar, O. M., Rubin, P., Feldstein, M. L., and Pizzutiello, R.,** High dose radiation therapy in the treatment of malignant gliomas: final report, *Int. J. Radiat. Oncol. Biol. Phys.,* 5, 1733, 1979.
8. **Salcman, M.,** Survival in glioblastoma: historical perspective, *Neurosurgery,* 7, 435, 1980.
9. **Terao, H.,** Intraoperative radiotherapy and conformation radiotherapy for malignant brain tumors, *Neo. Shinkei. Geka.,* 10, 119, 1982.
10. **Thomlinson, R. H. and Gray, L. H.,** The histological structure of some human lung cancers and the possible implications for radiotherapy, *Br. J. Cancer,* 9, 539, 1956.
11. **Yamashita, J., Handa, H., Keyaki, A., and Abe, M.,** Indication for Intraoperative Radiation Therapy (IOR) in the Treatment of Recurrent Malignant Gliomas, poster presented to the American Association of Neurological Surgeons, Atlanta, April 21 to 25, 1985.

Chapter 14

INTRAOPERATIVE RADIATION THERAPY FOR MALIGNANT BRAIN TUMORS

Masao Matsutani

TABLE OF CONTENTS

I. INTRODUCTION

Treatment results for the patient with a benign brain tumor have improved in the past decade, largely because of new diagnostic methods and the wide use of microsurgical techniques, but progress for the patient with a malignant glioma has been disappointingly slow. Among numerous clinical and laboratory research investigations conducted to improve the treatment results for malignant gliomas, intraoperative radiation therapy (IORT) is the most attractive one.

IORT has been developed in order to sterilize the remaining malignant remnants after surgery. Malignant gliomas belong to a group of radioresistant cancers, partly because high radiation doses are toxic to the normal brain tissue surrounding the tumor. IORT is quite applicable for radioresistant brain tumors because of precise demarcations of the target volume under direct vision, minimum damage to surrounding normal tissues, and a high target absorbed dose of 15 to 20 Gy/4 to 8 min. However, clinical trials of this therapy for malignant brain tumors are quite limited.[1,2] In this chapter, the present author reports the results of IORT for glioblastoma multiforme and metastatic brain tumors, which has been performed at Tokyo Metropolitan Komagome Hospital, and discusses the indications and the limitations of this therapy. Since little research has been done on how much radiation can be delivered to a normal brain, especially to the brain stem, the IORT was applied only to cerebral tumors in adults.

II. IORT FOR GLIOBLASTOMA MULTIFORME

A. BIOLOGY OF GLIOBLASTOMA MULTIFORME

Glioma, a neoplasm of neuroectodermal origin, is oncopathologically defined as carcinoma in the brain. Even the well-differentiated glioma in the adult cerebrum, astrocytoma, frequently undergoes dedifferentiation in the course of years, with the terminal histologic picture of poorly differentiated anaplastic astrocytoma or glioblastoma multiforme.

Glioblastoma multiforme usually grows in the deep white matter of the cerebrum, and rapid invasion in multiple directions along the white matter has already occurred by the time of diagnosis (Figure 1). Tumor cells infiltrate the surrounding brain tissue at least 3 cm distant from the margin of the enhanced tumor area on CT scan.[3] In advanced stages, the tumor infiltration in the white matter extends into the contralateral hemisphere, and finally to the brain stem or the cerebellum through the cerebral peduncle (Figure 2). Frequently, glioblastoma cells disseminate into the cerebrospinal fluid, causing carcinomatous meningitis. During surgery for such an invasive glioblastoma, most cases are beyond the point of removal of the tumors because of the risk of damage to the surrounding brain tissue. With surgery alone, followed by the best of conventional care, patients have a uniformly fatal course with a median survival of 17.0 weeks.[4] The restriction of the surgical treatment has inevitably required postoperative radiation therapy; this has been the most important treatment modality following surgery.

B. RADIATION THERAPY FOR GLIOBLASTOMA MULTIFORME

Although patients treated with postoperative radiation therapy showed significantly extended survival of about 20 weeks, as compared to those receiving surgical resection alone,[4,5] the median survival time has not exceeded 50.0 weeks, even in combination with chemotherapy,[6] as complete disappearance of the tumors on CT scan after conventional radiation therapy is obtained in only 5% of the cases.[7] The residual tumor at the primary site starts to regrow in most cases just after completing radiation therapy. This is shown by the fact that glioblastoma recurs within 2 cm of the primary site in more than 90% of the patients.[8,9] Histologic analysis of radiation effects for glioblastoma revealed that the extent to which

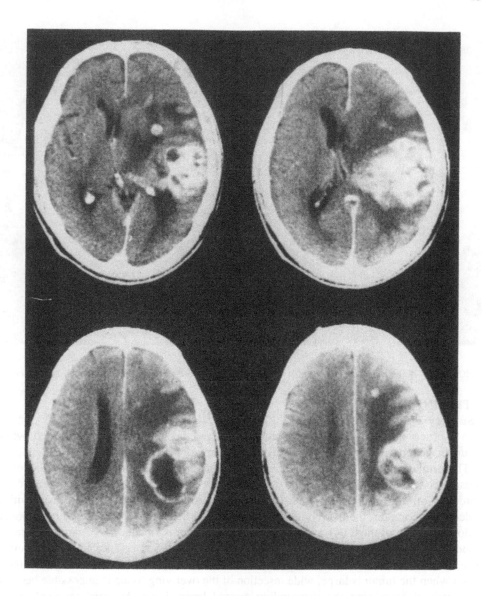

FIGURE 1.   The CT scan of glioblastoma multiforme is characterized by irregular outline with multiple buddings along the white matter and multilobular necrotic cysts.

tumor size was decreased depended upon the degree of ischemic necrosis due to the indirect effect of irradiation on tumor vessels, but not the direct lethal effect on tumor cells.[9] These clinical findings show that conventional external beam radiation therapy with a dose of 50 to 60 Gy did not result in local cure. However, Walker[10] showed that survival time was extended in proportion to the target absorbed dose and suggested that a higher localized radiation dose would improve the poor prognosis of patients with these tumors.

As a clinical approach to increasing the therapeutic ratio by developing a new irradiation technique, IORT was applied. After two pilot studies, our clinical approach was set up to maximize resectability and intensive irradiation of the tumor area. IORT was combined with a wide resection of the remnant tumor after conventional external radiation therapy. An extensive conformative irradiation controlled by computer was developed for treatment of glioblastoma multiforme.[1]

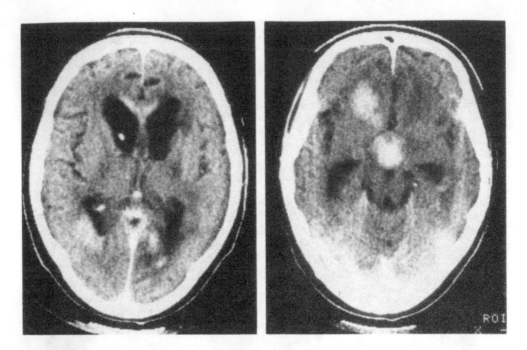

FIGURE 2.   Glioblastoma at the terminal stage. Tumor invasion is observed in both cerebral hemispheres.

C. TECHNIQUES
1. Surgery

All surgery is performed in the operating room, and then the patient is transported, while still under general anesthesia, to the radiation therapy department.

The primary objective of preparative surgery for IORT after conventional irradiation is to ensure complete resectability of the tumor remnants around the previous surgical margins in order to minimize the target area for irradiation. As glioblastomas usually grow within the deep white matter, the overlying cortical and subcortical brain tissue should be removed to allow insertion of the IORT applicator. When the tumor is smaller than 3 cm in diameter, a cone-shaped resection of the tumor with overlying brain tissue is possible, and the tumor tissue and tumor infiltrative area is then observed at the bottom of the resected region (Figure 3). But when the tumor is large, wide resection of the overlying tissue is impossible because of the risk of sacrificing the surrounding normal brain tissue. Minimal removal of the overlying tissue and intratumoral resection (U-shaped resection) is the usual procedure, and the tumor tissue or the infiltrative area remains beneath the surgical margin in these cases (Figure 3). These different kinds of operative procedures relate to the selection of treatment volume during IORT.

2. Anesthesia and Transportation of Patients

One of the most significant problems in performing IORT is the transportation of patients from the operating theater to the radiation therapy department. In the operating room in the first basement, a patient who receives preparatory surgery is moved, while still under general anesthesia, to the third basement where the betatron apparatus is.

The patient is laid on the mobile MAQUET 1120 operative bed (Figure 4A). As the IORT demands a precisely maintained position of the firmly fixed cranium, fixation is best achieved by a Sugita's pinion headholder (Mizuho Ika Co., Ltd.) (Figure 4B). An anesthetic gas tank with nitrous oxide and oxygen (1:1) is attached to the bed for transportation. Anesthesia is maintained with mixed nitrous oxide and oxygen at a flow rate of 6 l/min,

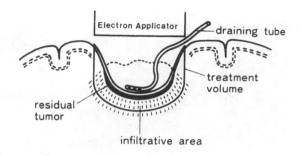

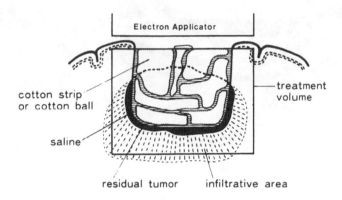

FIGURE 3. (Top) Cone-shaped resection for irradiation. By draining blood or cerebrospinal fluid with a thin ventricular draining tube, the dead space is kept dry. The treatment volume is calculated from the margin of dead space. (Bottom) In U-shaped resection, saline-saturated cotton balls fill in the dead space, and the treatment volume is designed to include them.

combined with a neuroleptic or a narcotic during transportation and IORT. In the radiation treatment room, electrocardiography, respiration rate, and the airway pressure of the patients are monitored by closed-circuit television.

After irradiation, the patient is returned to the operating room again for surgery. In close cooperation with neurosurgeons, anesthesiologists, radiotherapists, and nurses, the average time required is less than 30 min, until the final operation is started. No complications, including anesthesia problems or infection, have been encountered yet.

3. IORT Techniques

A Shimadzu 20-meV betatron used for IORT at our hospital has an energy range of 4 to 20 meV. Radiophysical details of this apparatus are described in chapter by Matsuda and Tanaka (Chapter 18).

As the head of the patient is fixed in place by a Sugita's pinion headholder, the designed radiation field is faced on the precise gantry angulation, allowing a precise beam alignment.

Saline-saturated cotton strips or cotton balls are inserted into the U-shaped surgical deficit as tissue-compensating material to maintain dose homogeneity. In the cone-shaped surgical defect, bleeding from the epidural space or cerebrospinal fluid from the brain tissues are drained continuously to keep the area dry using a ventricular drainage tube. This is because the treatment volume is designed as 1 to 2 cm below the marginal wall. The applicator size is determined to give a 1-cm perimeter of ''normal'' brain tissue. The electron beam energy is selected so that the 90% isodose line falls at least 1 to 2 cm below the deepest aspect of the tumor (Figures 3 and 9).

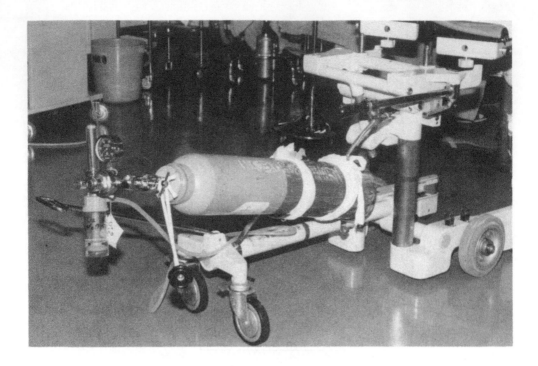

A

FIGURE 4.   (A) An anesthetic gas tank is attached to the mobile MAQUET 1120 operative bed for transporting a patient. (B) the head of patient is fixed with a Sugita's pinion headholder (Mizuho Ika Co., Ltd.). The removable holder (arrow) makes it possible to fix the head in an ideal position against the radiation applicator.

D. PATIENT SELECTION AND TREATMENT PROTOCOLS

From August 1975 to May 1985, 32 adult patients with cerebral glioma received IORT a total of 36 times. Of these, 24 patients had nonrecurrent tumors, and 8 patients had recurrent tumors. The histological diagnoses were 25 glioblastoma multiforme, 4 anaplastic astrocytomas, and 3 differentiated gliomas. The discussion of this chapter will primarily concern the treatment results for glioblastoma, and those other types of gliomas will only be briefly documented.

The clinical protocol of IORT was decided after two pilot studies. The first pilot study was performed on three patients in order to determine the proper dose to be delivered to patients. The second one was on four patients in order to select the best indication for this therapy.

The final protocol, started in April 1978, was based on the two pilot studies. Specific therapy is selected according to preceding therapy (Figure 5). In the first step of conservative surgery, the removal of the entire tumor, when practicable, is carried out to avoid intolerable functional disability. Following surgery, conventional external beam radiation therapy with 4-MV X-rays generated by the linear accelerator is automatically requested. The target volume, including presumed occult tumor involvement, is enclosed by a line 3 cm distal from the border of original tumor. Wide reresection of the tumor with or without IORT is applied to cases expected to be resectable after a total of 35 Gy or more, and over 50 Gy, respectively. Conformation radiation therapy to a total dose of 70 or 90 Gy was finally delivered to cases obtaining a marked reduction of tumor bulk.

Conformation radiation therapy by linear accelerator is a special moving-field therapy by which the dose is matched to the shape and size of the tumor, and dose is minimized to the tissue surrounding the tumor. The principle means of conforming to a complicated shape

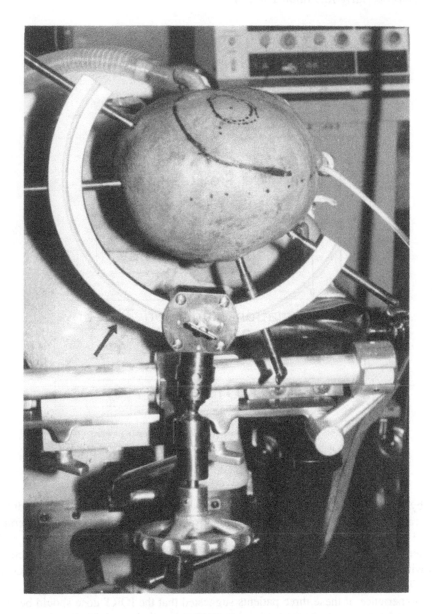

FIGURE 4B.

of target volume is to open five to eight pairs of collimators by computer control during rotation irradiation so that the photon beams are focused to the shape of the tumor.[11] After receiving the combination of surgery and radiation therapy, all patients receive chemotherapy.

Response to the IORT was evaluated using time-to-tumor progression (TTP) and survival. Determination of response was based on sequential evaluations performed every 8 weeks after the completion of all the radiation therapies. Tumor progression was defined as definite worsening in CT scan appearance and neurological examination. TTP was measured from the time of the first operation.

III. RESULTS

A. THE FIRST PILOT STUDY

As shown in Table 1, two patients with non-recurrent glioblastoma (Case 1 and 2) were

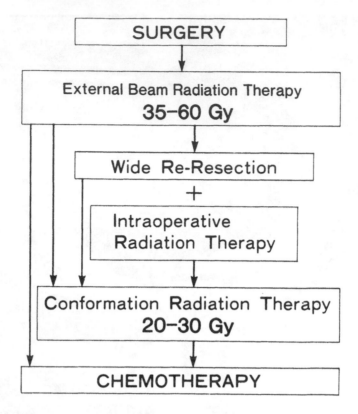

FIGURE 5.   Treatment course: after surgery and following external beam radiation therapy, wide resection of the tumor with or without IORT is performed. Conformation radiation therapy with 20 to 30 Gy is added to cases showing marked reduction of tumor.

treated by IORT with a dose of 30 Gy delivered to massive residual tumor bulk during the first operation without subsequent conventional radiation therapy. During the therapy, the irradiated brain tissue showed such marked edema that the bone flap could not be replaced. The patients deteriorated a few days later. The TTP was 9 and 19 weeks, respectively. A patient with recurrent oligodendroglioma (Case 3) was irradiated with a dose of 25 Gy during surgery. The irradiated brain was swollen, but he did not deteriorate, fortunately.

The experience of these three patients suggested that the IORT dose should be less than 25 Gy in order to avoid cerebral edema, and that irradiation of 30 Gy alone would not control the massive tumor bulk.

B. THE SECOND PILOT STUDY

As shown in Table 1, four patients with deep seated, widespread glioblastoma were treated with external beam therapy and IORT at a dose of 15 to 20 Gy. The location, size, and extent of the tumors restricted surgical resectability and IORT (Figure 6). The potential area of tumor involvement was beyond the extent of the IORT applicator. The enhanced tumor shadow on CT scan remained after therapy in all cases. The TTP was about 30 weeks in Cases 4 through 6, and 80 weeks in Case 7. The survival rate at 1 year was 50%, and no patient survived 2 years. Intraoperative or postoperative marked cerebral edema was not observed, but the large remnant tumor mass was not controlled, even by IORT doses of 15 or 20 Gy combined with external radiation therapy.

This study suggested that the IORT dose delivered during operation should be less than 20 Gy, and that the IORT should be applied as a boost therapy for minimum residual tumor or tumor infiltrative area, following the external radiation therapy.

TABLE 1

The First and Second Pilot Study

| Case no. | Patient | (Sex/age) | IORT | | | | External beam radiation therapy (Gy) | Outcome |
			Diameter (cm)	Depth (cm)	Energy (meV)	Dose (Gy)		
1	T.I.	(F/68)	4	4	14	30	None	Marked postoperative edema; TTP:[a] 9 weeks
2	T.H.	(F/50)	4	4	14	30	None	Marked postoperative edema; TTP: 19 weeks
3	T.S.	(M/50)[b]	4	2	8	25	None	TTP: 44 weeks
4	M.O.	(M/19)	6	3	12	18	34.5	TTP: 30 weeks
5	Y.K.	(M/52)	6	3	12	15	34.4	TTP: 34 weeks
6	Y.A.	(F/31)	5	3	12	20	40	TTP: 28 weeks
7	H.S.	(M/56)	4	2.5	8	15	60	TTP: 80 weeks

[a] TTP is time to tumor progression (weeks) and is measured from the time of first operation until the date of definite worsening in CT scan appearance and neurological examination.

[b] Recurrent oligodendroglioma.

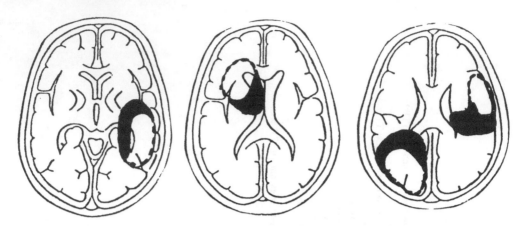

FIGURE 6.   Schematic drawings of the tumors in the second pilot study. Deep seated, widespread tumors are observed. Location, size, and extent of tumor restricted surgical resectability. Areas covered with dotted line show removed tumors, and black areas mean residual tumors.

C. FINAL PROTOCOL

Based on the experience of the first and the second pilot studies, the final protocol of IORT for glioblastoma was designed to irradiate areas adjacent to the margin of wide removal with a sufficient target volume (Figure 5). According to this plan (See Table 2), 15 patients were treated by IORT with a range of 8- to 20-meV beams to an absorbed dose of 10 to 20 Gy. External beam radiation therapy with doses between 35 and 70 Gy were given to all of the patients.

Complete resectability of the tumor was anticipated in 11 cases, and in 4 cases (Cases 11, 15, 21, 22), a small amount of remnant tumor tissue still remained after surgical intervention. The space wall, with presumed tumor remnants after the total removal of the tumor, was subjected to IORT.

For the patients who received cone-shaped resection (Cases 8 to 11, 14 to 16, 20, and 21), the energy of the electron beam was selected to place the 90% isodose line 1.5 to 2.0 cm below the surgical margin. In the other cases, the target volume included the dead space filled with saline-saturated cotton balls, and the 90% isodose line also fell 1.0 to 2.0 cm below the deepest aspect of the tumor (Figures 3 and 9).

Of the 15 patients, 8 have died, and 7 are alive. The median TTP from the first operation was 79.5 weeks (about 18 months), and the survival rate at 12 and 24 months was 100 and 61.1%, respectively (Figure 8). In seven patients, a recurrent tumor developed at the primary site, and at a remote site in three. Five patients have now been disease free for 25 to 56 weeks. Case 8 received IORT three times (Table 3) and is still alive 9 years after the first operation. His glioblastoma was an atypical one which always grew in the superficial temporal lobe; it was always removed completely. Case 12 deteriorated 45 weeks after the first operation. He received IORT for the recurrent tumor (Table 3). His disease-free period from the second treatment has already exceeded that of the first treatment.

Three patients (Cases 22 to 24) received brachytherapy with ^{192}Ir seeds combined with IORT. This will be described in the summary.

D. RESULTS FOR RECURRENT GLIOBLASTOMA

As shown in Table 3, eight patients with recurrent glioblastoma received IORT. Four of them had already received it as a first therapy, and two of those have alrady been described. All of the patients had macroscopic total removal of their recurrent tumors. The delivered dose was between 10 and 20 Gy. The median TTP — from the therapy to the recurrent tumor — was 30 weeks.

TABLE 2
Results of Final Protocol

Case no.	Patient	(Sex/age)	IORT Diameter (cm)	Depth (cm)	Energy (meV)	Dose (Gy)	External beam radiation therapy[a] (Gy)	TTP[b] (weeks)	Survival
8[c]	J.K.	(M/29)	3	1.5	8	10	40	69	9 years, alive
9	T.N.	(M/43)	5	1.5	8	20	60	137	37 months
10	E.N.	(M/45)	3	2.0	10	10	38	146	36 months
11	M.K.	(M/56)	8	2.0	20	20	35	90	24 months
12[c]	T.K.	(M/38)	6	4.0	14	15	70	45	25 months, alive
13	M.M.	(F/32)	5	3.0	12	15	72	48[d]	22 months
14[c]	S.Y.	(F/63)	3	2.0	10	15	50	68	24 months
15	K.S.	(F/68)	5	2.0	8	15	40	34+	8 months, alive
16	N.Y.	(F/34)	4	2.0	8	15	70	61	17 months
17	T.T.	(M/43)	4	3.0	12	20	60	56+	13 months, alive
18	N.K.	(M/50)	5	3.5	14	15	70	43+	10 months, alive
19	H.K.	(M/42)	5	3.5	14	15	70	25+	6 months, alive
20[e]	M.A.	(F/52)	3	1.5	8	15	62	31[d]	13 months
21[e]	S.K.	(M/55)	3 × 4	1.5	8	15	70	52[d]	20 months
22[e]	M.J.	(M/60)	5	4.5	18	20	50	56+	13 months, alive

[a] High-dose external beam irradiation was made possible using conforming techniques of external beam.

[b] TTP: time to tumor progression.

[c] Patients who received IORT again at the time of recurrence (Table 3).

[d] Recurrence at remote site, not at primary site.

[e] These three patients also received ^{192}Ir brachytherapy combined with IORT.

TABLE 3
Results of Recurrent Glioblastoma Multiforme

| | | | IORT | | | | External beam radiation therapy (Gy) | TTP[a] (wks) |
			Diameter (cm)	Depth (cm)	Energy (meV)	Dose (Gy)		
Case no.	Patient	(Sex/age)						
5[b]	Y.K.	(M/52)	6	3	12	15	None	26
8[b]	J.K.	(M/29)	4	2	10	15	None	82
			5	1	8	15	None	34
12[b]	T.K.	(M/38)	5	1	6	10	None	56 +
14[b]	S.Y.	(F/63)	5	3	12	20	None	17[c]
23	Y.T.	(F/31)	2	3	20	10	None	13[c]
24	T.S.	(F/58)	5	1.5	8	10	30	34
25	H.I.	(F/60)	4	1.5	6	15	None	39
26	J.T.	(M/72)	4	1	6	15	None	13[c]

[a]   TTP: time to tumor progression.
[b]   These four patients received IORT at the first therapy (Table 2).
[c]   These 3 patients died of other causes without tumor recurrence.

E. RESULTS FOR OTHER GLIOMAS

As shown in Table 4, three patients with recurrent anaplastic astrocytoma, one with nonrecurrent anaplastic astrocytoma and two with differentiated astrocytoma, were treated with IORT. The indication for this therapy for anaplastic astrocytoma is the same as that for glioblastoma multiforme. One patient (Case 28) survived 24 months without tumor recurrence. Three patients with recurrent anaplastic astrocytoma did not show good results from this therapy. One of them deteriorated only 12 weeks after the therapy, and two of them died 1 month after surgery.

The reasons for IORT for differentiated astrocytoma are based on the facts that even the well-demarcated and histologically differentiated astrocytoma shows some evidence of diffuse infiltration into the adjacent tissues (Figure 7). Differentiated tumor cells in the infiltrative area, which frequently remain after macroscopic total removal, are generally resistant to conventional radiation therapy and chemotherapy. They become the source of recurrence. This is based on the fact that the survival rate of differentiated cerebral astrocytoma in adults is about 50% at 5 years.[12] In order to suppress the remaining infiltrative cells in astrocytoma and to obtain a cure, IORT would be logical. Two patients with differentiated astrocytoma treated in this study are surviving for more than 2 and 6 years without recurrence.

F. COMPLICATIONS

Any troubles, including anesthesia problems and infection, have not yet been encountered with IORT. Two patients died postoperatively. One (Case 27) suffered from acute hepatic failure unrelated to the therapy; the other (Case 30), however, showed marked brain swelling just after the completion of surgery. Computed tomography scan showed no hematoma in the surgical area. The tumor lay in the subcortical area in the frontal lobe, and the target volume was irradiated with an applicator 4 cm in diameter, to a dose of 15 Gy at 4 cm depth. These conditions were much the same as for the other patients treated. As no autopsy was performed, the cause of cerebral edema remains unresolved.

IV. SUMMARY

In order to evaluate the effect of IORT for glioblastoma, it is necessary to compare the treatment results of different treatment modalities. Since April 1978, 66 patients with non-

TABLE 4
Results of Other Gliomas

Case no.	Patient (Sex/age)	Histological diagnosis[a]	IORT					External beam radiation therapy (Gy)	Outcome[b]
			Diameter (cm)	Depth (cm)	Energy (meV)	Dose (Gy)			
27	M.S. (M/41)	r-AA	4	2	10	20	None	Postoperative death (1)
28	T.S. (M/56)	AA	5	2	8	15	60	24 months, died (2)
29	K.M. (M/57)	r-AA	3	4	20	20	None	TTP:[c] 12 weeks
30	H.M. (M/35)	r-AA	4	4	20	15	None	Postoperative death (3)
31	H.M. (F/20)	DA	2	1	6	12	42	6 years, alive
32	H.M. (M/42)		4	1.5	8	15	30	2 years, alive

[a] r: recurrent; AA: anaplastic astrocytoma; DA: differentiated astrocytoma.

[b] (1) postoperative death: acute hepatic failure; (2) death due to acute hepatic failure without tumor recurrence; (3) postoperative death: acute intracranial hypertension.

[c] TTP: time to tumor progression

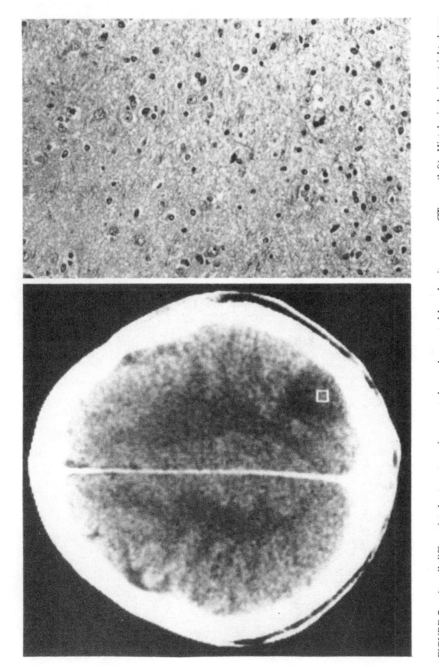

FIGURE 7.   A well-differentiated astrocytoma is presented as a demarcated low-density area on CT scan (left). Histological view (right shows the infiltration of tumor cells (lower half) into the surrounding white matter (upper half).

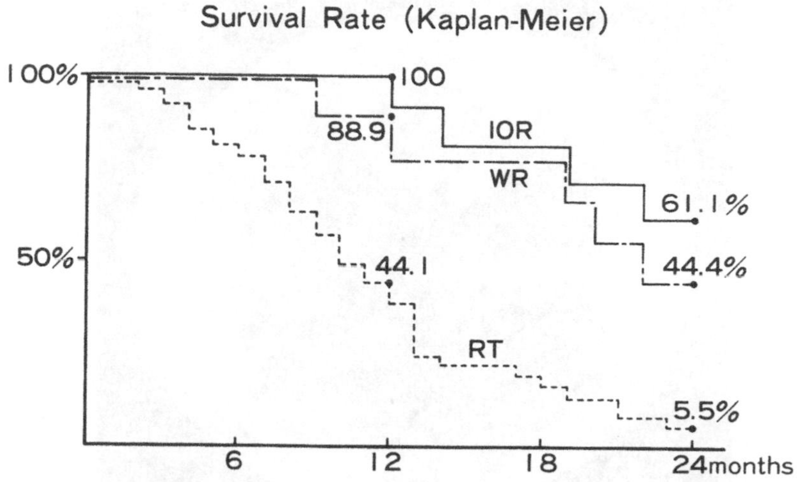

Survival Rate (Kaplan-Meier)

FIGURE 8. Survival (Kaplan-Meier). IOR: intraoperative radiation therapy (15 cases); WR: wide resection (9 cases); and RT: conventional external radiation therapy (42 cases).

recurrent glioblastoma multiforme were treated according to the final treatment protocol described above (Figure 5). A total of 15 patients were selected for IORT (Table 2); 9 patients received wide tumor resection after external beam radiation therapy;[13] a wide resection made it possible to minimize the tumor mass by removing areas of ischemic necrosis produced by irradiation. IORT, however, was inapplicable to the deep-seated tumors, because there would have been mechanical damage to surrounding tissues by insertion of a radiation cone. The median survival was 21.0 months and the 2-year survival rate was 14.4% (Figure 8).

External beam radiation therapy alone was performed in 42 patients with doses of 50 to 70 Gy. These tumors were too large for wide resection and IORT (Figure 1). The median survival was 11.0 months and the 2-year survival rate was 5.5% (Figure 8).

The results of these treatment comparisons have demonstrated that the significant difference between a 2-year survival rate of 44.4% for wide resection, and that of 5.5% for conventional external irradiation, is closely correlated with the extent to which the tumor mass was surgically removed. It is generally accepted that patients with a successful removal of tumor have a prolonged survival. The difference in the survival rates between IORT of patients and those treated by wide resection might be related to the intensive absorbed dose at the operation. The results apparently indicate that areas adjacent to the margin of almost complete removal should be irradiated with a sufficient dose to sterilize the remaining malignant tumor remnants. In summary, for patients treated by radiation therapy combined with chemotherapy the median survival was reported to be 40.5 to 50 weeks, the median TTP was 31.0 to 41.0 weeks, and the 2-year survival rate was less than 40%.[4,6,14] It can be said that IORT is the best treatment at present for glioblastoma multiforme; but, the true indications for this therapy are quite limited. As glioblastoma generally grows in the deep white matter, the number of patients suitable for IORT is restricted. Only 15 of 66 patients (23%) in this study were candidates for IORT.

Although these patients survived longer than those treated by external beam radiation therapy and subsequent chemotherapy (mainly with nitrosourea compounds), local recurrence developed in seven of eight patients who received IORT alone (Cases 8 to 19). Also, when a large tumor mass remained, such advanced cancer was not controlled even by IORT. Failures of this kind are considered to be due to inadequate radiation dose and inadequate treatment volume. The recurrent tumor in Case 12 developed at the surgical margin (Figure 9). If glioblastoma cells infiltrate into an area 3 cm distant from the margin of the tumor

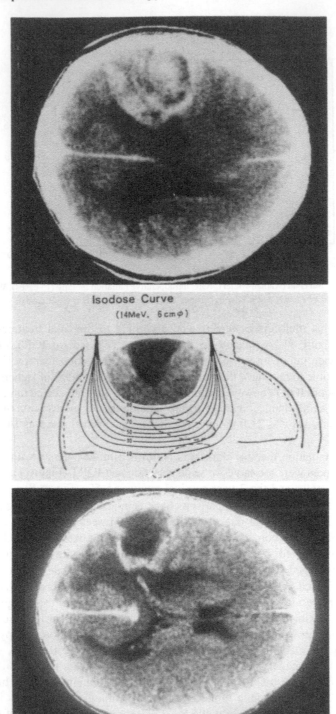

FIGURE 9.   CT scan of Case 12 (glioblastoma) at the time of diagnosis (top). Isodose curves generated by a 14-meV betatron (6-cm applicator with a 4-cm depth) are superimposed on the schematic drawing of CT scan after wide resection (middle). No visual tumor is observed. The recurrent tumor develops along the surgical margin (bottom).

bulk, the treatment volume for the typical case, designed for the 90% isodose line 1.5 cm from the tumor margin, might be inadequate. The determination of an optimum dose of 20 Gy or less in this protocol was based on the experience that administration of 30 Gy resulted in marked cerebral edema in three patients in whom resections were complete. It might be possible to increase the dose to 25 Gy because with experiments in dogs, there appeared to be little difficulty in the toleration of doses of 30 Gy for the retroperitoneal organs including blood vessels.[15]

The fact that Case 12's disease-free period from the second IORT procedure has already exceeded that from the first surgery strongly suggests the necessity of increasing doses with bigger treatment volumes without damaging the surrounding normal brain. As for the enlargement of the radiation field in Case 12, the treatment volume which would cover the whole infiltrative area using an 8-cm applicator with a 6-cm depth of the 90% isodose line, would affect the posterior part of the thalamus and the upper brain stem. The question of how much radiation can be delivered to a normal brain, especially to the brain stem, still remains in doubt, and is a major problem for this therapy as a curative form of treatment for glioblastoma multiforme.

In order to cover the limitations of this therapy at present, brachytherapy, using ^{192}Ir, was developed as a boost radiation treatment. For three patients (Cases 20 to 22), ^{192}Ir seeds were inserted into the peritumoral area which the IORT field could not cover (Figure 10). In two patients, local tumor control was obtained without recurrence at the primary site. This new combination therapy could be an attractive one in the near future.

For a local cure of glioblastoma, a cancer invasive in multiple directions, the first step of therapy should be an intensive local treatment. IORT is obviously one of the logical treatments, as is brachytherapy.[16]

The effect of IORT on recurrent glioblastoma multiforme is summarized as 30 weeks being the median TTP (range 13 to 82 weeks); this is better than that achieved by conventional treatment (radiation and chemotherapy), which is reported as 22 to 26 weeks median TTP.[17,18]

The indication for this therapy for anaplastic astrocytoma is considered to be the same as that for glioblastoma multiforme, but the indication for well-differentiated astrocytoma has not been established. These tumors, even though their histological characteristics are well differentiated, show malignant transformation in their clinical course and therefore demand intensive treatment for remnant tumor cells after surgery. IORT would be a logical treatment for such cases.

V. IORT FOR METASTATIC BRAIN TUMORS

A. INTRODUCTION

Therapy for metastatic brain tumors should be considered according to the patient's general condition. It is generally accepted that aggressive therapy for intracerebral metastasis should be applied only to patients without systemic metastases in order to obtain a "local cure".[19,21] For a single intracerebral metastasis without systemic metastases, the general form of treatment is surgical removal, followed by radiation therapy, but for multiple intracerebral metastases radiation therapy is performed. The median survival of the former group is reported to be 6 to 14 months,[19-22] whereas that of the latter is 7 months.[20] Steroid therapy alone is applied only for patients with advanced systemic metastases.

In order to improve the patient's survival in both quality and longevity and to provide significant palliation, surgical removal combined with intensive radiation therapy should be attended to in selected patients.

As metastatic brain tumors usually grow at the corticomedullary junction of the brain, they are more suited for IORT than malignant gliomas growing deep in the white matter. As the area of local invasion might be considered to be smaller (less than 1 cm from the

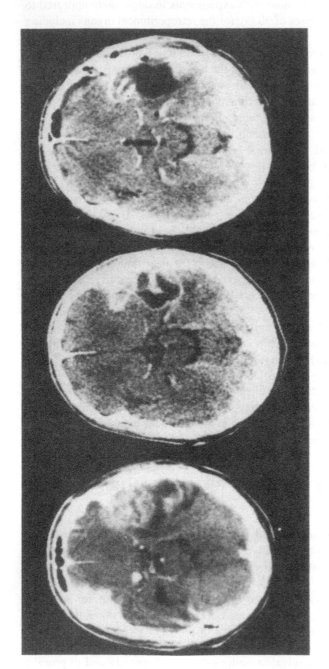

FIGURE 10. The CT scans of Case 21 (glioblastoma) treated by the combination of IORT and ^{192}Ir brachytherapy. The tumor located in the middle fossa (left) and a small residual tumor are observed at the tip of temporal lobe at the time of IORT (center). Two ^{192}Ir seed-containing tubes are inserted there, where the electron beam missed (right).

TABLE 5
IORT for Metastatic Brain Tumors from Lung Cancer

| | | | IORT | | | | |
| | | Histologic | Diameter | Depth | Energy | Dose | |
Case no.	Patient (Sex/age)	Diagnosis[a]	(cm)	(cm)	(meV)	(Gy)	Outcome
1	K.N. (F/41)	Ad	4	2.5	10	16	19 months, dead
2	M.S. (M/52)	Ad	3	2.0	10	15	11 months, dead[b]
3	R.T. (M/56)	Ad	4	1.0	6	15	15 months, dead[b]
4	T.K. (F/58)	Ad	4	1.5	8	20	
			3	1.5	8	20	15 months, dead[b]
5	M.S. (M/71)	Mx	4	1.0	6	15	17 months, dead
6	H.Y. (M/56)	Mx	3	1.0	8	15	34 months, alive
7	K.H. (M/67)	Mx	3	1.0	8	15	8 months, dead
8	T.Y. (M/68)	Ep	3	1.5	8	15	5 months, dead[b]
9	T.H. (M/68)	Lc	3	1.5	8	15	8 months, alive
10	T.I. (F/58)	Ad	3	1.5	8	15	10 months, dead[b]
11	S.H. (M/72)	Ad	3	1.5	8	15	6 months, dead
12	S.S. (M/47)	Ad	4	1.5	6	20	12 months, alive
13	K.O. (M/48)	Mx	4	2.0	8	20	4 months, dead
14	T.N. (M/61)	Ep	3	2.5	12	20	6 months, alive
15	J.K. (F/30)	Ad	5	1.0	6	15	14 months, alive
16	M.K. (F/41)	Ad	3	2.5	14	20	12 months, alive
			4	3.0	14	20	
17	H.Y. (M/55)	Ad	5	1.0	4	20	9 months, alive
18	M.I. (F/72)	Ad	3	3.0	16	15	8 months, alive
19	K.K. (F/66)	Ad	4	2.5	10	20	8 months, alive
20	M.F. (M/60)	Ad	5	3.0	12	20	5 months, alive

[a]   Ad adenocarcinoma; Mx: mixed carcinoma; Ep: epidermoid carcinoma; Lc large cell carcinoma.
[b]   Died of other causes without intracerebral recurrence.

margin of the tumor) than that of malignant glioma, the effect of localized intraoperative irradiation may be expected to be better than that for malignant gliomas. In addition, high-dose irradiation during surgery will shorten the period of external beam treatment that will, in most cases, be beneficial for patients with a limited life span.

B. PATIENT SELECTION AND METHOD

From January 1976 until May 1980, 20 patients with metastatic brain tumors from lung cancer and eight from other cancers were treated by IORT (see Table 5). All but two patients (Cases 4 and 16) had a single metastasis in the brain without systemic metastases or primary tumor recurrence. Metastases in the posterior fossa were excluded from study because brain stem irradiation has not been studied. Metastases at the thalamus and the basal ganglia were also excluded because extensive removal of the tumor and wide resection of overlying brain tissue for insertion of the radiation cone are not usually acceptable.

Histologic diagnoses of patients with metastases from lung cancer were as follows: 13 adenocarcinomas, 4 mixed carcinomas, 2 epidermoid carcinomas, and 1 large cell carcinoma. It was not unusual that there were some differences in the histologic pictures between the primary cancer and the metastatic foci. Generally, a progressive loss of differentiation was observed. Well-differentiated carcinomas changed into poorly differentiated ones.

As the response to IORT for various subtypes of intracerebral metastases is almost the same,[20] the treatment protocol was uniformly applied to all histoiogical types.

C. TREATMENT PROTOCOL

IORT for metastatic tumors is performed during the first surgery, which is different from the protocol for malignant gliomas. Total or extensive removal of the tumor produces a cone-shaped dead space, where minimum tumor remnant or invading tumor cells remain in the marginal wall. The appropriate radiation cone diameter is chosen to give a 1-cm perimeter around the surgical defect, and the electron beam energy is selected so that the 90% isodose line falls 1 cm below the deepest aspect of the tumor. The dose delivered is 15 to 20 Gy. After the IORT, patients receive whole-brain irradiation to a dose of 30 Gy.

In cases where the patient has to wait more than 2 weeks for the operation, whole-brain irradiation is performed prior to surgery and IORT. In both pre- and postoperative irradiation, the tumor area receives 30 Gy via conventional external irradiation plus 15 to 20 Gy of IORT. The other part of the brain received 30 Gy of conventional radiation therapy as a prophylactic treatment against existing silent metastases.

D. RESULTS

As shown in Table 5, 20 patients with intracerebral metastasis from lung cancer received IORT. Two patients (Cases 4 and 16) received it twice for two metatstic tumors at different sites (Figure 11). Other patients had single metastasis in the brain and had no signs or symptoms of systemic metastases.

Five patients died within 1 year; 3 of them received surgery for primary lung cancer after brain surgery and died of postoperative complications (Cases 8, 10, and 13). They had no recurrent cerebral metastasis at the time of death. One patient (Case 2) died of systemic metastases without a recurrent brain tumor 11 months after the IORT. In another patient (Case 7) a new intracerebral metastasis was the cause of death.

Among four patients who survived more than 1 year, two had new intracerebral metastasis and two showed systemic metastases without intracerebral recurrence. Four patients are still living and well, without recurrence, after more than 1 year. The 6- and 12-month survival rates were 90 and 65%, respectively. If the three patients who died of postoperative complications following pulmonary surgery are excluded, the 6- and 12-month survival rates would be 100 and 79%. These results are better than those obtained by conventional surgery and radiation therapy.[19-23]

As the survival rate of patients with intracerebral metastases largely depends on systemic conditions, the evaluation of treatment should examine the success of local control of cancer foci, which could prolong survival for patients without systemic metastases. The results of IORT in this study are manifested in the low local recurrence rate in the brain, that is, of course, related to the excellent 1-year survival rate of 65%. The results for eight patients with other primary cancer sites were also excellent, the same as those for lung cancer, with no intracerebral recurrence for 6 to 15 months. Only one patient died of recurrent intracerebral metastasis 24 months after IORT. In the treatment of metastatic brain tumors, IORT could be the most effective treatment in prolonging the useful life of selected patients.

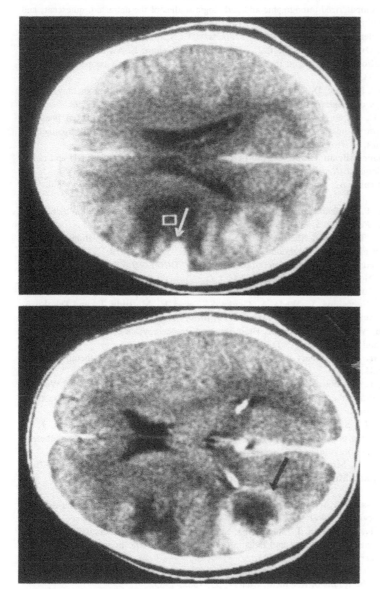

FIGURE 11. Double metastatic tumors (arrows) in Case 4 are also treated by IORT.

REFERENCES

1. **Matsutani, M., Matsuda, T., Nagashima, T., Kohno, T., Hoshino, T., and Terao, H.,** Surgical treatment and radiation therapy for glioblastoma multiforme with special reference to intraoperative radiotherapy, *Jpn. J. Cancer Clin.,* 30, 325, 1984.
2. **Goldson, A. L., Streeter, O. E., Jr., Ashayeri, E., Collier-Manning, J., Barber, J. B., and Fan, K.-J.,** Intraoperative radiotherapy for intracranial malignancies, *Cancer,* 54, 2807, 1984.
3. **Burger, P. C., Dubois, P. J., Schold, S. C., Jr., Smith, K. R., Jr., Odom, G. L., Crafts, D. C., and Giangaspero, F.,** Computerized tomographic and pathologic studies of the untreated, quiescent, and recurrent glioblastoma multiforme, *J. Neurosurg.,* 58, 159, 1983.
4. **Walker, M. D., Alexander, E., Jr., Hunt, W. E., MacCarty, C. S., Mahaley, M. S., Jr., Mealey, J., Jr., Norrell, H. A., Owens, G., Ransohoff, J., Wilson, C. B., Gehan, E. A., and Strike, T. A.,** Evaluation of BCNU and/or radiotherapy in the treatment of anaplastic gliomas. A cooperative clinical trial, *J. Neurosurg.,* 49, 333, 1978.
5. **Jellinger, K., Kothbauer, R., Volc, D., Vollmer, R., and Weiss, R.,** Combination chemotherapy (COMP protocol) and radiotherapy of anaplastic supratentorial gliomas, *Acta Neurochir.,* 51, 1, 1979.
6. **Levin, V. A., Wilson, C. B., Davis, R., Wara, W. M., Pischer, T. L., and Irwin, L.,** A phase III comparison of BCNU hydroxyurea, and radiation therapy to BCNU and radiation therapy for treatment of primary malignant gliomas, *J. Neurosurg.,* 51, 526, 1979.
7. **Takakura, K. and Japanese Brain Tumor Chemotherapy Study Group,** Effects of ACNU and radiotherapy on malignant glioma, *J. Neurosurg.,* 64, 53, 1986.
8. **Hochberg, F. H. and Pruitt, A.,** Assumption in the radiotherapy of glioblastoma, *Neurology,* 30, 907, 1980.
9. **Matsutani, M., Kohno, T., Matsuda, T., and Seto, T.,** Histological evaluation of radiation therapy for glioblastoma multiforme, *Radiother. Syst. Res.,* 2, 63, 1985.
10. **Walker, M. D., Strike, T. A., and Sheline, G. E.,** An analysis of dose-effect relationship in the radiotherapy of malignant gliomas, *Int. J. Radiat. Oncol. Biol. Phys.,* 5, 1725, 1979.
11. **Matsuda, T.,** Computer controlled conformation radiotherapy, in *MEDINFO 80,* Lindberg, D. A. B. and Kaihara, S., Eds., North-Holland, Amsterdam, 1980, 14.
12. The Committee of Brain Tumor Registry in Japan, Brain Tumor Registry in Japan, 5, 1984.
13. **Matsutani, M., Hori, T., Nagashina, T., Ikeda, A., Genka, S., Terao, H., Matsuda, T., and Takakura, K.,** Extensive surgical removal of gliomas after radiotherapy, *Brain Nerve,* 33, 811, 1981.
14. **Edwards, M. S., Levin, V. A., Wilson, C. B.,** Brain tumor chemotherapy: an evaluation of agents in current use for phase II and III trials, *Cancer Treat. Rep.,* 64, 1179, 1980.
15. **Tepper, J. and Sindelar, W.,** Summary of the workshop on intraoperative radiation therapy, *Cancer Treat. Rep.,* 65, 911, 1981.
16. **Gutin, P. H., Phillips, T. L., Wara, W. M., Leibel, S. A., Hosobuchi, Y., Levin, V. A., Weaver, K. A., and Lamb, S.,** Brachytherapy of recurrent malignant brain tumors with removable high-activity iodine-125 sources, *J. Neurosurg.,* 60, 65, 1984.
17. **Levin, V. A., Edwards, M. S., Wright, D.C., Seager, M. L., Schimberg, T. P., Townsend, J. J., and Wilson, C. B.,** Modified procarbazine, CCNU, and Vincristine (PCV 3) combination chemotherapy in the treatment of malignant brain tumors, *Cancer Treat. Rep.,* 64, 237, 1980.
18. **Young, B., Oldfield, E. H., Markesbery, W. R., Haack, D., Tibbs, P. A., McCombs, P., Chin, H. W., Maruyama, Y., and Meacham, W. F.,** Reoperation for glioblastoma, *J. Neurosurg.,* 55, 917, 1981.
19. **Galicich, J. H., Sundaresan, N., Arbit, E., and Passe, S.,** Surgical treatment of single brain metastasis: factors associated with survival, *Cancer,* 45, 381, 1980.
20. **Matsutani, M., Kohno, T., Nagashima, T., Nagayama, I., Hoshino, T., Ikeda, T., Sakai, T., Matsuda, T., and Takakura, K.,** Surgical treatment and radiation therapy for metastatic brain tumors from lung cancer, *J. Jpn. Soc. Cancer Ther.,* 18, 1979, 1983.
21. **Sundaresan, N. and Galicich, J. H.,** Surgical treatment of brain metastases. Clinical and computerized tomography evaluation of the results of treatment, *Cancer,* 55, 1382, 1985.
22. **Gagliardi, F. M. and Mercuri, S.,** Single metastasis in the brain: late results in 325 cases, *Acta Neurochir.,* 68, 253, 1983.
23. **White, K. T., Fleming, T. R., and Laws, E. R., Jr.,** Single metastasis to the brain. Surgical treatment in 122 consecutive patients, *Mayo Clin. Proc.,* 56, 424, 1981.

Chapter 15

INTRAOPERATIVE RADIATION THERAPY FOR ADVANCED OR RECURRENT HEAD AND NECK MALIGNANCIES

Peter Garrett, Newell Pugh, David Ross, Ron Hamaker, and Mark Singer

TABLE OF CONTENTS

I. INTRODUCTION

The patient with locally advanced or recurrent head and neck cancer remains a difficult problem for the practicing oncologist. Patients with advanced nodal disease are difficult to control with radiation alone.[7] Once recurrence takes place, surgery is difficult in the presence of fixed disease; and long-term prognosis is poor.[4] After initial reports of encouraging results, most chemotherapeutic regimens have failed to alter the course of this advanced disease dramatically.[10]

To combat the problem of advanced or marginally resectable disease in the abdomen, the use of radiation at the time of surgery has become popular.[1,2,6,9,11] Intraoperative radiation therapy (IORT) allows the radiation oncologist to give a high single dose of radiation to the tumor volume. The tumor can be visualized directly and normal critical structures can be moved from the field. A large single fraction on the order of 15 to 20 Gy can overcome the initial shoulder of repair and produce tumor cell kill of several logs. We began a pilot project in 1982 to treat advanced or recurrent head and neck cancer with resection combined with IORT. The head and neck tumor sites are ideally suited for this type of treatment. The surgical field is easily visualized, and normal tissue such as the skin and soft tissue can be moved out of the radiation field. The spinal cord is avoided by using electrons of appropriate energies. There are no other reports of IORT in the head and neck region, and this chapter reports our initial results.

II. METHODS AND MATERIALS

Between May 1982 and October 1984, we treated 41 patients with advanced head and neck malignancies with IORT. All surgery was performed by one surgical team, and the IORT was administered by one group of radiation oncologists. One patient was treated on two separate occasions, and a second had two separate sites treated concurrently. There were 43 sites for analysis in 41 patients.

An analysis was done of local tumor control and survival. Comparisons between the treatment groups were done using the log-rank method.[8] The actuarial method was used to calculate survival,[3] and survival was calculated from the time of IORT.

There were 28 males and 13 females in the study (ratio of 2.2:1). The age range was 15 to 81 years with a median of 60 years. There were 10 treated in 1982, 13 in 1983, and 18 in 1984. The minimum follow-up was 9 months.

The neck was the most common site treated (19 patients). There were seven parotid malignancies and seven maxillary cancers. A complete breakdown of the sites treated is shown in Table 1.

Prior full-course external beam irradiation had been given to 18 patients. The previous dose of radiation ranged from 45 to 70 Gy with a median of 60 Gy. Between 40 and 54 Gy was given after IORT with a median of 50 Gy. In three patients, only IORT was used. As expected, the most common histologic type was squamous cell carcinoma (28 cases). We had seven cases of adenoidcystic carcinoma. Table 2 shows the pathology for the remaining cases.

All the patients were transported from the operating room to the radiation therapy department for treatment. This involved transportation through two long corridors and down four floors by elevator. The IORT was given at the end of the treatment day and did require some rescheduling of patients.

All therapy was given using a Siemens® Mevatron XII linear accelerator. Most of the patients (35) were treated with a 4-meV electron beam. Seven were treated with 7-meV electrons and one was treated at 11 meV electron energy. The dose was prescribed at 100% (D_{max}). The median dose was 20 Gy with a range of 10 to 100 Gy (Table 3). The field sizes

TABLE 1
Distribution of Sites Treated
by IORT

Site treated	Number
Neck	19
Maxilla	7
Parotid	7
Floor of mouth	4
Pterygoid-base of skull	2
Temporal bone	2
Submandibular gland	1
Tongue	1
Total	43

TABLE 2
Histopathology of Tumors
Treated

Pathology	Number
Squamous cell CA	28
Adenoidcystic CA	7
Mucoepidernoid CA	3
Adenocarcinoma	1
Oncocytic carcinoma	1
Osteogenic sarcoma	1

TABLE 3
Dose of IORT Used for Head
and Neck Cancer

IORT dose (Gy)	Number
10	3
15	14
20	23
25	1
30	1
100	1
	43

TABLE 4
Analysis of Failure for the Three Groups of
Patients Treated for Cancer of the Head and
Neck

	Close margins	Microscopic residual	Gross disease
In-field failures	1	1	4
Surgical field outside IORT field	1	1	4
Number at risk	21	11	8

were 4.4 cm (13 sites), 5.1 cm (10 sites), 6.3 cm (16 sites), and 9.5 cm (4 sites). Individualized lead shields were used to block critical tissue (i.e., skin edges).

We used IORT when the surgeon could not obtain an acceptable margin of normal tissue around the tumor or if residual tumor was left after surgery. For the purpose of analysis, the indications were classified as (1) gross residual disease (10 sites), (2) microscopic residual disease (12 sites), and (3) close surgical margins (21 sites). During the same time period there were 24 cases where IORT was initially considered, but either inoperable disease was found at the time of surgery or an acceptable margin of normal tissue was achieved during surgery ending that consideration.

III. RESULTS

The results of treatment in terms of local control were analyzed by disease group (Table 4). There were 21 sites treated in the close-margins group with one failure in the IORT treatment field and one failure in the surgical field, but outside to the IORT field.

There were 12 sites treated in the microscopic residual group; one patient died 3 weeks after treatment of pulmonary fibrosis secondary to bleomycin. This patient is not included in our analysis. There was 1 failure within the IORT field and 1 failure outside the IORT field, but within the surgical field among the 11 patients at risk.

Ten patients were treated with gross residual disease. One patient died of airway obstruction by a mucous plug 2 days postoperatively. The second patient died of a carotid rupture 1 month following IORT. These patients died too early to be included in local control analysis, but are included in the survival data analysis. All eight patients treated for gross disease have failed locally. There have been four failures in the IORT field and four failures beyond the field, but within the surgical margins.

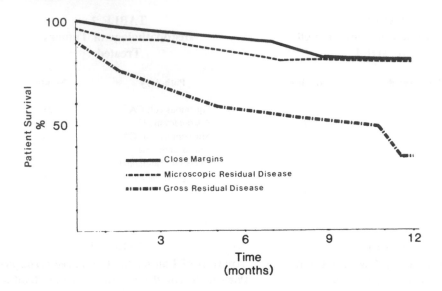

FIGURE 1.   The 1-year patient survival rate following IORT for head and neck tumors.

There is a statistically significant difference in local failure (p <0.001) between the close margin (2 of 11) and gross residual disease patients (8 of 8). There were also statistically significant differences (p <0.001) in local failure between the microscopic residual disease group (2 of 11) and gross residual disease group (8 of 8). There were essentially no differences in local failure between the close margin group (2 of 21) and microscopic residual disease group (2 of 11).

The overall patient survival from the time of IORT was 70% at 1 year for all the patients treated. The survival for the close margins group was 83%, and for the microscopic residual disease group it was 82%. Those patients with gross residual disease had a survival of only 36% at 1 year (Figure 1).

No complications were associated with patient transit to and from the radiation therapy department or with treatment of the anesthetized patient. The major morbidity associated with treatment of these patients with advanced head and neck malignancies was carotid rupture. This occurred in three patients and proved fatal in each case.

The first patient had gross disease left in the carotid artery at the time of surgery. This area received 20 Gy in a single fraction. At 1 month following treatment, the patient died of a carotid rupture. A post-mortem examination was not performed.

The second case of carotid rupture was in a patient treated with microscopic disease around the carotid artery. He died 3 months after IORT. Post-mortem examination revealed necrotic tumor in the treatment field. This patient did not have muscle coverage of the carotid at the time of surgery.

The final case occurred in a patient treated for close margins. This patient received 15 Gy at the time of IORT followed by postoperative irradiation with an additional 50 Gy in 24 treatments. Subsequent to this, an ulcer appeared in the pyriform sinus secondary to irradiation. This progressed to a sinus formation with infection and a carotid rupture occurred 9 months after the IORT. Post-mortem examination showed no local tumor, but did show radiation effect in the carotid artery.

One other major complication occurred, this being osteonecrosis of the mandible. This patient had a carcinoma of the floor of the mouth, treated by a composite resection of the floor of the mouth, partial glossectomy, marginal mandibulectomy, and radical neck dissection. Microscopic residual disease remained in the mandible, and this area received 100 Gy intraoperatively followed by 60 Gy in 30 treatments postoperatively. At 2 months after the IORT, a fistula developed and subsequently exposed bone was visible. The mandible was removed and focal necrotic debris found.

IV. DISCUSSION

The patient with advanced or recurrent head and neck cancer has an extremely poor prognosis. The disease may be disfiguring and cause a painful and distressing demise. Ulceration of tumor nodules with associated infection and bleeding creates difficult nursing problems.

We have treated this group of patients with combined surgery and IORT. The procedure has been relatively safe and adaptable to a tertiary-care general hospital. Patient transport was not a problem. Because patients were treated with the same accelerator used to treat the daily load of outpatients, scheduling of the IORT had to be done with great care. On the day of IORT, outpatients were scheduled earlier than usual and generally finished by 4 pm. Surgery was scheduled for the afternoon, and the IORT was usually not done until 5 or 6 p.m.

The results of treatment were excellent for the group with close margins or microscopic residual disease. Failure in the operative field was uncommon, and over 80% are alive 1 year after treatment. Patients with gross disease remain a problem. The survival is poor and all the patients at risk have failed locally. Thus, it appears that for IORT to be successful in head and neck cancer, all gross disease must be resected.

The major complication observed was carotid rupture. The three cases of this all occurred in the early part of the series. After these cases, we took two precautions to try to prevent this catastrophic event from recurring: if disease was removed from the region of the carotid, a flap with a myocutaneous graft was placed covering the surgical defect — this improved the vascularity of the region and provided extra protection to the carotid; also, if gross disease was left on the carotid, IORT was not given. Shrinkage of the tumor may weaken the carotid wall or result in a direct ulceration leading to a rupture. Since we have adopted these measures we have had no more of these complications.

We are encouraged by the preliminary results with IORT in head and neck cancer. Further patient accrual is required to confirm these results with large numbers of patients. It will be necessary to study this treatment in a randomized multicentric trial in the future. The addition of radiosensitizers to IORT is an interesting possibility. By treating with IORT at peak serum levels, some of the dose-related toxicity of radiosensitizers may be avoided.[5] Hopefully, these new treatments will benefit the unfortunate patient with advanced head and neck cancer.

V. SUMMARY

Between 1982 and 1984, we treated 41 patients with advanced head and neck malignancies with surgery and IORT. Of these, 1 patient had 2 separate sites treated, and a second was treated on 2 separate occasions, giving 43 sites for analysis. The overall survival for the patients treated was 70% at 1 year. Those treated for close surgical margins had a 1-year survival of 83%, and for microscopic residual disease the survival was 82%. Only 36% of gross residual disease patients were alive at 1 year. Local failure occurred in 2/21 in the close margins group and 2/11 in those with microscopic residual disease. In gross residual disease, patients (8/8) had local failure. The major complication of treatment was carotid rupture. Measures taken to prevent this complication seem effective. We believe intraoperative irradiation is an effective treatment for advanced or recurrent head and neck cancer.

REFERENCES

1. **Abe, M. and Takahashi, M.**, Intraoperative radiotherapy: the Japanese experience, *Int. J. Radiat. Oncol. Biol. Phys.*, 7, 863, 1981.
2. **Abe, M., Takahashi, M., Yabumoto, E., Adachi, H., Yoshi, M., and Mori, K.**, Clinical experience with intraoperative radiotherapy of locally advanced cancers, *Cancer*, 45, 40, 1980.
3. **Cutler, S. J. and Ederer, F.**, Maximum utilization of the life table method in analyzing survival, *J. Chronic Dis.*, 8, 699, 1958.
4. **Garrett, P., Beale, F., Cummings, B., Harwood, A., Keane, T., Payne, D., and Rider, W.**, Cancer of the tonsil: results of radical radiation with surgery in reserve, *Am. J. Surg.*, 146, 432, 1983.
5. **Gray, A., Dische, S., Adams, G., Flockhart, I., and Foster, J.**, Clinical testing of the radiosensitizer Ro-07-0582. I. Dose, tolerance, serum and tumor concentrations, *Clin. Radiol.*, 27, 151, 1976.
6. **Gunderson, L., Cohen, A., Doseretz, D., Shipley, W., Hedberg, S., Wood, W., Rodkey, G., and Suit, H.**, Residual, unresectable, or recurrent colorectal cancers: external beam irradiation and intraoperative electron beam boost ± resection, *Int. J. Radiat. Oncol. Biol. Phys.*, 9, 1597, 1983.
7. **Harwood, A., Beale, F., Cummings, B., Keane, T., Payne, D., Rider, W., Rawlinson, E., and Elhakim, T.**, Supraglottic laryngeal carcinoma: an analysis of dose-time-volume factors in 410 patients, *Int. J. Radiat. Oncol. Biol. Phys.*, 9, 311, 1983.
8. **Peto, R., Poke, M., and Armitage, P.**, Design and analysis of randomized clinical trials requiring prolonged observation of each patient. I. Analysis and examples, *Br. J. Cancer*, 35, 1, 1977.
9. **Shipley, W., Wood, W., Tepper, J., Warshaw, A., Orlow, E., Kaufman, S., Battit, G., and Nardi, G.**, Intraoperative electron beam irradiation for patients with unresectable pancreatic cancer, *Ann. Surg.*, 200, 289, 1984.
10. **Vogel, S., Schoenfield, D., Kaplan, B., Lerner, H., Engstrom, P., and Horton, J.**, A randomized prospective comparison of methotrexate with a combination of methotrexate, bleomycin and cisplatin in head and neck cancer, *Cancer*, 56, 432, 1985.
11. **Wood, W., Shipley, W., Gunderson, L., Cohen, A., and Nardi, G.**, Intraoperative irradiation for unresectable pancreatic carcinoma, *Cancer*, 49, 1272, 1982.

Chapter 16

INTRAOPERATIVE RADIATION THERAPY FOR GASTRIC CANCER

Mitsuyuki Abe

TABLE OF CONTENTS

I. INTRODUCTION

Most of the published data concerning incidence and patterns of failure for gastric cancer patients after surgery suggest that local and regional control is important in the improvement of prognosis.[1-5] Surgeons have exerted much effort in performing larger, more extensive resection for the treatment of gastric cancer.[6,7] However, except for early gastric cancer in which tumor invasion is limited to the mucosa or submucosa, operative results are not satisfactory. Significant improvement in the cure rate of locally advanced gastric cancer has not been achieved by surgery for many years. The 5-year survival rate of patients subjected to curative operation is only about 40%.[8]

One of the reasons for the limited success of gastric cancer surgery is the high incidence of metastasis to the lymph nodes along the left gastric and common hepatic arteries and around the celiac axis.[9,10] Complete elimination of microscopic disease around these blood vessels is difficult to attain with a surgical procedure. The possibility always exists too that microscopic lesions remain in the tumor bed, even after what is believed to be a curative operation.

On the other hand, radiotherapy has not played a major role in the treatment of gastric cancer because adenocarcinoma is relatively radioresistant and high-dose external irradiation to the gastric region can cause intestinal damage. This damage is often a serious limiting factor in the delivery of a complete course of radiation therapy. In intraoperative radiation therapy (IORT), a cancericidal dose can be delivered safely to the unresectable tumor remnants because normal organs, such as the small intestine or liver, can be shifted from the field so that the lesion is exposed directly to radiation. The rationale for IORT is the possibility of sterilizing residual tumors or tumor cells around the celiac axis, which are hard to eliminate by surgical procedures.[11]

II. TECHNIQUES

A. SELECTION OF ELECTRON ENERGY

IORT can be performed best with an electron beam, since the appropriate beam energy can be chosen to produce the desired depth of tissue penetration with sharp fall-off, thereby avoiding the potential problem caused by exposure of normal structures under the tumor. The electron energy is selected so that whole lesion is included by the 90% isodose curve. The dose is measured at the reference depth described in ICR Report No. 35,[12] that is, at 1.0 cm depth from the tissue surface when the electron energy used is less than 10 meV, and 2.0 cm depth when it is more than 10 meV but less than 20 meV.

B. RADIATION DOSE

Of particular importance in IORT is the determination of the optimal cancerocidal dose given in a single irradiation. Based on many experimental and clinical investigations of cellular lethality, it is clear that the dose required to eradicate a tumor depends upon the number of tumor cells, the fraction of hypoxic cells, and their pathologic type.[13] In fractionated irradiation, the hypoxic portion of the tumor decreases after each irradiation, thus making successive irradiation more effective. This is because of improved vascularization following tumor regression and increased availability of oxygen resulting from its reduced consumption by the damaged cells. In single-dose irradiation, however, one cannot utilize this reoxygenation effect. Accordingly, a single dose cannot be extrapolated from a simple time-dose graph, such as Strandqvist curves.[14]

Radiobiology does not, at present, give us the necessary information for determining a reasonable single dose for IORT. The optimal single dose must therefore be estimated from an analysis of clinical results and post-mortem examinations. From the clinical results of

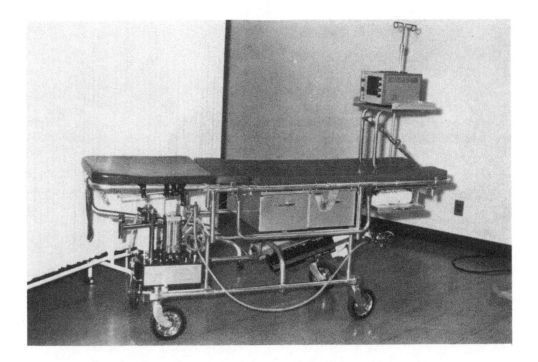

FIGURE 1. A stretcher with a portable anesthesia machine for transportation of patients from an operating theater to a radiation therapy room.

IORT, the biologic effectiveness of a single dose may be estimated to be equivalent to a conventionally fractionated dose 2 to 2.5 times as large. That is, a single dose of 20 Gy given by IORT may be biologically equivalent to a total dose of 40 to 50 Gy given at the usual 1.8 to 2.0 Gy per fraction.[15-17]

For IORT to unresectable lymph node metastases, a single dose of 30 to 35 Gy, increasing with tumor size up to approximately 3 cm in diameter, is considered potentially curative. To eradicate microscopic or clinically undetectable lesions, 28 to 30 Gy may be sufficient.

C. ANESTHESIA

The IORT is performed easily if all surgical procedures can be carried out in a radiation therapy room. When the operating theater is separated from the radiation therapy suite, the abdomen is temporarily closed with nylon stay sutures. The patient is then covered with sterile sheets and transported to the radiation therapy room under general anesthesia. Figure 1 demonstrates a stretcher furnished with a portable anesthesia machine for transportation of patients. During irradiation, the patient is observed by an anesthesiologist outside the radiation therapy room on closed circuit television. Vital signs, including EKG, pulse, and respiration are monitored by television and by a multichannel oscilloscope in the control room.

D. RADIATION FIELD

When IORT is applied during a curative operation, the radiation field is positioned over the lymph node groups around the celiac axis, which most frequently contain metastatic cancer and are difficult to remove surgically. When the posterior wall of the stomach is grossly adherent to the pancreas, this is encompassed by the radiation field also (Figure 2).

The pentagonal stainless steel cones which fit the costal arch and encompass the area stated above are specially made (Figure 3). These cones are of various sizes and shapes to

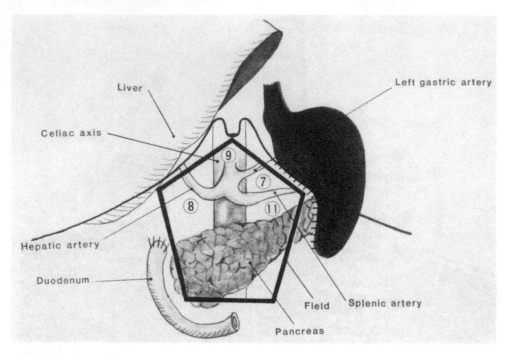

FIGURE 2.   Field for gastric cancer with invasion of the pancreas. The field covers lymph node groups which most frequently contain metastasis and are hard to eliminate by surgery. (7) Lymph nodes along the left gastric artery; (8) lymph nodes along the common hepatic artery; (9) lymph nodes around the celiac artery; and (11) lymph nodes along the splenic artery.

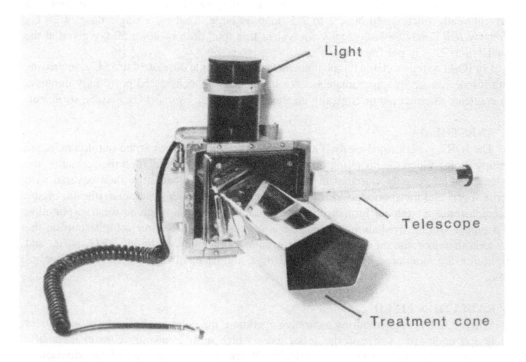

FIGURE 3.   Pentagonal treatment applicator with an electric lamp and telescope to observe the field.

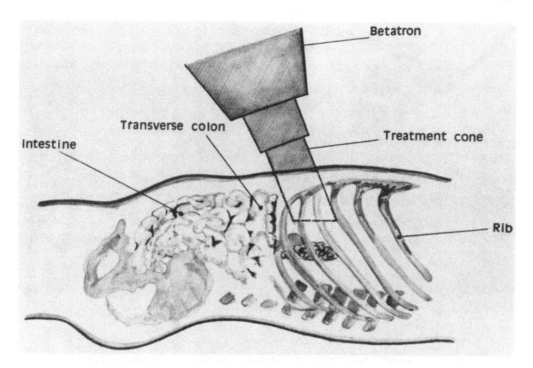

FIGURE 4.   IORT for gastric cancer. A treatment applicator is inserted into the abdominal cavity, inclining about 15° so that the celiac axis is sufficiently covered.

work in various anatomic situations. The field is illuminated by an electric lamp fixed to the telescope. The cone is inserted into the abdomen inclining about 15°, so that the celiac axis is sufficiently covered (Figures 4 and 5).

E. PROCEDURE FROM OPERATION TO IRRADIATION

In an operating theater, gastrectomy is performed and as much tumor tissue as possible is extirpated; this is because larger tumors require higher doses of radiation than smaller ones to produce the same degree of regression. Following tumor regression, the abdomen is temporarily closed and draped in a sterile fashion. The patient is then covered with sterile sheets so he/she can be transported to the radiation therapy room through nonsterile areas. In preparing the radiation therapy room for IORT, special room sterilization may not be necessary. At Kyoto University Hospital, two ultraviolet lamps in the radiation therapy room are turned on during the night.

In the radiation therapy room, the abdomen is reopened and a treatment cone is inserted over the unresectable tumor or sites suspected of containing residual tumor cells before gastroenterostomy, because at this stage the site to be irradiated can be adequately exposed and the organs to be protected pulled outside. The entire small intestine and liver are packed out of the radiation field. The treatment cone and the operation wound are covered by a sterilized sheet to prevent the possibility of any stray material from the machine falling directly into the abdomen. After irradiation, the cone is removed from the abdomen and the gastroenterostomy is made. The abdomen is then closed using standard techniques.

III. STAGING AND RESULTS

A. STAGING FOR GASTRIC CANCER

All patients described in this chapter are classified according to *The General Rules for Gastric Cancer Study in Surgery and Pathology,* issued by the Japanese Research Society

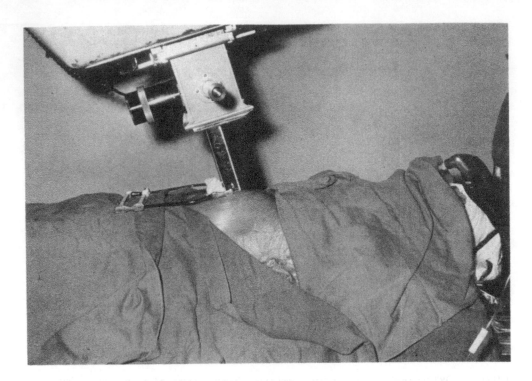

FIGURE 5. Intraoperative electron beam irradiation in gastric cancer under general anesthesia.

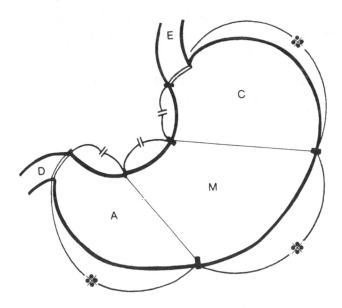

FIGURE 6. Location of gastric cancer (see text).

for Gastric Cancer.[18] The rules have been widely accepted in most medical centers in Japan and international gastric cancer registration with the World Health Organization is also conducted using descriptions based on these rules. The rules are summarized below.

1. Location of Gastric Cancer and Primary Cancer Site

The stomach is separated into the upper, middle, and lower portions by drawing lines between the corresponding trisecting points on the greater and lesser curvatures (Figure 6).

If the lesion extends across these lines, the more extensively involved portion is listed first, followed by the less involved portion(s).

2. Classification of Serosal Invasion Based on Gross Findings

S_0 — no serosal invasion.
S_1 — suspected serosal invasion.
S_2 — definite serosal invasion.
S_3 — invasion of contiguous structures.

3. Classification of Lymph Nodes Based on Gross Findings

The regional lymph nodes of the stomach are designated as shown in Table 1 and Figure 7. The lymph nodes of Groups 1, 2, and 3 are referred to as N_1, N_2, and N_3, respectively. Distant lymph nodes located beyond Group 3 (N_3) are referred to as N_4.

N $(-)$ — no suspected lymph node metastasis.
N_1 $(+)$ — metastasis to lymph nodes of Group 1.
N_1 $(-)$ — no metastasis to lymph nodes of Group 1.
N_2 $(+)$ — metastasis to lymph nodes of Group 2.
N_2 $(-)$ — no metastasis to lymph nodes of Group 2.
N_3 $(+)$ — metastasis to lymph nodes of Group 3.
N_3 $(-)$ — no metastasis to lymph nodes of Group 3.
N_4 $(+)$ — metastasis to lymph nodes located beyond Group 3.
N_4 $(-)$ — no metastasis to lymph node located beyond Group 3.

Use of the designation Group 1, 2, 3 (N_1, N_2, N_3) indicates the anatomical position of the lymph nodes. These designations do not imply that the respective lymph nodes are primary, secondary, or tertiary lymph nodes. For example, lymph nodes 8, 10, and 11 of Groups 2 and 3 are primary regional lymph nodes.

4. Classification of Disseminating Peritoneal Metastases Based on Gross Findings

P_0 — no metastases to the gastric serosa, greater and lesser omentum, mesentery, visceral, and parietal peritoneum, and retroperitoneum.
P_1 — metastases to the adjacent peritoneum (above the transverse colon and including the greater omentum) without metastasis to the distant peritoneum, i.e., the peritoneum below the transverse colon and the abdominal surface of the diaphragm.
P_2 — a few to several scattered metastases to the distant peritoneum. This classification is applicable to cases in which there is only ovarian metastasis.
P_3 — numerous metastases to the distant peritoneum.

5. Classification of Liver Metastasis Based on Gross Findings

H_0 — no liver metastasis.
H_1 — metastasis is limited to one of the lobes.
H_2 — few scattered metastases to both lobes.
H_3 — numerous scattered metastases to both lobes.

6. Stage Grouping of Gastric Cancer

The cancer stage is expressed according to Table 2. The stage to be recorded is that under which there is the highest degree of metastasis or invasion. For example, P_0, H_0, N_3, S_1 is to be recorded as stage IV.

TABLE 1
Grouping and Lymph Node Designations Used in the
Japanese Research Society for Gastric Cancer

	Location			
Group	AMC, MAC MCA, CMA	A, AM	MA, M MC	C, CM
Group 1 (N_1)	1	3	3	1
	2	4	4	2
	3	5	5	3
	4	6	6	4s
	5		1	
	6			
Group 2 (N_2)	7	7	2	4d
	8	8	7	7
	9	9	8	8
	10	1	9	9
	11		10	10
			11	11
				5
				6
Group 3 (N_3)	12	2	12	12
	13	10	13	13
	14	11	14	14
	110	12		110
	111	13		111
		14		

1 — right cardial lymph node.
2 — left cardial lymph node.
3 — lymph node along the lesser curvature.
4 — lymph node along the greater curvature.
4s — (Left group) lymph node along the left gastroepiploic artery and short gastric arteries.
4d — (right group) lymph node along the right gastroepiploic artery.
5 — suprapyloric lymph node.
6 — infrapyloric lymph node.
7 — lymph node along the left gastric artery.
8 — lymph node along the common hepatic artery.
9 — lymph node around the celiac artery.
10 — lymph node at the splenic hilus.
11 — lymph node along the splenic artery.
12 — lymph node in the hepatoduodenal ligament.
13 — lymph node at the posterior aspect of the pancreas.
14 — lymph node at the root of the mesentery.
110 — lower thoracic paraesophageal lymph node.
111 — diaphragmatic lymph node.

B. CLINICAL RESULTS

1. Survival

At the start of investigations at Kyoto University Hospital, patients with no hope of cure because of liver or peritoneal metastases were treated in an effort to determine the effectiveness and safety of IORT. The total number of patients treated was 14, and resections could not be performed since all patients had advanced stage disease. The radiation field for IORT was limited to the primary tumor and regional lymph node metastases in order to alleviate symptoms. A single dose ranging from 18 to 40 Gy was delivered.

The following information was obtained:

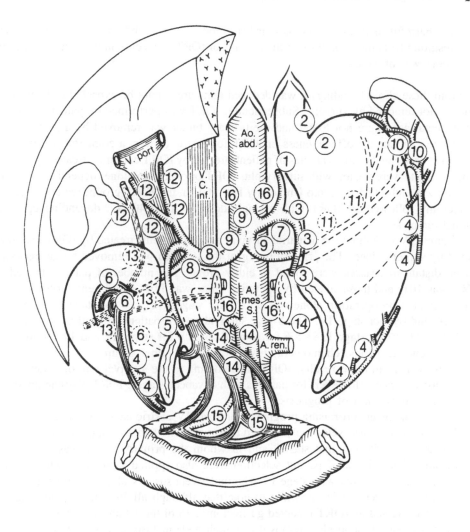

FIGURE 7.   Lymph node designation used in the Japanese Research Society for Gastric Cancer.

TABLE 2
Staging for Gastric Cancer Based on Gross Findings

Stage	Peritoneal metastasis	Liver metastasis	Lymph node metastasis	Serosal invasion
I	P_0	H_0	$N(-)$	S_0
II	P_0	H_0	$N_1(+)$	S_1
III	O_0	H_0	$N_2(+)$	S_2
IV	P_1, P_2, P_3	H_1, H_2, H_3	$N_3(+), N_4(+)$	S_3

1. Marked palliation, such as relief of obstruction of the stomach from a large tumor mass was obtained about 2 weeks after irradiation in patients who received more than 20 Gy. All the patients died. The mean survival time was 6.2 months.

2. Post-mortem examination revealed that a single dose of more than 40 Gy is necessary to erradiate gross gastric cancer, since remaining cancer cells were still sporadically found by histological examination in the radiation field in patients who received 40 Gy. However, it was demonstrated that lymph node metastases which were about 3 cm in diameter were eliminated by a single dose of 35 Gy.

3.   No harmful morbidity, such as diarrhea, bloody stools, abdominal pain or infection resulting from transportation of the patients or IORT procedure in the radiation therapy room was observed.

From these clinical findings it was deduced that cure cannot be expected if the primary tumor is not removed by surgery. Subsequently, IORT was performed on patients in whom distant metastases were not found and the primary tumor was removed by a gastrectomy. In order to evaluate the effectiveness of IORT for gastric cancer, a comparative study was performed between the survival rates of patients treated by IORT and those treated by surgery alone. Patients were treated with surgery plus IORT or operation alone, depending upon the day they were admitted to Kyoto University Hospital. In the IORT group, patients received gastrectomy followed by IORT with a single dose of 20 to 40 Gy, depending upon the residual tumor size.

Figures 8A to D show the actuarial survival rates of patients treated by IORT and those treated by surgery alone. The primary tumor of the stomach was removed by gastrectomy, and no distant metastases were found in either group. The number of patients treated by IORT was 101, and those treated by operation alone was 110. The 5-year survival rate of patients treated by operation alone was 93.0% for stage I, 61.8% for stage II, 36.8% for stage III, and 0% for stage IV. The 5-year survival rate of patients treated by surgery plus IORT was 87.2% for stage I, 83.5% for stage II, 62.3% for stage III, and 14.7% for stage IV. With few exceptions, chemotherapy was not used in either group.

As is clear from these results, IORT adds nothing to the survival rate of patients with stage I gastric cancer. However, for patients with advanced stages, IORT plays an important role in the improvement of prognosis.

The reason for the promising prognosis for stage IV gastric cancer treated by IORT is that this radiotherapy was selectively applied to patients who had no distant metastases, such as liver and/or peritoneal metastases, and in whom the primary tumor was resected by gastrectomy. The criteria of patient selection were also applied to patients who received surgery alone. No patients with stage IV who underwent surgery alone survived more than 2 years after treatment. It is important to note that although all 19 patients with stage IV gastric cancer treated by IORT received gastrectomy, 15 of the 19 underwent a noncurative operation because of incomplete removal of lymph node metastases and/or lesions directly invading the pancreas. The details of three patients who underwent noncurative surgery with incomplete excision of tumors, but who have survived more than 5 years after IORT, are described below.

Case 1 — A 60-year-old female. The primary tumor was located in the gastric antrum and penetrated through the serosa with direct invasion of the pancreas. Metastases were found in the lymph nodes $N_{7,8,11,13}$. The patient was classified as $P_0H_0N_3S_3$, stage IV. The primary tumor was remove by subtotal gastrectomy and a single dose of 30 Gy with 8-meV electrons was delivered through a pentagonal cone which encompassed the invaded part of the pancreas and the unresectable lymph node metastases. The patient has survived with no evidence of disease more than 8 years after treatment.

Case 2 — A 64-year-old male. The primary tumor was found in the M and A portions of the stomach. Metastatic lesions were located around the celiac axis and invaded directly into the liver. The patient was classified as $P_0H_1N_2S_3$, stage IV. The primary tumor as well as the invaded part of the liver was removed, but elimination of metastatic lymph nodes around the celiac axis was incomplete. A single dose of 30 Gy with 8-meV electrons was delivered through a cone which encompassed the residual tumors. The patient is well and free from recurrence more than 7 years after treatment.

Case 3 — A 64-year-old male. The primary tumor was located in the A and M portions of the stomach and invaded the pancreas. Metastases to the lymph nodes $N_{7,8,9,11,13}$ was

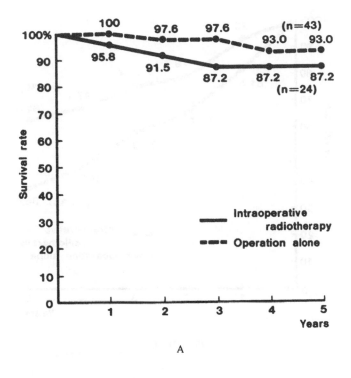

A

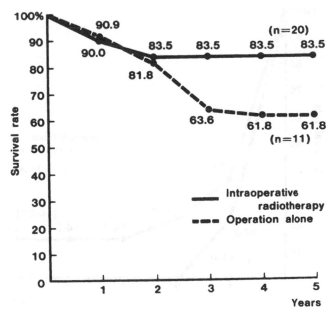

B

FIGURE 8. Actuarial survival curves of gastric cancer patients treated by IORT and those treated by surgery alone. (A) Survival rates of stage I gastric cancer; (B) survival rates of stage II gastric cancer; (C) Survival rates of stage III gastric cancer; and (D) Survival rates of stage IV gastric cancer.

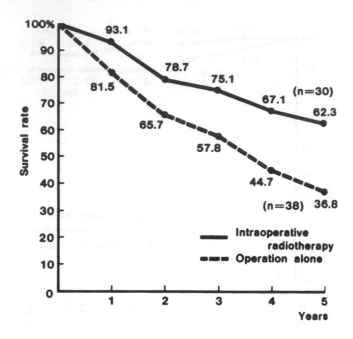

FIGURE 8C.

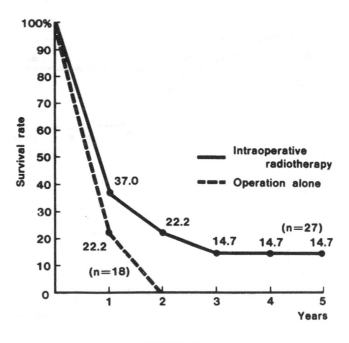

FIGURE 8D.

evident (Figure 9a). The patient was classified as $P_0H_0N_3S_3$, stage IV. The primary tumor was resected by subtotal gastrectomy and a single dose of 35 Gy with 12-meV electrons was delivered to the unresectable lymph node metastases (Figure 9b). The patient has survived more than 8 years after treatment with no evidence of disease.

2. Complications

In IORT of gastric cancer, irradiation of the pancreas cannot be avoided; but less than

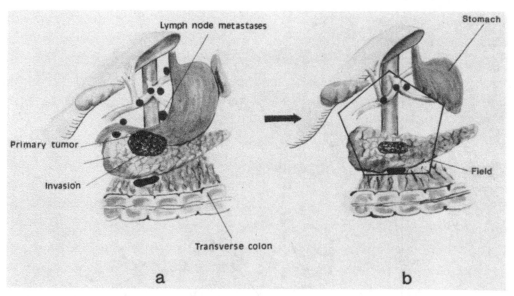

FIGURE 9. A patient with gastric cancer underwent IORT as a result of incomplete removal of neoplasms. (a) The primary tumor located in the gastric antrum penetrated through the serosa with invasion of the pancreas. Lymph node metastases were found mainly around the celiac axis. (b) The primary tumor was removed by subtotal gastrectomy. The invaded part of the pancreas and unresectable lymph node metastases were covered by a pentagonal treatment cone.

40% of the whole pancreas is generally included in the radiation field. Acute and late damage of the pancreas was examined by changes in serum amylase and blood sugar after IORT in 11 patients. Figures 10 and 11 show the changes of serum amylase and blood sugar, respectively. Preirradiation levels of serum amylase and blood sugar were determined and changes in mean values after IORT were plotted as percentages of preirradiation levels. A temporary increase in serum amylase and blood sugar occurred after IORT, but these returned to preirradiation levels within a week. Neither significant late complications, such as diabetes mellitus, nor deviation from the usual postoperative courses was observed. A definite difference from conventional external beam radiotherapy is that almost no patients developed leukopenia following IORT. This is due to the reduced treatment volume. There were no instances of delayed wound healing, and experiences to date with IORT have shown that no complications have occurred as a result of infection.

IV. INDICATIONS

Indications for IORT in gastric cancer are summarized as follows:

1. The primary tumor must be located in the lower two thirds of the stomach. When it is located in the upper third, the left costal arch prevents a treatment cone from covering enough of the regional lymph nodes in the splenic hilum and around the splenic artery.
2. The primary tumor must be resected. If not, large single doses more than 40 Gy and high-energy electrons will be required for tumor control. This will result in a high risk of harmful side effects to the normal structures which cannot be shifted from the field.
3. There must be no distant metastases to the liver or the peritoneum. Since IORT is a local or regional treatment, cure cannot be expected in patients with distant metastasis.
4. All residual lesions must be included within the treatment cone.

Intraoperative electron beam therapy seems quite promising as an adjuvant to partial gastrectomy in the management of selected gastric cancers.

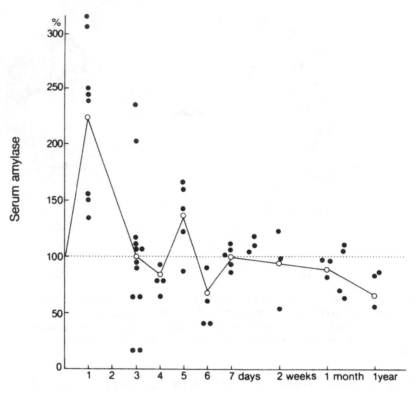

FIGURE 10.   Changes in serum amylase as a function of time after intraoperative irradiation of pancreas.

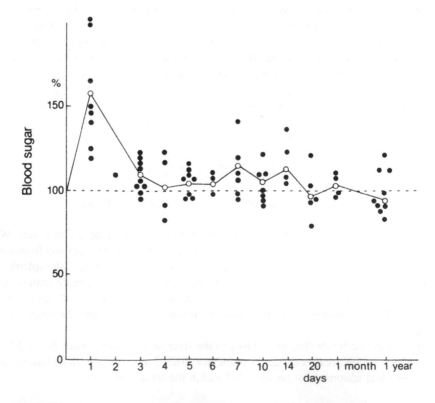

FIGURE 11.   Changes in serum amylase as a function of time after intraoperative irradiation of pancreas.

REFERENCES

1. **McNeer, G., Vandenberg, H., Jr., Donn, F. Y., and Bowden, L.,** A critical evaluation of subtotal gastrectomy for the cure of cancer of the stomach, *Ann. Surg.,* 134, 2, 1951.
2. **Thomson, F. B. and Robins, R. E.,** Local recurrence following subtotal resection for gastric carcinoma, *Surg. Gynecol. Obstet.,* 95, 341, 1952.
3. **Horn, R. C.,** Carcinoma of the stomach: autopsy findings in untreated cases, *Gastroenterology,* 29, 515, 1955.
4. **Fujimaki, M., Soga, J., Wada, K., Tani, H., Aizawa, O., Kawaguchi, M., Ishibashi, K., Maeda, M., Kanai, T., Omori, Y., and Muto, T.,** Total gastrectomy for gastric cancer. Clinical considerations on 431 cases, *Cancer,* 30, 660, 1972.
5. **Gunderson, L. L. and Sosin, H.,** Adenocarcinoma of the stomach. Areas of failure in a reoperation series (second or symptomatic look). Clinicopathologic correlation and implications for adjuvant therapy, *Int. J. Radiat. Oncol. Biol. Phys.,* 8, 1, 1982.
6. **Appleby, L. H.,** The coeliac axis in the expansion of the operation for gastric carcinoma, *Cancer,* 6, 704, 1953.
7. **Gilbertsen, V. A.,** Results of treatment of stomach cancer — an appraisal of efforts for more extensive surgery and a report of 1983 cases, *Cancer,* 23, 1305, 1969.
8. **Maruta, K. and Shida, H.,** Some factors which influence prognosis after surgery for gastric cancer, *Ann. Surg.,* 167, 313, 1968.
9. **Berry, R. E. L. and Rottschafer, W.,** The lymphatic spread of cancer of the stomach observed in operative specimens removed by radical surgery including total pancreatectomy, *Surg. Gynecol. Obstet.,* 104, 269, 1957.
10. **Sunderland, D. A., McNeer, G., Ortega, L. G., and Pearce, L. S.,** The lymphatic spread of gastric cancer, *Cancer,* 6, 987, 1953.
11. **Abe, M., Yabumoto, E., Takahashi, M., Tobe, T., and Mori, K.,** Intraoperative radiotherapy of gastric cancer, *Cancer,* 34, 2034, 1974.
12. Radiation Dosimetry: Electrons with Initial Energies Between 1 and 50 MeV, ICR Rep. No. 35, International Commission on Radiation Units and Measurements, Washington, D.C., 1984.
13. **Nice, C. M. and Kurz, J.,** Relation of the tumor size to radioresistance, *Radiology,* 60, 555, 1957.
14. **Strandqvist, M.,** Studien über die kumulative Wirkung der Röntgenstrahlen bei Fraktionierung, *Acta Radiol. Suppl.,* 55, 1944.
15. **Abe, M., Takahashi, M., Yabumoto, E., Onoyama, Y., Torizuka, K., Tobe, T., and Mori, K.,** Techniques, indications and results of intraoperative radiotherapy of advanced cancers, *Radiology,* 116, 693, 1975.
16. **Abe, M., Takahashi, M., Yabumoto, E., Adachi, H., Yoshii, M., and Mori, K.,** Clinical experiences with intraoperative radiotherapy of locally advanced cancers, *Cancer,* 45, 40, 1980.
17. **Gunderson, L. L., Shipley, W. U., Suit, H. D., Epp, E. R., Nardi, G., Wood, W., Cohen, A. M., Nelson, J., Battit, G., Biggs, P. J., Russell, A., Rockett, A., and Clark, D.,** Intraoperative irradiation. A pilot study combining external beam photons with "boost" dose intraoperative electrons, *Cancer,* 49, 2259, 1982.
18. **Japanese Research Society for Gastric Cancer,** The general rules for gastric cancer in surgery and pathology, *Jpn. J. Surg.,* 11, 127, 1981.

Chapter 17

INTRAOPERATIVE RADIATION THERAPY FOR PANCREATIC CANCER IN JAPAN

Takehisa Hiraoka, Ikuo Nakamura, Seiki Tashiro, and Yoshimasa Miyauchi

TABLE OF CONTENTS

I. INTRODUCTION

Despite recent advances in diagnostic and surgical techniques, the results of treatment for carcinoma of the pancreas are discouraging. Because tumors are not found early, pancreatectomy is possible in only 20% to 30% of the patients at presentation, and even if radical resection for pancreatic carcinoma is performed, local recurrence is very often found at autopsy. Since 1970, we have applied intraoperative radiation therapy (IORT) for patients in the advanced stages of pancreatic cancer, and since 1976, we have been combining IORT with resection for patients with pancreatic cancer. Our results for cancer of the pancreas are presented in this chapter.

II. IORT FOR UNRESECTABLE PANCREATIC CANCER

A. MATERIALS AND METHODS
1. Patient and Tumor Characteristics

From January 1969 to March 1986, we saw 153 patients with cancer of the pancreas at our clinic. The cases in which resection could be performed accounted for only 51 of the 153 patients. We have applied IORT to 30 out of 102 patients in the advanced stages of pancreatic cancer when no resection was performed (Table 1). There were 30 patients (13 women and 17 men) with a mean age of 57.4 years (range: 43 to 78) treated with IORT for unresectable cancer of the pancreas. Of the 30 patients, 18 underwent surgical bypass procedures with IORT. During this time interval, IORT was not applied to 40 other patients with unresectable tumors. The selection criteria for patients to be eligible for inclusion in this study were (1) biopsy-proven adenocarcinoma of the pancreas, (2) a localized unresectable tumor that could be included in a high-dose intraoperative "boost" volume, (3) no distant metastatic disease (except metastases to the liver), and (4) no contraindications to a surgical exploration.

The primary tumor was located in the head of the pancreas in 10 patients, in the body and tail of the pancreas in 19 patients, and in the entire pancreas of the remaining patient; 10 patients presented with jaundice and 26 with pain. All 30 patients had evidence of extrapancreatic spread on surgical evaluation, and all had lymph node metastases. A total of 16 had direct invasion of the retroperitoneal soft tissues, including the portal vein, and 10 had liver metastases. The surgical criteria for unresectability were fixation to major vessels (16), extrapancreatic tumor extension (13), and medically unfit (1). In these 30 patients, the largest tumor diameter was between 6 and 10 cm. There were 11 patients who received adjunctive chemotherapy with 5-fluorouracil and mitomycin C following IORT. Neither intravenous hyperalimentation nor elemental diet were applied in the postoperative course.

2. Electron Beam IORT Technique

Under general anesthesia, the pancreatic tumor was exposed and a needle or incisional biopsy performed to obtain an histological confirmation of the diagnosis. The extent of the tumor and its local spread were defined. This required taking down the gastrocolic omentum, reflecting the stomach superiorly, and performing a Kocher maneuver. When the tumor was situated at the head or body of the pancreas, gastrectomy by means of the Billroth II method was carried out to facilitate adequate exposure of the tumor, as well as to reroute the alimentary tract. Biliary diversion procedures were also done if necessary. In our clinic, patients in the operating room were then transferred to a cleaned radiation room. Remote physiological monitoring was carried out during irradiation. The electron beam was delivered from a linear accelerator. After the adjacent normal tissues and organs were displaced outside of the planned radiation field, an applicator from the linear accelerator was placed on the

TABLE 1
Patients with Cancer of the Pancreas

site of lesion	number of patients	number of resections	operative procedure			no resection
			pancreato-duodenectomy	distal pancreatectomy	total pancreatectomy	
Head	90	40(44.4%)	32(15)	0	8	50(10)
Body & Tail	57	10(17.5%)	0	8(1)	2(1)	47(19)
Entire pancreas	6	1(16.7%)	0	0	1(1)	5(1)
Total	153	51(33.3%)	32(15)	8(1)	11(2)	102(30)

( ) number of patients with intraoperative radiation
from January 1966 to March 1986

surface of the lesions. The energy of the electron beam was selected on the basis of the thickness of the tumor. The energy ranged from 10 to 18 meV. The range of radiation dose was from 25 to 40 Gy.

B. RESULTS
1. Patient Survival

All 30 patients who underwent IORT died. Of the 30, 26 died of cancer, 3 died due to treatment complications, and 1 died of another disease. The postoperative survival times of these patients ranged from 1 to 15.4 months. The mean survival of all the patients was 4.8 ± 3.4 months. The mean survival was 3.4 ± 1.9 months in cancer of the head of the pancreas and 5.6 ± 3.8 months in cancer of the body and tail. The survival time of the one case with cancer of the entire pancreas was 3.5 months. In spite of palliative benefits, the survival time of patients treated with IORT was not prolonged compared to that of patients without IORT. The survival results of patients with liver metastases were especially poor (Table 2).

In the case of one patient who had a tumor of the pancreatic body and tail and received 40 Gy with 40-meV electrons, stenosis due to invasion of the common hepatic artery and superior mesenteric vein was shown to be improved on an angiogram taken 1 month after IORT, at a second operation total pancreatectomy was performed. As the tumor could not be completely removed, a second dose of IORT was delivered to the remaining tumor. This patient died of idiopathic perforation of the ileum 10 months after the second operation.

2. Palliative Benefits

The most obvious merit of IORT in cancer of the pancreas is the alleviation of pain. Of the 20 patients who complained of abdominal and/or back pain and whose treatment was not combined with celiac ganglion block, 16 patients (80%) experienced pain relief within 4 weeks of irradiation. These patients showed subjective improvements lasting from 3 weeks up to 8 months, and a distinctly remarkable effect was found in patients with cancer of the body and/or tail of the pancreas. However, in the late stages of the progress of the cancer, all of these patients had recurrent pain.

A decrease in size of the tumor was found in most cases, this being evaluated by palpation, CT, and/or autopsy (Figure 1).

TABLE 2
Effects of IORT on Unresectable Pancreatic Cancer

Clinical Site Effect of Lesion	Survival Time after IORT			Relief of Pain	Decrease in Tumor Size	Side Effect
	mean value	with liver meta	without liver meta			
Head 10 cases	3.4 ± 1.9 months	2.0 m.	4.4 m.	5 / 7 (3)	5 / 6 (4)	3 / 10
Body & Tail 19 cases	5.6 ± 3.8 months	3.2 m.	6.9 m.	11 / 13 (6)	12 / 14 (5)	1 / 19
Entire 1 case	3.5 months	3.5 m.		(1)	(1)	0 / 1
Total 30 cases	4.8 ± 3.4 months	2.8 m.	6.1 m.	16 / 20 80.0 %	17 / 20 85.0%	4 / 30 13.3%

( ): Unevaluable case   March, 1986

On the angiogram of two cases, both with cancer of the body and tail of the pancreas, stenosis of the splenic artery was significantly improved after the radiation treatment with a dose of 40 Gy with 12-meV electrons for periods of 1 and 5 months, respectively (Figure 2).

3. Treatment Complications

There have been neither anesthetic complicatios nor perioperative wound infections in these patients. Of the 16 patients given IORT doses of less than 40 Gy, 5 patients had treatment complications, 4 had intestinal bleeding, and 1 developed a fistula. Intestinal bleeding developed 12 to 30 d after the treatment. In all four cases, infiltration of the cancer was found in the duodenum. Three of the four patients died of complications due to the intestinal bleeding. A fistula developed 23 d after IORT in a patient who had a tumor in the pancreatic head and received 30 Gy with 10-meV electrons. The fistula persisted during her terminal hospital admission. Autopsy disclosed that radiation necrosis of the tumor was followed by abscess formation.

In the cases of 14 patients with IORT doses of 40 Gy, 3 patients had radiation treatment complications; stricture of the jejunum occurred in 1 patient, diarrhea in another, and serious anorexia occurred in 2 patients. Stricture of the jejunum developed 1.5 months after accidental bowel irradiation during IORT in a patient who had a tumor in the pancreatic body. Consequently, a jejunostomy was performed. In this case, before the IORT procedure was started, we believed that we had verified that the jejunum was fully excluded from the irradiation field. However, at the end of the IORT procedure, it was confirmed that a part of the jejunum had been included within the field.

In a few cases, transient slight elevations of fasting blood sugar and serum amylase levels were observed subsequent to the treatment; but they returned to their normal range within a few days. In a few cases, glucose tolerance tests performed 1 month after treatment showed improvement.

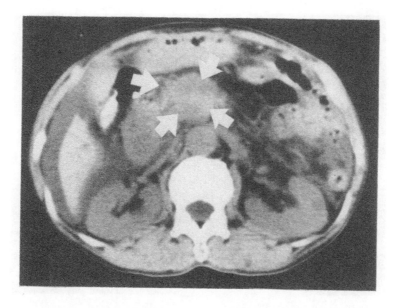

A

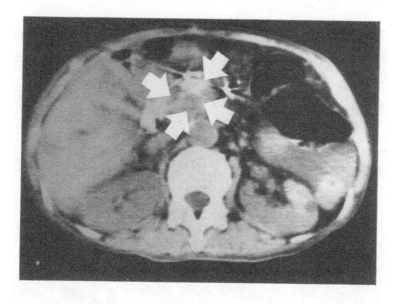

B

FIGURE 1. Computed tomogram of 72-year-old man with cancer of the body of the pancreas. (A) Before IORT; (B) 4 months after IORT (30 Gy, 18 meV, 8 × 5 cm).

4. Pathological Findings

Post-mortem examinations were performed on 11 of the 30 patients and compared with those of nonirradiated patients. The size of the tumor in 9 of the 11 patients had become smaller that it was before irradiation. In all 11 patients, microscopic examination showed cancerous tissues completely replaced by connective tissues in wide areas of the central portions of the tumor, to which a dose of 30 Gy had been administered. However, there were a few recognizable tumor cells in the superficial and deep portions of the tumor. The

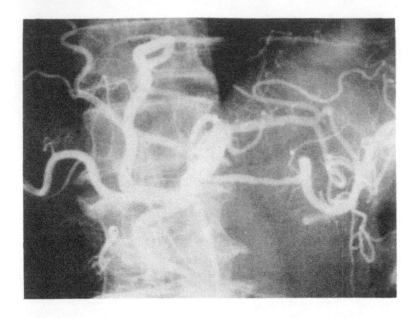

A

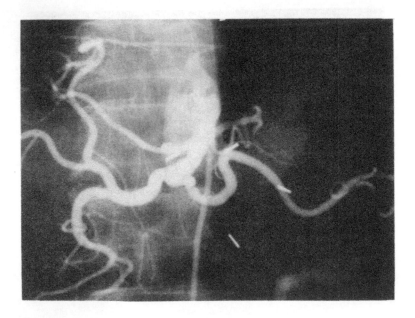

B

FIGURE 2.   Angiogram of 63-year-old man with cancer of the body and tail of the pancreas. (A) Before IORT; (B) 5 months after IORT (40 Gy, 12 meV, 8 cm 0).

extent of damage to the tumor cells caused by the irradiation corresponded well with the distribution of the radiation dose. In one case, in which a fistula developed 23 d after IORT, massive radiation necrosis was followed by abscess formation sharply delimited from the nonirradiated area.

As for the effect of IORT on normal tissue at the periphery of the irradiated area, it usually caused destruction and marked atrophy of the glandular cells in pancreatic parenchyma. Interstitial fibrosis was seen in parts of the atrophied glandular tissue, and glandular tissues were replaced by connective tissues. The islet tissue remained normal in the irradiated field. Fibrous thickening of the walls of arteries in the irradiated field resulted in luminal narrowing of the blood vessels.

No remarkable changes were detected in the neighboring organs, such as the liver, kidney, stomach, or aorta, except for the jejunum irradiated accidentally in the one case.

III. IORT COMBINED WITH RESECTION FOR PANCREATIC CANCER

Based on our clinical expeiences with IORT for unresectable pancreatic cancer, in 1976 we began combining resection with IORT as an adjunctive therapeutic procedure to prevent local recurrence.

A. MATERIALS AND METHODS
1. Patient and Tumor Characteristics

From January 1969 to March 1986, resection was performed on 51 patients about 34% of the cases in this report. Of the 51 cases, 40 underwent resection for cancer of the head of the pancreas; 32 of these patients underwent pancreatoduodenectomy, and 8 underwent total pancreatectomy with extended dissection of the lymph nodes. Studies on the patients with cancer of the head of the pancreas are presented in this chapter.

Of the 32 patients who underwent pancreatoduodenectomy, 15 also had IORT; 11 (7 women and 4 men) of the 15 patients, with a mean age of 63.8 years (range 51 to 72), were irradiated following pancreatoduodenectomy with 30 Gy (electron beams) to the operative field; this included the celiac axis and the superior mesenteric artery (standard IORT group). Of this 11, 7 patients underwent "curative" resection and 4 of the 15 patients (1 woman and 3 men), with a mean age of 54.5 years (range 37 to 68), were irradiated with 30 Gy to a more extended operative field including the para-aortic area from the diaphragm above to the inferior mesenteric artery below (extended IORT group). Out of these four patients, three underwent "curative" resection and one underwent noncurative resection.

Of the 32 patients, 17 (5 women and 12 men), with a mean age of 57.5 years (range 50 to 77), were treated by pancreatoduodenectomy alone. Of these patients, 13 underwent "curative" resection and 4 underwent noncurative resection. Almost all of these patients underwent resection before 1976.

The effect of IORT on the surgical treatment of cancer of the head of the pancreas was evaluated by comparing the two groups with combined pancreatoduodenectomy and IORT to the group with pancreatoduodenectomy alone.

Pancreatic cancer was classified from stage I to III, according to the Vermont Tumor Registry system: stage I, tumor apparently localized in the pancreas; stage II, local extension of the tumor to the regional lymph nodes; and stage III, distant metastases.[1]

2. Electron Beam IORT Combined with Pancreatoduodenectomy

The method of IORT was as follows: in 11 patients (standard IORT group), resection of the pancreatic lesion and dissection of the lymph nodes around the celiac axis and superior mesenteric artery were performed. Then a dose of 30 Gy of 8-meV electrons from a linear accelerator was administered to the operative field, including the celiac axis and superior mesenteric artery, using a 6- to 8-cm circular applicator.[2] In four patients (extended IORT group), a dose of 30 Gy of 9-meV electrons was administered to the operative field, including the para-aortic area from the diaphragm above to the inferior mesenteric artery below, using a special applicator (Figure 3). For expansion of the IORT portal, we made a special applicator which we could vary in size according to the patient's body size to irradiate around the aorta

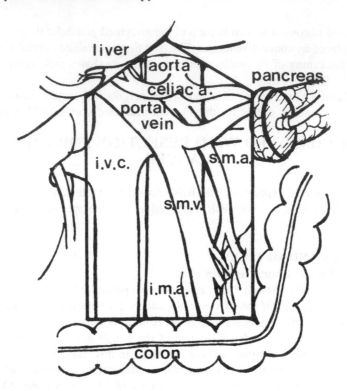

FIGURE 3.   The pentagon indicates the borders of the radiation field.

from the diaphragm above to the inferior mesenteric artery below. This applicator is metallic and pentagonal, 6 cm in width by 10 to 18 cm in length. The field to be irradiated could be confirmed by observation through the window at the side of the adaptor of the applicator.

Isodose curves for the electron beams are shown in Figure 4. The pancreatic remnant and the bile duct were kept outside of the irradiation field. The electron beam can be sharply focused and concentrated within a depth of approximately 5 cm from the surface, thus minimizing unnecessary exposure to adjacent normal tissue. A sterilizing, cancericidal dose can be administered to the target volume with sharp limitation. Patients were anesthetized with either epidural anesthesia or endotracheal anesthesia with nitrous oxide and oxygen.

B. RESULTS
1. Patient Survival

Of the 32 patients with pancreatoduodenectomy, there were 4 operative deaths for a 14% mortality rate due to failure of the pancreaticojejunostomy. None were in the combined therapy group. One patient in the pancreatoduodenectomy-only group died of another disease 2.2 months after operation. There were no postoperative complications due to IORT in the combined therapy group. In the combined therapy group for cancer of the distal common bile duct or papilla of Vater, there weren't any complications in the postoperative course for more than 5 years.

At present, two patients with extended IORT are still alive without evidence of the disease 17 and 25 months postreatment, respectively. A total of 25 patients died of recurrence of cancer within 25 months, regardless of having IORT or not. The remaining case with extended IORT died of sepsis 8 months postoperatively. As shown in Figure 5, the cumulative survival rate of the seven patients who were treated by radical pancreatoduodenectomy and standard IORT was compared to that of the eight patients with radical pancreatoduodenectomy. It showed a markedly higher survival rate, 75% at 1 year in the combined therapy

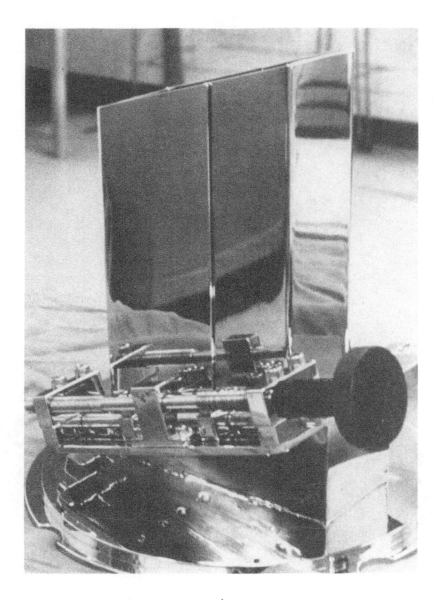

A

FIGURE 4. (A) Variable applicator and its isodose curve. (B) 6 × 10 cm, 18 meV; (C) 6 × 18 cm, 18 meV.

group, but did not show any difference between the two groups at 2 years. Additionally, there was no difference between the cumulative survival rates of the three patients with and the two groups without standard IORT after palliative pancreatoduodenectomy. Regarding survival time related to therapy and to state of disease, in 16 patients with the radical operation, in the stage II group, a significant (p <0.01) prolongation of the mean survival time was found in the combined therapy group.[2] Of the four patients who underwent extended IORT, two are still alive. One of the other two patients died of recurrence (peritoneal seeding) 11 months postoperatively. The remaining one had a nutrition disorder during the postoperative course and died of sepsis 8 months posttreatment.

2. Pathological Findings

Autopsies of the four patients who underwent only pancreatoduodenectomy showed

FIGURE 4B.

FIGURE 4C.

recurrence in the pancreatic remnant in one patient and liver metastases in three patients. All the patients, in spite of dissection of the lymph nodes, showed involvement of the lymph nodes along the mesenteric artery, and celiac axis, and around the aorta. The autopsies of the three patients who underwent pancreatoduodenectomy combined with standard IORT showed recurrence in the pancreatic remnant in one patient. All the patients showed liver metastases and involvement of the lymph nodes around the aorta, outside of the radiation field. Two patients showed involvement of lymph nodes in the mesentery of the jejunum. Involvement of the lymph nodes and local recurrence were seldom found within the radiation field for 5.2 to 21 months after combined therapy; but recurrences were found outside the radiation field. Post-mortem examination of the two patients who underwent pancreato-

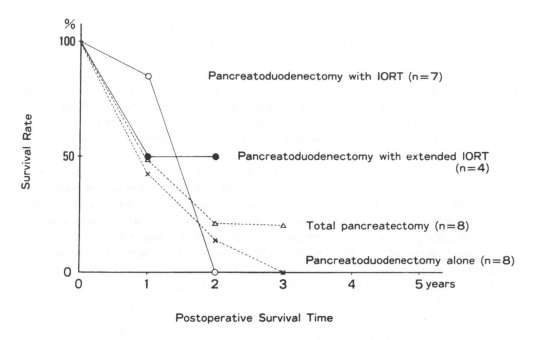

FIGURE 5. Cumulative survival rate of patients with radical resection for cancer of the head of the pancreas.

duodenectomy combined with extended IORT showed peritoneal seeding in one patient, but no recurrence within the radiation field. There was no recurrence in the other patient.

On the other hand, the autopsies of two patients who underwent total pancreatectomy with almost complete dissection of the involved lymph nodes around the mesenteric arteries, the celiac axis, and the aorta, without any IORT, showed local recurrence around the celiac axis, the superior mesenteric artery, and the aorta from the diaphragm to the inferior mesenteric artery in one patient and recurrence at the mesentery of the jejunum in the other.

VI. DISCUSSION

If direct irradiation can be applied to advanced pancreas cancer while sparing the normal tissues as much as possible, some clinical benefits can be expected. In our series with IORT for unresectable pancreatic cancer, prolongation of survival was not observed; but palliation effects, such as relief of pain, decrease in tumor size, and improvement in the general condition due to the remarkable local effect on macroscopic and microscopic lesions were obtained. Such palliative effects are generally recognized, as reported in a collective review by Abe.[3]

Duodenal ulceration must be expected in IORT for patients with cancer of the head of the pancreas. In our series, intestinal bleeding developed 12 to 30 d after IORT in four patients in whom infiltration of the cancer was found in the duodenum. Therefore, it was not clear that the intestinal bleeding was due to radiation. However, when the duodenum is included within the radiation field and high doses of more than 30 Gy are used, gastrectomy by the Billroth II method might be advisable. We saw stricture of the jejunum due to accidental irradiation in one case. Our study with dogs showed that a dose of 30 Gy always caused ulceration of the jejunum. The jejunum should always be kept outside the radiation field. A fistula developed 23 d after IORT in one case. This was due to the formation of abscesses following rapid radiation necrosis of the tumor. On the other hand, this suggests a remarkable anticancer effect of IORT.

Autopsy of patients who underwent IORT for resectable pancreatic cancer showed remarkable local anticancer effects. In the central portion of the tumor, subjected to the peak absorbed dose of 25 to 40 Gy with 10- to 18-meV electrons, cancerous tissues were almost completely replaced by connective tissues. This may indicate that the dose of 30 Gy is suitable as a cancericidal dose.

Many patients with unresectable pancreatic cancer will fail outside the primary treatment area, even if that area is sterilized. Thus, it may be unfortunately necessary to approach patients having pancreatic cancer with palliation as the primary objective. We thought that if combined with radical operations, such as pancreatoduodenectomy, IORT might be of help in improving results. Therefore, we have had only three cases with IORT for unresectable pancreatic cancer since 1976.

The prognosis for patients with resectable pancreatic cancer has consistently been poor, offering at best only the expectations of modest prolongation of survival or temporary palliation of symptoms. There is not much agreement among surgeons as to the proper therapeutic approach for this type of cancer. Total pancreatectomy[4,5] and regional pancreatectomy, including resection and reconstruction of the portal vein and/or superior mesenteric artery,[6] were suggested recently, but there still remain many problems in evaluating the results of these operations.[7-10]

The results of pancreatoduodenectomy for pancreatic cancer have been unsatisfactory.[11] One of the reasons for these disappointing results, as noticed from autopsy findings, is local recurrence around the celiac axis and the mesenteric vessels. In this case, involved lymph nodes and single cancer cells or cancer cell aggregates cannot always be removed by the surgical procedure alone. Therefore, as the first step, we have applied IORT to the celiac axis and mesenteric region following pancreatoduodenectomy. However, remarkable prolongation of survival in patients with pancreatic cancer did not result from this combined therapy, in spite of the local effects of IORT. We found that no in-field local recurrences developed in the areas where IORT was administered, but recurrences developed outside the radiation field. This represents a significant step forward in designing treatment strategies for pancreatic cancer. As a next step, we expanded the IORT portal from the 6- to 8-cm circular applicator utilized initially to a larger radiation field, encompassing the area from the diaphragm to the level of the inferior mesenteric artery. A special variable applicator was made to irradiate around such areas according to the body size.

On the other hand, during the same time, we performed extended operations with almost complete dissection of the lymph nodes around the mesenteric vessels, celiac axis, and aorta, from the diaphragm to the level of the inferior mesenteric artery, without IORT. However, such extended surgery resulted in nutritional disturbances with diarrhea and fatty liver and did not improve survival time. Autopsy of a patient who underwent such extended operation showed local recurrence of cancer around the aorta from the celiac axis to the level of the inferior mesenteric artery. This suggests that clearance of the involved lymph nodes, single cancer cells, or cancer cell aggregates in such areas is impossible by surgery alone.

At present, we have followed four patients who underwent extended IORT after pancreatoduodenectomy. Two patients are still alive and free from the disease 17 and 25 months postoperatively. Autopsy in the remaining two cases showed no recurrence in one case. The other case showed no in-field local recurrence, but peritoneal seeding of the tumor was evident. Expansion of the IORT portal resulted in improvement of local control rates. These preliminary observations suggest that aggressive radiotherapy may play a beneficial role in the treatment of pancreatic cancer.

It is unrealistic to believe that surgery and radiation will cure large numbers of patients with pancreatic cancer. However, stepwise evaluations of the therapeutic modalities may have considerable merit. If the strategy of combined surgery and irradiation does improve local control, then the next logical step in the sequence of therapeutic attack on pancreatic cancer would be the addition of systemic chemoimmunotherapeutic adjuvants in the hopes of controlling disseminated disease that results in the eventual demise of the vast majority of patients with pancreatic malignancy.

No treatment complications were noticed postoperatively in patients who underwent standard IORT or extended IOKT following pancreatoduodenectomy. However, when irradiation is given over a more extended field, some consideration should be given to the low tolerance of the ureter to a dose of 30 Gy, as indicated by Sindelar et al.[12]

The present study was not randomized for the purpose of studying the influence of IORT on the survival rate of the resections for cure of pancreatic cancer, and so far, reaching conclusions cannot be drawn. However, the material might yet give valuable information as the groups are comparable and suitable for statistical analysis. To obtain potentially unbiased information on the utility of IORT as an adjuvant to the surgical resection of pancreatic cancer, a prospective randomized trial would have to be undertaken with a large number of patients.

Based on our clinical experience and the added benefits from expanding the IORT portal, we were encouraged to continue this approach, after resection, for the cure of pancreatic cancer and the control of local recurrence.

REFERENCES

1. **Leadbetter, A., Foster, R. S., and Haines, C. R.,** Carcinoma of the pancreas. Results from the Vermont Tumor Registry, *Am. J. Surg.,* 129, 356, 1975.
2. **Hiraoka, T., Watanabe, E., Mochinaga, M., Tashiro, S., Miyauchi, Y., Nakamura, I., and Yoko-yama, I.,** Intraoperative irradiation combined with radical resection for cancer of the head of the pancreas, *World J. Surg.,* 8, 766, 1984.
3. **Abe, M. and Takahashi, M.,** Intraoperative radiotherapy: the Japanese experience, *Int. J. Radiat. Oncol. Biol. Phys.,* 7, 863, 1981.
4. **Pliam, M. D. and ReMine, W. H.,** Further evaluation of total pancreatectomy, *Arch. Surg.,* 110, 506, 1975.
5. **Ihse, I., Lilja, P., Arnesjö, B., and Bengmark, S.,** Total pancreatectomy for cancer, *Ann. Surg.,* 186, 675, 1977.
6. **Fortner, J. G., Kim, D. K., Cubilla, A., Turnbull, A., Pahnke, L., and Shill, M. E.,** Regional pancreatectomy: en bloc pancreatic, portal vein and lymph node resection, *Ann. Surg.,* 186, 42, 1977.
7. **Cooperman, A. M., Herter, F. P., Marboe, C. A., Helmreich, Z. V., and Perzin, K. H.,** Pancreatoduodenal resection and total pancreatectomy: an institutional review, *Surgery,* 90, 707, 1981.
8. **Longmire, W. P., Jr.,** Cancer of the pancreas: palliative operation, Whipple procedure, or total pancreatectomy, *World J. Surg.,* 8, 872, 1984.
9. **Heerden, J. A.,** Pancreatic resection for carcinoma of the pancreas: Whipple versus total pancreatectomy — an institutional perspective, *World J. Surg.,* 8, 880, 1984.
10. **Moossa, A. R., Scott, M. H., and Lavelle-Jones, M.,** The place of total and extended total pancreatectomy in pancreatic cancer, *World J. Surg.,* 8, 895, 1984.
11. **Mongé, J. J., Judd, E. S., and Gage, R. P.,** Radical pancreatoduodenectomy: a 22-year experience with complications, mortality rate and survival rate, *Ann. Surg.,* 160, 711, 1964.
12. **Sindelar, S. F., Tepper, J., Travis, E. L., and Terill, R.,** Tolerance of retroperitoneal structures to intraoperative radiation, *Ann. Surg.,* 196, 601, 1982.

Chapter 18

INTRAOPERATIVE RADIATION THERAPY IN COMBINATION WITH COMPUTER-CONTROLLED CONFORMATION RADIOTHERAPY FOR PANCREATIC CANCER

Tadayoshi Matsuda and Yoshiaki Tanaka

TABLE OF CONTENTS

I. INTRODUCTION

Pancreatic cancer is not generally considered an indication for radiation therapy and is hardly ever dealt with in radiation therapy textbooks.[1] The reason for this is that pancreatic cancer, a somewhat radioresistant tumor, is surrounded by radiosensitive organs, such as the stomach, small intestine, liver, kidney, and spinal cord.[2] Pancreatic cancer is seldom excisable, even with the most advanced surgical techniques, and even if resected, the prognosis is not satisfactory.[3-5] Recently a new method of radiation therapy for this disease has been developed, primarily in the U.S., and the preconception regarding the optimum method of treatment is now changing.[2]

In Japan, we have developed a method of intraoperative radiation therapy (IORT) combined with conformation therapy. It is becoming evident that this is an effective treatment for pancreatic cancer.[6] This report describes our clinical experience with this new modality.

II. IORT FOR PANCREATIC CANCER

A. RADIATION THERAPY APPARATUS

We use a Shimadzu 20-meV betatron (Figure 1) for IORT. This machine generates high-energy electron beams with a selection of nine energy levels from 4 to 20 meV. The electron beam output is high and stable. For example, 1-min output levels for a treatment applicator of 1 cm in diameter are: 4 meV, 4.4 Gy; 6 meV, 4 Gy; 8 meV, 6.5 Gy; 10 meV, 8.5 Gy; 14 meV, 9.5 Gy; 16 meV, 11 Gy; 18 meV, 14 Gy; and 20 meV, 17 Gy. The high output electron beam enables IORT to be completed in a short time. Treatment applicators of several sizes and shapes were manufactured, and the percentage depth-dose curves were drawn for each. Figure 2 shows the depth-dose curves for the 5-cm-diameter applicator for the energy range 4 to 20 meV. The depths for 90% attenuation are: 4 meV, 1.1 cm; 6 meV, 1.5 cm; 8 meV, 2.0 cm; 10 meV, 2.6 cm; 13 meV, 3.3 cm; 14 meV, 3.6 cm; 16 meV, 3.8 cm; 18 meV, 4.4 cm; and 20 meV, 4.6 cm. Depth-dose curves are provided for each treatment applicator.

B. TRANSPORTATION OF THE PATIENT

The operating room is located on the first below ground floor, the betatron room on the third below ground floor. Preparation for IORT is made in the operating room, and then the patient is transported to the betatron room. In surgery, the patient and mattress are tranferred to the stretcher. This stretcher was designed and manufactured on the basis of a 5-year clinical study; it is almost free from vibration while in motion. Fine adjustments of vertical and horizontal movements and rotation are possible when the stretcher is placed under the irradiation port of the betatron (Figure 3). After IORT, the patient is returned to surgery for anastomoses or any other necessary procedures.

The times required for IORT and the stay in the betatron room were recorded for 75 cases during the past 3 years (Table 1). Only 30 min or less were needed for 65 cases, or

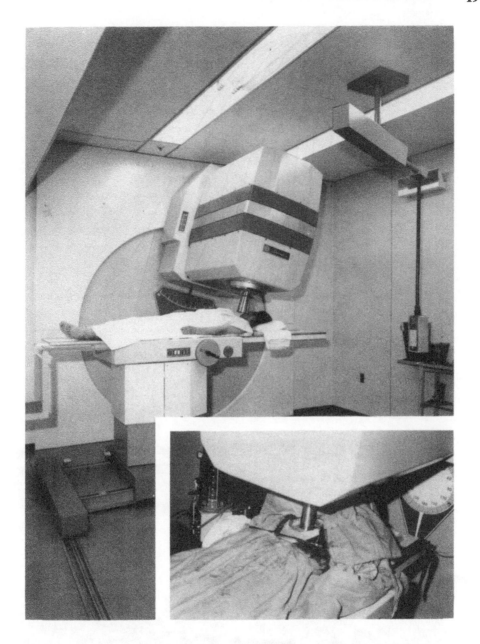

FIGURE 1. Shimadzu 20-meV betatron. (Inset) Actual view of IORT for pancreatic cancer.

87%; 40 min or longer were required for 3 cases of rectal cancer because of the considerable time taken to insert and set the applicator precisely into the pelvis; 51 min were required for 1 case of urinary bladder cancer (for a 25-min treatment of 4 meV, 30 Gy with the 3-cm-diameter applicator) because the urine was drained during surgery; 25 to 60 minutes are required for a patient to leave the operating room, move to the betatron room, and return to surgery after IORT. Surgeons, radiotherapists, anesthetists, and nurses form a 9- to 11-member team. In our experience, 178 sessions of IORT have been performed without any problems.

C. CASES OF IORT

We performed IORT 170 times from August 1975 through March 1985. The cases were classified as follows: 59 cases of brain tumor, 54 cases of pancreatic cancer, 26 cases of

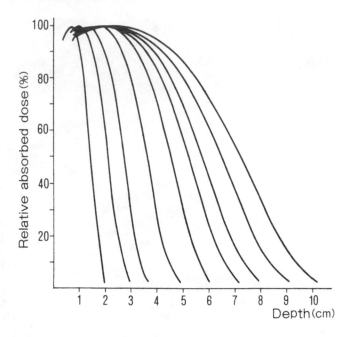

FIGURE 2.   Depth dose curves for electron beams from 4 to 20 meV.

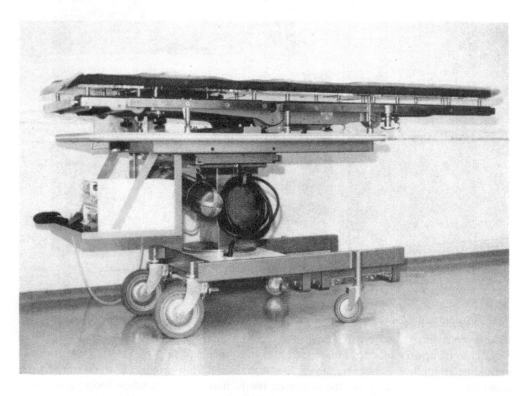

FIGURE 3.   Stretcher modified for patient transport and IORT.

bile duct cancer, 8 cases of head and neck cancer, 7 cases of metastasis of esophageal cancer into abdominal lymph nodes, 5 cases of rectal cancer, 4 cases of urinary bladder cancer, 3 cases of uterus cancer, a 4 other cases (Table 2). This report describes the 54 cases of pancreatic cancer.

TABLE 1
Patient Time in Radiotherapy Room

	10 to 19 min	20 to 29 min	30 to 39 min	40 to 49 min	50 to 59 min	Total
Brain tumor	13	19	3			35
Pancreatic cancer	8	11				19
Esophageal cancer	1	5	1			7
Bile duct cancer	2	3	1			6
Rectal cancer		2		3		5
Others	24	1	1		1	3
Total		41	6	3	1	75

Note: From operating room to betatron room, 5 to 7 min; stay in betatron room, 10 to 40 min; and from betatron room to operating room, 6 to 9 min.

TABLE 2
Number of Cases of IORT from August 1975 Through January 1985

Brain tumors	59 (5)[a]
Pancreatic cancer	54 (2)[a]
Bile duct cancer	26
Head and neck cancer	8
Esophageal cancer[b]	7
Rectal cancer	5
Urinary bladder cancer	4
Uterine cancer	3
Others	4
Total	170 (7)[a]

TABLE 3
IORT of Pancreatic Cancer Patient Age and Sex

Age (years)	Sex		Total
	Male	Female	
40 to 49	6	1	7
50 to 59	12	8	20
60 to 69	9	7	16
70 to 79	3	6	9
80 to 89	1	1	2
Total	31	23	54

[a] Number of cases indicated in parentheses are multiple irradiation.
[b] Metastasis of esophageal cancer to abdominal lymph nodes.

D. CASES OF PANCREATIC CANCER TREATED BY IORT

The 54 cases comprised 31 males and 23 females. The ages ranged from 44 to 86 years. The 50 to 59 age group held the largest percentage, 37%, or 20 cases; followed by the 60 to 69 age group which represented 16 cases (30%) (Table 3). On the basis of findings during surgery, the location and stage of the cancer were classified according to the American Joint Committee for Cancer Staging 1981,[7] as shown in Table 4. There were 28 cases (52%) of cancer of the pancreatic head, 11 cases (20%) of cancer of the pancreatic head and body, 5 cases of cancer of the pancreatic body, and 9 cases of cancer of the pancreatic tail. Stage classifications were 4 cases (8%) of stage I, 11 cases (20%) of stage II, 28 cases (52%) of stage III, and 11 cases (20%) of stage IV. Three cases of stage I were given preventive irradiation after duodenopancreatectomy. Of the 11 cases in stage IV, 7 were given palliative treatment in the first 3-year period. Currently, stage IV cases are excluded from consideration for IORT.

The cases of pancreatic cancer treated by IORT have been classified according to stage and into three 3-year periods (Table 5). In the early and middle periods, IORT was applied to stage IV cases where metastasis was found in the liver or Virchow's node, and so on. This had palliative effects, but did not prolong life. Therefore, stage IV cases were excluded in the later period of our clinical experience.

TABLE 4
Site and Stage, Pancreatic Cancer

	Stage I $T_1T_2N_0M_0$	Stage II $T_3N_0M_0$	Stage III $T_{1-3}N_1M_0$	Stage IV $T_{1-3}N_{0-1}M_1$	Total
Head	4	9	15		28
Head-body		1	6	4	11
Body		1	2	2	5
Body-tail			4	5	9
Head-tail			1		1
Total	4	11	28	11	54

TABLE 5
Number of Cases of IORT for Cancer of the Pancreas

	Number of cases	Stage				Number of cases of adjuvant IORT
		I	II	III	IV	
Early period, 1976 to 1979	17		2	8	7	
Middle period, 1979 to 1982	18	3	6	6	3	2
Later period, 1982 to 1985	19	1	3	14	1	4
Total	54	4	11	28	11	6

After pancreatectomy, six cases were treated by IORT. These included five cases of duodenopancreatectomy and one case of total pancreatectomy.

E. DETERMINATION OF IORT FACTORS FOR PANCREATIC CANCER
1. Selection of Applicators

A total of 56 treatments of IORT were performed in 54 cases of pancreatic cancer. The applicator sizes and electron beam energies varied widely with the shape and size of the lesion (Table 6). In five cases, applicators of 4 cm diameter or less, and in five cases, applicators of 10 cm or larger were utilized in our first 3-year period. This was due to our lack of experience in selection of patients and treatment factors; 47 times (or 84%), applicators ranging in diameter from 5 to 8 cm were used.

2. Electron Beam Energy

Energies were selected from the range of 10 to 20 meV; 18 and 20 meV were most frequently used (Table 6). In three of the four cases utilizing 10-meV, duodenopancreatectomy was performed and IORT was used as an adjuvant.

3. Radiation Dose

In most cases, either 20 or 30 Gy was selected. The dose was classified according to three 3-year periods; early, middle, and late (Table 7). The dose of 30 Gy was dominant in the early period, and 20 Gy in the late period, with less dominance noticed in the middle period. This trend is due to our experience that IORT sometimes results in ulceration of the duodenum and stomach. When the duodenum is located within the irradiation field, the dose was limited to 20 Gy. When the dueodenum, stomach, and jejunum are completely located outside the radiation field, and the pancreatic body and tail are irradiated, the dose was 30 Gy. In five cases where doses of 15 and 18 Gy were employed, treatment was delivered to invasive tumors around great vessels after duodenopancreatectomy, or a part of the pyloric antrum was located within the radiation field. The two listed as 40 Gy were actually two treatments, each 20 Gy, with intervals of less than a month.

TABLE 6
Electron Beam Energy and Electron Applicator Size and Shape

Electron energy (meV)	3 × 4 cm ellipse	4 cm circle	5 cm circle	6 cm circle	4 × 8 cm rectangle	6 × 8 cm rectangle	6 × 10 cm rectangle	5 cm pentagon	7 cm circle	8 cm circle	10 cm circle	7 × 12 cm rectangle	12 × 12 cm square	Total
10				2		1		1						4
12		2	2	2										6
14	1	1		3	1						1			7
16				1				2		1				4
18				7						2				9
20		1	1	2		2	3		1	12	2	1	1	26
Total	1	4	3	17	1	3	3	3	1	15	3	1	1	56

Note: Two cases were double counted for IORT (see text).

TABLE 7
Radiation Dose

Duration	Number of IORT	15 Gy	18 Gy	20 Gy	25 Gy	30 Gy	35 Gy	40 Gy
1976.4 to 1979.3	17	1		3		10	1	2
1979.4 to 1982.3	18			9	3	6		
1982.4 to 1985.3	19		4	12	1	2	1	
Total	54	1	4	24	4	18	2	2

TABLE 8
Dose Data in Other 14 Medical Facilities for 94 Cases as of July 1979

Dose	10 Gy	15 Gy	20 Gy	25 Gy	28 Gy	30 Gy	35 Gy	40 Gy
No. of cases	1	1	10	25	3	40	3	11

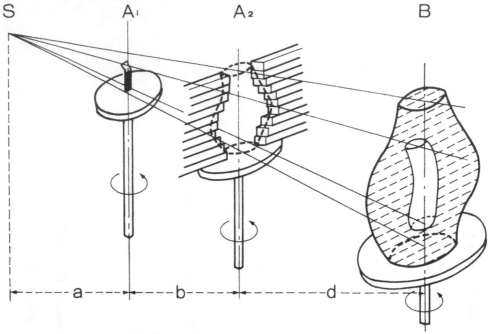

FIGURE 4.   Principle of conformation radiotherapy (I).

The radiation dose data as of July 1979 have been tabulated with respect to 14 medical facilities in Japan where IORT is performed[6] (Table 8). There, 54 cases (or 57%), received doses of 30 Gy or higher, which is much higher than in our proposed protocol.

III. CONFORMATION RADIOTHERAPY FOR PANCREATIC CANCER

A. PRINCIPLES OF CONFORMATION RADIOTHERAPY
Conformation radiotherapy is rotation radiotherapy coordinated with a mechanism for changing the collimator opening to collimate the radiation beam according to the three-dimensional shape and size of the tumor. The principle of conformation radiotherapy is illustrated by Figure 4 and also explained in the textbook by Takahashi, a pioneer in the development of this technique.[8]

In Figure 4, rotating disks, A2 and B, rotate in the same direction at identical speed. The radiation source, S, is located on a line which connects the two rotation axes. A multileaf collimator is on the rotation disk A2. While the disk is rotating, each leaf of the collimator opens or closes independently. Thereby the beam is brought to a shape which is analogous to the contour of the collimator opening. This is called the beam focus. Two opposing leaves of the collimator collimate the beam so that it may strike the target. The contour of the lesion is drawn by the margin of the beam. During a 360° rotation, the opening and closing of the collimator results in a beam collimation which forms a shape analogous to the lesion (Figure 5). This collimation is done at other cross-sections, and it is possible to obtain a beam shape which conforms to the geometrical shape of the lesion. For example, the CT outline of cancer of the pancreatic head was used to form a beam focus which looks like an oval with a 6-cm major axis and a 4-cm minor axis. The direction of the long axis is inclined to form an angle of 60° against the median line of the body (Figure 6). Figure 7 is a beam focus radiograph taken using this method of computer-controlled conformation radiotherapy. This radiograph shows that the radiation is well concentrated to the target volume. A beam focus of any shape and inclination can be formed for any desired position in the body. This is possible only by conformation radiotherapy.

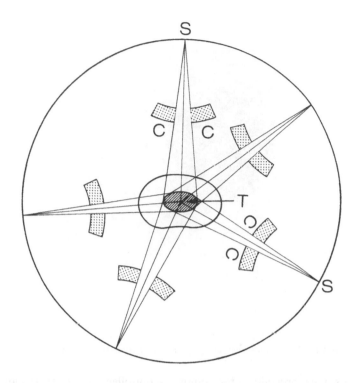

FIGURE 5. Principle of conformation radiotherapy (II). (S) Beam source; (C) collimator; (T) target volume.

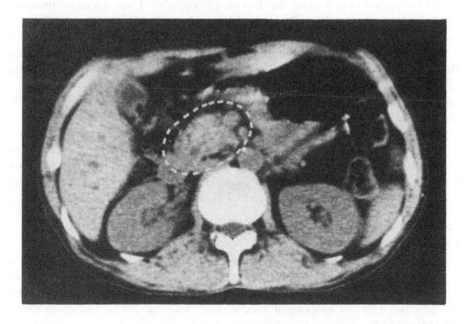

FIGURE 6. CT image of pancreatic cancer.

B. COMPUTER-CONTROLLED CONFORMATION RADIOTHERAPY

We have developed and constructed a computer-controlled conformation radiotherapy apparatus for the first time in the world.[9-11] The multiple-leaf collimator consists of five pairs of tungsten leaves. It is mounted to the X-ray head of a 4-meV linear accelerator for clinical use (Figure 8).

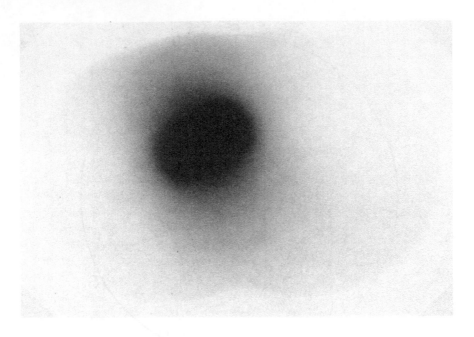

FIGURE 7.   Beam focus radiograph taken by conformation radiotherapy.

The mechanism and procedures for computer-controlled conformation radiotherapy are as follows: Figure 9 is a block diagram of the apparatus. Five CT image slices are used to select the radiation field for each slice. This is input to a computer which calculates radiation parameters for each slice and stores the data on a floppy disk. Once a rotation treatment by the linear accelerator starts, the collimator leaves are driven by signals from the floppy disk, opening or closing every 1° of rotation. After rotation is completed, the opening and closing movements of the collimator are recorded for comparision with the planned parameters.

The features of computer application to conformation radiotherapy founded on fundamental study and a 390-case clinical experience of this method are as follows: (1) it is very easy to plan and prepare for conformation radiotherapy, (2) automatic control by computer is accurate, and conformation radiotherapy can be made as planned, (3) when a treatment-planning computer is used, it is possible to select treatment parameters most suited to each case, (4) CT finding can clearly define the position, size, and shape of the lesion and are therefore very useful for planning and execution of conformation radiotherapy, and (5) application of the computer and CT scanner contributes to expanded use and popularization of conformation radiotherapy.

C. FEATURES OF THE CLINICAL APPLICATION OF CONFORMATION RADIATION THERAPY

Since treatment was started by a computer-controlled conformation radiotherapy apparatus, 390 cases have been treated over a 7-year period. They are classified as follows: 126 cases (32%) of brain tumor, 60 cases (15%) of uterine cancer, 53 cases (14%) of prostatic cancer, 14 cases (4%) of esophageal cancer, and small number of malignant tumors in various regions of the body.

In conformation radiotherapy, healthy tissues are protected, as the radiation beam is concentrated to the lesion, thus decreasing the injury of normal tissues.[8] This is the most important advantage of conformation radiotherapy.

The purposes of conformation radiotherapy are to protect normal tissues, to provide the highest possible dose to the target lesion, and to improve the local control rates. The treatment results of lung cancer, prostatic cancer, and esophageal cancer are available.[12]

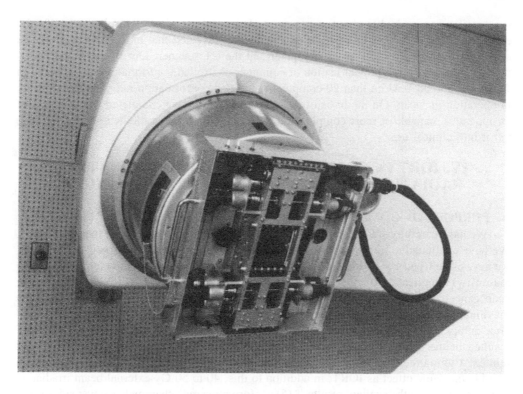

FIGURE 8. Multileaf collimator (mounted on irradiation port of linear accelerator).

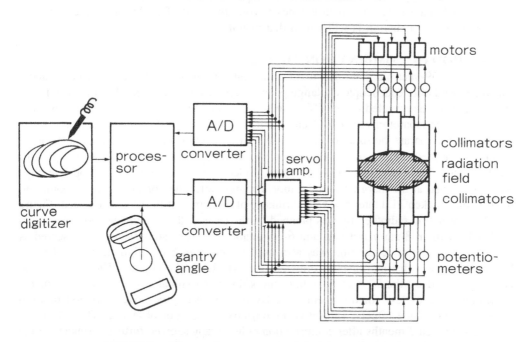

FIGURE 9. Diagram of computer-controlled conformation radiotherapy.

D. ADOPTION OF COMPUTER-CONTROLLED CONFORMATION RADIATION THERAPY

Despite the fact that conformation radiotherapy is an ideal method of treatment, it is not yet popular. The reasons include apparent difficulty of treatment planning and execution for specific cases, doubts about accuracy, and the lack of clinical results to justify the efficacy of this method.[13] Our 7-year experience has revealed that most of these problems are resolved by application of the computer and the CT scanner. Our research and development have motivated popularization of computer-controlled conformation radiotherapy in Japan and abroad.[14] More than 20 computer-controlled conformation radiotherapy units are in operation in Japan. On the basis of past experience, we have completed a new design of an apparatus, capable of more complex and precise conformation radiotherapy, and we have put it into clinical use.

IV. IORT IN COMBINATION WITH CONFORMATION RADIATION THERAPY FOR PANCREATIC CANCER

A. PURPOSE OF COMBINATION

We have carefully studied each case of IORT for pancreatic cancer over the past 9 years. We have continued to improve in order to attain a higher efficacy of treatment. As a result, we have established a combination of IORT with conformation radiotherapy for the following reasons: (1) application of IORT alone does not prolong survival, (2) IORT of pancreatic head cancer often includes the duodenum in the irradiation field; in our experience, the maximum allowable dose to the duodenum is 20 Gy, (3) we studied pathological findings after autopsy of pancreatic cancer treated by IORT and found that 20 to 30 Gy of IORT resulted in the destruction of cancerous cells, but there were also many cells which still remained uninjured,[15] (4) 120 Gy interstitial irradiation by ^{125}I seeds was carried out to provide the same effect as IORT; in addition to this, 40 to 50 Gy external beam irradiation was carried out, with excellent results,[16] (5) conformation radiotherapy has fewer side effects than opposing two-port irradiation, and (6) postoperative irradiation is combined with IORT to cover malignant invasion which extends beyond the field of IORT; therefore, the field of postoperative irradiation is wider than that of IORT.

B. METHOD OF COMBINATION THERAPY

Case 1: a 59-year-old male. His main complaint was jaundice. A pancreatic head cancer was diagnosed after endoscopic cholangiopancreatography and angiography. Localized pancreatic cancer was revealed by the CT images at 90 and 100 mm below the xiphoid process (Figure 10). At laparotomy, a 4 × 4-cm tumor was palpated in the pancreatic head. It was impossible to separate the superior mesenteric arteries and veins from the lesion, so excision was not attempted. Intraoperative irradiation was applied with the 5-cm-diameter applicator on the tumor. The dose was 30 Gy of 14-meV electrons. After IORT, radio-opaque clips were positioned at the margins of the tumor. Progress after the operation was smooth, and the CT image taken 31 d later revealed shrinkage of the tumor of the pancreatic head (Figure 11). Conformation radiotherapy was planned on the basis of this CT image. We selected an oval field with an 8-cm major axis and 6-cm minor axis. The radio-opaque clips served as a guide. A simulator X-ray film was also used to select an 8-cm high field of radiation. Figure 12 is a dose distribution chart drawn by the THERAC-III computer. The target volume is encompassed by the 90% isodose line; the kidney and spinal cord receive 30% of the maximum dose or less. In this method, 2 Gy/fraction was given over a period of 21 d totaling 30 Gy. Side effects, subjective or objective, were not observed. The CT image (Figure 13) taken 2 months after conformation radiotherapy showed further shrinkage of the tumor.

C. COMBINATION METHOD

Postoperative irradiation was applied to 30 of 54 cases of pancreatic cancer which had received IORT. The frequency of combined postoperative irradiation follows: 3 cases out

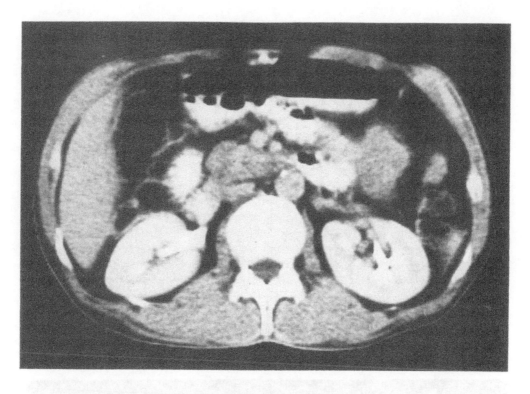

FIGURE 10. CT image of Case 1 before treatment.

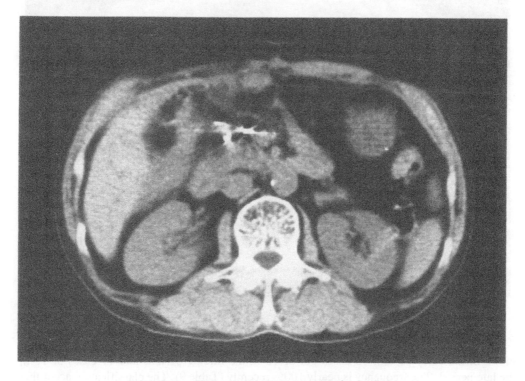

FIGURE 11. CT image after 30 Gy intraoperative irradiation.

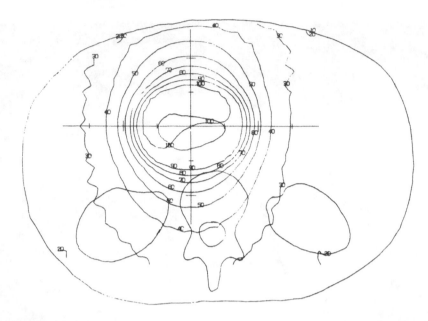

FIGURE 12. Dose distribution of conformation radiotherapy. Planned on CT outline of tumor as shown in Figure 11 and plotted by THERAC-III.

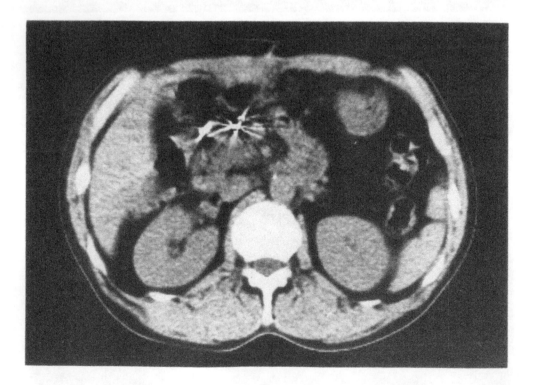

FIGURE 13. CT image 2 months after 30-Gy conformation radiotherapy.

of 17 in the early period, 10 cases out of 18 in the middle period, and 17 cases of 19 in the late period. The frequency is nearly 100% recently (Table 9). The classification according to stage is 2 cases of stage I, 7 cases of stage II, 18 cases of stage III, and 3 cases of stage IV. The three cases of stage IV were exceptional. In the late period, we had four cases of the combined application of IORT and postoperative radiotherapy after duodenopancreatectomy or total pancreatectomy. We had two cases which received duodenopancreatectomy and IORT alone, and both resulted in recurrence and death within 1 year. Therefore, our treatment protocol recommends the addition of conformation radiotherapy to pancreatectomy and IORT.

The radiation field should be selected very carefully for external beam radiation therapy after IORT. Radio-opaque clips are inserted during surgery. The patient is X-rayed in the operation posture, and the clips shown on simulation films will serve as a guide. The radiation position and volume are decided after considering the CT images before and after surgery, surgical findings, anatomical drawing of the pancreatic lymph nodes, and so on. The radiation area on a cross-section was set to be 1 cm larger than the target volume. In 70% of cases there was metastasis to lymph nodes. In order to cover these, the treated volume was made larger in the longitudinal direction of the body. There were 17 cases of postoperative irradiation classified as follows in terms of the length of longitudinal direction: 8 cm for four cases, 9 cm for four cases, 10 cm for seven cases, and 11 and 12 cm for one case each. The postoperative irradiation was classified into 6 cases of two-opposed field irradiation and 24 cases of conformation radiotherapy. In terms of radiation dose, they were classified as follows: 30 Gy or less for 3 cases, 30 to 39 Gy for 5 cases, 40 to 49 Gy for 16 cases, 50 to 59 Gy for 5 cases, and 60 Gy for 1 case. During the 9-year period, 40 or 50 Gy conformation irradiation was most frequent; this is our present protocol (Table 9).

D. RESULTS OF TREATMENT

1. Pain Relief

The remarkable palliative effect of IORT on pancreatic cancer has been pointed out by many researchers.[15,17] We have treated 48 cases of pancreatic cancer which were too advanced to be excised. Of these cases, 16 had serious pain requiring 3 doses of analgesic per day and another 16 cases had moderate pain requiring 1 or 2 doses per day. The pain disappeared in 24 cases, or 86%, of the 28 patients (Table 10). In four cases the palliative effect could not be estimated because death occurred within 1 month of the surgical operation. This result is favorable compared with other reports of palliation of pain resulting from radiotherapy of pancreatic cancer[18-21] (Table 11). The relationship between pain relief and the radiation dose is not clear (Table 10).

2. Side Effects Accompanying Combination Method

IORT was applied to pancreatic cancers which could not be excised. Several of these patients suffered radiation sickness. These were assessed according to the severity of their radiation sickness.

Out of the six cases of the two-opposed field irradiation, the severity of radiation sickness was mild in two cases and severe in four. Two patients complained of severe sickness, and radiation was interrupted when the dose reached 9 Gy (Table 12). Out of 24 cases of conformation radiotherapy, sickness was absent in 7 cases, mild in 8 cases, moderate in 6, and severe in 3. In 15 cases, representing 67% of the 24, radiation sickness was absent or mild. Side effects were much less than with two-opposed field irradiation. One patient treated with 12 Gy irradiation transferred his care to another hospital of his own volition (Table 12).

3. Results of Clinical Laboratory Tests

Periodic tests of blood, liver function, and renal function were made for those cases which had been treated by a combination of IORT and postoperative irradiation. There were no adverse findings.[6]

4. Complications

The most frequent complication of the combination of IORT and postoperative radiation

TABLE 9
Cases of Pancreatic Cancer Treated with Combination of IORT and Postoperative Irradiation (RTx)

Time period	Number of patients treated with		RTx technique		Dose (Gy)					Number of patients that survived more than 1 year
	IORT	Postop RTx	Fixed	Conformation	<30	30—39	40—49	50—59	60	
1976 to 1979	17	3	3		1		1		1	2 (12%)
1979 to 1982	18	10	1	9	2	4	4			3 (16%)
1982 to 1985	19	17	2	15		1	11	5		8 (42%)
Total	54	30	6	24	3	5	16	5	1	13 (24%)

TABLE 10
Pain Relief by IORT: Pancreatic Cancer

Severity of pain	Number of cases	Effect of IORT on pain			Radiation dose producing complete pain relief (Gy)				
		Complete relief	No change	Difficult to decide	15	20	25	30	35
Severe	16	10	3	3	—	5	1	3	1
Moderate	16	14	1	1	1	8	2	3	—
Total	32	24	4	4	1	13	3	6	1

TABLE 11
Pain Relief After Radiation Therapy for
Pancreatic Cancer

Treatment	Authors	Pain relief
Telecobalt + 5FU	Haslam[19]	Good, 45 %
		Fair, 24 %
PHD technique, 45-meV betatron	Dobelbower[20]	10/13, 77%
125I implant + external beam irradiation	Hilaris[21]	25/27, 93%
IORT	Matsuda	24/28, 86%

TABLE 12
Incidence of Radiation Sickness: Pancreatic Cancer

IORT plus two-opposed field irradiation (6 cases)		IORT plus conformation irradiation (24 cases)	
IORT dose (Gy)	Two-opposed field dose (Gy)	IORT dose (Gy)	Conformation irradiation dose (Gy)
15 (1)[a]	9 (2)	18 (3)	12 (1)
18 (1)	32 (1)	20 (16)	30 (4)
20 (3)	40 (2)	25 (1)	40 (14)
30 (1)	60 (1)	30 (3)	50 (5)
		35 (1)	

Radiation Sickness			
Moderate	2 cases	None	7 cases
Severe	4 cases	Mild	8 cases
		Moderate	6 cases
		Severe	3 cases

[a]   Numbers in parentheses represent number of cases.

therapy of pancreatic cancer is injury to the superior parts of the digestive tract. In 54 patients with pancreatic cancer treated by IORT, there were 3 cases of duodenal ulcer and 2 cases of stomach ulcer. Ulcers were not found in 30 cases treated by a combination of IORT and postoperative irradiation. It is not certain whether the IORT is directly related to stomach ulceration. Duodenal ulcer was found in 3 cases 1.5, 10, and 13 months, respectively, after IORT. This was confirmed by endoscopic and X-ray examination (Table 13). All three cases were pancreatic head cancer. The 20-Gy dose was given in two cases, and the 30-Gy dose in one case. When the duodenum is located in the radiation field, we consider that the dose should be limited to a 20-Gy maximum. Decreasing the dose given via IORT and increasing the number of treatments of postoperative irradiation seems to contribute to a decreased possibility of ulcer formation.

E. PROGNOSIS AND SURVIVAL RATE

The actuarial survival rate for the 54 cases of pancreatic cancer treated by IORT was calculated at the end of July 1985 and is shown in Figure 14. All of the 24 patients treated by IORT alone died within 15 months; the average survival period being 3 months. In contrast, 13 patients or, 43%, of 30 patients treated by a combination of IORT and post-operative radiation therapy survived beyond 1 year; the average survival period being 11

TABLE 13

Bleeding in the Digestive Tract After IORT for Pancreatic Cancer

Case	Site of tumor	Conditions of irradiation	Time of bleeding	Degree of bleeding	Confirmation of lesion
Age 47, male	Head	5 cm, 12 meV, 20 Gy	After 10 months	Small amount	Confirmed duodenal ulcer by endoscope and X-ray exam
Age 66, male	Head	4 cm, 12 meV, 30 Gy	After 10 d	Large amount	Confirmed ulcer by endoscope
Age 57, male	Head	8 cm, 20 meV, 30 Gy	After 18 d	Small amount	Confirmed ulcer by autopsy
Age 59, male	Head	4 cm, 12 meV, 30 Gy	After 13 months	Small amount	Confirmed duodenal ulcer by endoscope and X-ray exam
Age 56, male	Uncus	8 cm, 12 meV, 20 Gy	After 1.5 months	Small amount	Confirmed duodenal ulcer by endoscope and X-ray exam

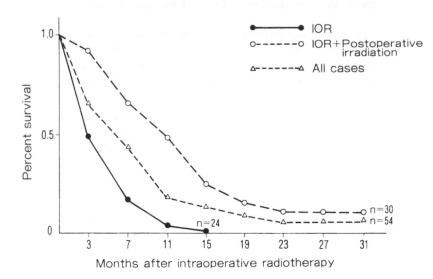

FIGURE 14.   Comparison of actuarial survival of 24 patients with pancreatic cancer treated by IORT only and survival of 30 patients treated by combination IORT and conformation radiotherapy.

months. Compared with the use of IORT alone, the survival rate is obviously longer. The median survival time for the cases treated by IORT was 3.2, 6.2 and 11.2 months, respectively, for the cases treated in the early, middle, and late periods (Figure 15).

Survivorship beyond 1 year for patients treated by combined therapy increased in each successive period (Table 9). The main reason for the improvement are proper selection of indications for treatment and an increase in the dose administered by postoperative irradiation. All 11 stage IV cases died within 6 months, and 3 cases treated by combined irradiation died within 4 months. When the pancreatic cancer had evidently metastasized to the liver, IORT did not prolong survival. The longest patient survival observed in our experience was 4 years and 3 months after IORT. In this case, a large tumor 10 × 8 × 8 cm, was found extending from the pancreatic body to its tail; 20 Gy IORT and 41 Gy external irradiation were applied, and systematic chemotherapy was also used over a prolonged period.

New radiotherapeutic methods for treating pancreatic cancer have been developed, and the clinical results of the typical methods are tabulated[16,22-25] (Table 14). The median survival is around 12 months, although generalization is not necessarily justifiable due to the difference in stage composition of the cases.

TABLE 14
Survival of Patients with Localized Pancreatic Carcinoma

Institution	Year	Therapeutics	Number of patients	Median survival (months)	Ref.
Massachusetts General Hospital	1980	^{125}I implant external beam irradiation	12	11	16
Thomas Jefferson University	1981	45-meV betatron PHD technique	48	10	22
		^{125}I implant + PHD technique	18	12	
Lawrence Berkeley Laboratory	1982	Helium and heavy ions	94	10	23
Massachusetts General Hospital	1982	IORT + external beam irradiation	11	15	24,25
Tokyo Metropolitan Komagome Hospital	1985	IORT + external beam irradiation	30	11	

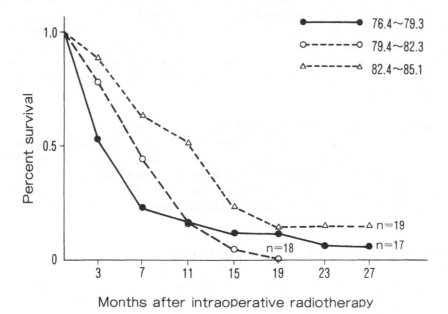

FIGURE 15.   Comparison of actuarial survival of the cases treated in the early, middle, and late periods.

A combination of IORT and conformation external beam radiotherapy was just as successful as other developed modalities for pancreatic cancer (Table 9 and Figure 15).

In our experience, the yearly clinical results have been more satisfactory due to the improvement of this combination method (Figure 14), and future development is expected (Table 9).

V. SUMMARY AND DISCUSSION

The high-energy electron beam IORT method developed in Japan[26,27] finds its best indications in pancreatic cancer. It is being performed in many facilities.[17] Reports concerning pancreatic cancer treated by IORT state that it produced remarkable pain relief (Table 10), but does not lengthen survival. On the other hand, the computer-controlled conformation radiotherapy pioneered by us seems the ideal method of external beam irradiation because it concentrates the radiation beam on the tumor, and healthy tissues surrounding the organ are protected.[9,10,12] Our 9 years of research have established the protocol for IORT combined with conformation radiotherapy. The details follow.

A. ESTABLISHMENT OF INDICATIONS

In the first half of this series, stage IV pancreatic cancer was also treated by IORT for the purpose of palliation, but improved survival was not observed.[6] Therefore, stage IV pancreatic cancer was excluded in the latter half of this series (Table 5). Intraoperative and conformation radiotherapy were applied after noncurative surgery for pancreatic cancer. In other words, the indication for this combined radiation therapy is pancreatic cancer of stage I through stage III. Out of 19 cases treated by IORT during the last 3 years, 17 received conformation external beam radiotherapy.

B. ESTABLISHMENT OF TREATMENT PROTOCOL

The irradiation conditions were established almost completely. When the duodenum and stomach fell within the radiation field, the dose was limited to 20 Gy. When they were outside the field, the dose was increased to 30 Gy. The dose by conformation radiotherapy was 40 to 50 Gy. Wood et al.[24] reported the longest median survival so far using IORT for pancreatic cancer. Their technique is a combination of 15 to 18 Gy IORT and 45.67 Gy mean total external beam irradiation. The target volume of conformation irradiation was more extensive than that of IORT. The length of the field should be sufficient to cover the regional lymph nodes.

C. MINIMIZING SIDE EFFECTS AND COMPLICATIONS

Radiation sickness is less severe in conformation radiotherapy than in two-opposed field irradiation, so an adequate dose can be given (Table 12). By decreasing the dose of IORT and increasing the dose of conformation radiotherapy, stomach and duodenal ulcers were prevented. Side effects are most frequent in postoperative irradiation of the superior abdominal area. For such cases, the computer-controlled conformation radiotherapy is most effective.

D. IMPROVEMENT OF TREATMENT RESULTS

The median survival time of the 24 cases of pancreatic cancer treated by IORT alone was only 3 months. In contrast, the median survival time of the 30 cases of pancreatic cancer treated by combined radiation therapy was 11 months. Furthermore, the survival period of the cases treated by combined radiotherapy increased in the latter period (Table 9). It is suggested that the effect of combined radiation therapy is significant and that the improvement of the treatment protocol contributes to better clinical results.

In recent years, new therapeutic methods for pancreatic cancer have been developed, mainly in the U.S., with excellent results.[5] They are the Precision High Dose (PHD) technique by Dobelbower et al.,[20,22,28] [125]I implant combined with external irradiation by Shipley et al.,[16,21] and the treatment with heavy charged particles by Castro et al.[23,29,30] These have been as effective as surgery. Our results are comparable to theirs (Table 14).

VI. CONCLUSION

From April 1976 through March 1985, 54 cases of pancreatic cancer were treated by IORT. Of these cases, 30 were treated additionally by postoperative external beam irradiation. The consistent research to improve the treatment protocol for pancreatic cancer established the combination of IORT and conformation radiotherapy.

In summary, the ideal radiation conditions for high-energy electron beam therapy for pancreatic cancer and criteria for patient selection are given. We describe the introduction of conformation radiotherapy and explain how computer control is most effective for ideal conformation radiotherapy.

The combination of IORT and conformation radiotherapy reduces the side effects and complications significantly. The combination of IORT and conformation radiotherapy evidently prolongs survival time in pancreatic cancer. The improved protocol of combined treatment contributes to its success.

REFERENCES

1. **Leadbetter, A., Foster, R. S., and Haines, C. R.,** Carcinoma of the pancreas. Results from the Vermont Tumor Registry, *Am. J. Surg.,* 129, 356, 1975.
2. **Hiraoka, T., Watanabe, E., Mochinaga, M., Tashiro, S., Miyauchi, Y., Nakamura, I., and Yokoyama, I.,** Intraoperative irradiation combined with radical resection for cancer of the head of the pancreas, *World J. Surg.,* 8, 766, 1984.
3. **Najera, M. E. and White, R. R., III,** Carcinoma of the pancreas, *Arch. Surg.,* 106, 293, 1973.
4. **Tepper, J., Nardi, G., and Suit, H.,** Carcinoma of the pancreas: review of MGH experience from 1963 to 1973 analysis for radiation therapy, *Cancer,* 27, 1519, 1976.
5. **Cubilla, A. L., Fitzgerald, P. J., and Fortner, J. G.,** Pancreas cancer-duct cell adenocarcinoma: survival in relation to site, size, stage and type of therapy, *J. Surg. Oncol.,* 10, 465, 1978.
6. **Matsuda, T.,** Multi-disciplinary therapy for unresectable pancreatic cancer with special reference to intraoperative irradiation, *Jpn. J. Cancer Clin.,* 26, 988, 1980.
7. Cancer of the pancreas task force: staging of cancer of the pancreas, *Cancer,* 47, 1631, 1981.
8. **Takahashi, S.,** Conformation radiotherapy rotation techniques as applied to radiography and radiotherapy of cancer, *Acta Radiol. Suppl.,* 242, 1965.
9. **Matsuda, T. and Inamura, K.,** Computer controlled conformation radiotherapy, *Nippon Acta Radiol.,* 39, 1088, 1979.
10. **Matsuda, T. and Inamura, K.,** Computer controlled multi-leaf conformation radiotherapy, *Nippon Acta Radiol.,* 41, 965, 1981.
11. **Matsuda, T.,** Computer controlled conformation radiotherapy, in *MEDINFO 80, IFIP,* Lindberg, and Kaihara, Eds., North-Holland, Amsterdam, 1980, 14.
12. **Matsuda, T.,** Clinical significance of computer controlled conformation radiotherapy from seven years experience, in *Proc. 8th Int. Conf. on the Use of Computers in Radiation Therapy,* IEEE Computer Society Press, Los Angeles, 1984, 474.
13. **Rosenbloom, M. E.,** Treatment monitoring, verification recording and automated set-up, in *Proc. 6th Int. Conf. on the Use of Computers in Radiation Therapy,* IEEE Computer Society Press, Los Angeles, 1978, 300.
14. **Ishigaki, T., Sakuma, S., Banno, T., Imazawa, M., Tanaka, T., and Araki, K.,** Computer-assisted conformation radiotherapy system, *Eur. J. Radiol.,* 3, 367, 1983.
15. **Nishimura, A., Nakano, M., Otsu, H., Nakano, K., Iida, K., Sakata, S., Iwabuchi, K., Maruyama, K., Kihara, M., Okamura, T., Todoroki, T., and Iwasaki, Y.,** Intraoperative radiotherapy for advanced carcinoma of the pancreas, *Cancer,* 54, 2375, 1984.
16. **Shipley, W., Nardi, G., Cohen, A. M., and Ling, C. C.,** Iodine-125 implant and external beam irradiation in patients with localized pancreatic carcinoma, *Cancer,* 45, 709, 1980.
17. **Abe, M. and Takahasi, M.,** Intraoperative radiotherapy: the Japanese experience, *Int. J. Radiat. Oncol. Biol. Phys.,* 7, 863, 1981.
18. **Green, N.,** Carcinoma of pancreas-palliative radiotherapy, *Radiology,* 117, 620, 1973.
19. **Haslam, J. B., Cavanaugh, P. J., and Stroup, S. L.,** Radiation therapy in the treatment of unresectable adenocarcinoma of the pancreas, *Cancer,* 32, 1341, 1973.
20. **Dobelbower, R. R., Jr., Borgelt, B. B., Strubler, K. A., Kutcher, G. J., and Stuntharalingam, N.,** Precision radiotherapy for cancer of the pancreas; technique and results, *Int. J. Radiat. Oncol. Biol. Phys.,* 6, 1127, 1980.
21. **Hilaris, B. S. and Moorthy, C. R.,** Radiotherapeutic management of pancreatic cancer at Memorial Sloan-Kettering Cancer Center, in *Pancreatic Cancer,* Cohn, I., Eds., Masson, New York, 1981, 43.

22. **Whittington, R., Dobelbower, R. R., Jr., Mohiuddin, M., Rosato, F. E., and Weiss, S. M.,** Radiotherapy of unresectable pancreatic carcinoma: a six year experience with 104 patients, *Int. J. Radiat. Oncol. Biol. Phys.*, 7, 1639, 1984.

23. **Castro, J. R., Saunders, W. M., Tobias, C. A., Chen, G. T. Y., Curtis, S., Lyman, J. T., Collier, J. M., Pitluck, S., Woodruff, K. A., Blakely, E. A., Tenforde, T., Char, D., Phillips, T. L., and Alpen, E. L.,** Treatment of cancer with heavy charged particles, *Int. J. Radiat. Oncol. Biol. Phys.*, 8, 2191, 1982.

24. **Wood, W. C., Shipley, W. U., Gunderson, L. L., Cohen, A. M., and Nardi, G. L.,** Intraoperative irradiation for unresectable pancreatic carcinoma, *Cancer*, 49, 1272, 1982.

25. **Rich, T. A.,** Radiation therapy for pancreatic cancer: eleven year experience at the JCRT, *Int. J. Radiat. Oncol. Biol. Phys.*, 11, 759, 1985.

26. **Abe, M., Fukuda, M., Yamano, K., Matsuda, S., and Handa, H.,** Intraoperative irradiation in abdominal and cerebral tumors, *Acta Radiol.*, 10, 408, 1971.

27. **Abe, M., Takahasi, M., Yabumoto, E., Adachi, H., Yoshi, M., and Mori, K.,** Clinical experiences with intraoperative radiotherapy of locally advanced cancers, *Cancer*, 45, 40, 1980.

28. **Dobelbower, R. R., Jr., Borgelt, B. B., Suntharalingam, N., and Strubler, K. A.,** Pancreatic carcinoma treated with high-dose small-volume irradiation, *Cancer*, 41, 1087, 1978.

29. **Castro, J. R. and Quivey, J. M.,** Clinical experience and expectations with helium and heavy ion irradiation, *Int. J. Radiat. Oncol. Biol. Phys.*, 3, 127, 1977.

30. **Al-Abdulla, A. S., Hussey, D. H., Olson, M. H., and Wright, A. E.,** Experience with fast neutron therapy for unresectable carcinoma of the pancreas, *Int. J. Radiat. Oncol. Biol. Phys.*, 7, 165, 1981.

Chapter 19

INTRAOPERATIVE RADIATION THERAPY FOR BLADDER CANCER

Keiichi Matsumoto

TABLE OF CONTENTS

I. INTRODUCTION

The problems in treating superficial bladder cancer are the prevention of heterotopic recurrence in the bladder and preservation of vesical function. Transurethral resection is the most popular treatment at the present time; however, the recurrence rate within 5 years after initial resection is reported as high as 80%[5] with 40 to 50% of the recurrences occurring within the first year. To avoid recurrence, investigators have tried a local prophylactic treatment using intravesical instillation of thiothepa[7,17,20] or Bacillus Calmette-Guerin,[3,9,13] or a number of other agents,[12,17,20] but the results were unsatisfactory.

Radiation therapy has also been used for the treatment of bladder cancer. Van der Werf-Messing[18] reported that the 5-year survival rate for T1 and T2 lesions after external supervoltage irradiation was 50 and 45%, respectively. Suprapubic radium implantation with or without additional external beam irradiation were 12 and 20%, respectively.

To obtain high curability and retain the normal function of the urinary bladder, single-dose irradiation with electrons was tried on patients with bladder cancer. This author reported the results of intraoperative radiation therapy (IORT) using single-fraction, high-dose electron irradiation as a radical means of treatment for bladder cancer.[10] From previous discussions in that report, the sequelae may be predictable.

II. INTRAOPERATIVE IRRADIATION TECHNIQUES

A. OPERATIVE PROCEDURE

The tumor was exposed by opening the bladder with an incision approximately 5 cm in length at the dome of the bladder under spinal anesthesia (Figure 1). When the tumor was located high in the lateral or anterior wall, the incision point of the bladder was appropriately shifted. After careful observation of the tumor and surrounding area, the irradiation was planned. A collimating cylindrical electron applicator was inserted into the bladder cavity to cover the tumor (Figure 2). Immediately after the irradiation, the bladder was closed with absorbable suture material; the suprapubic wound was primarily closed; a balloon catheter remained in place for approximately 7 d.

B. SELECTION OF IRRADIATION FIELD, ELECTRON ENERGY, AND RADIATION DOSE

An irradiation field was selected to cover the tumor with a 1.5-cm margin around it. Three sizes of electron applicators (i.e., 4, 5, and 6 cm in diameter) were used.

Electron beam energy was selected according to the thickness of the tumor and the dose distribution (Figure 3). A total dose of 25 to 30 Gy of 4- to 6-meV electrons was delivered in one fraction in about 10 min.

C. ADDITIONAL EXTERNAL BEAM IRRADIATION

After 3 or 4 weeks, additional fractionated external beam irradiation was given to most of the patients with linear accelerator supervoltage X-ray to cover the whole bladder so that the radicality of local treatment could be increased and heterotopic recurrences could be prevented in the bladder. The additional dose was between 30 and 40 Gy within 15 to 20 d. After completion of treatment, all the patients were submitted to regular follow-up examinations. Cystoscopy was performed every month for the first year and every 3 months thereafter. No patient was lost to follow-up.

III. IORT FOR BLADDER CANCER

A. SUBJECTS

There were 117 patients treated by this method; a combination of patients treated at the

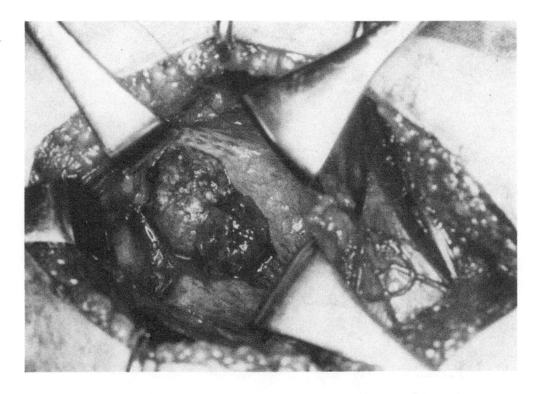

FIGURE 1. Tumor is exposed by opening the bladder at the dome. Tumor and adjacent mucosa are carefully observed.

National Cancer Center Hospital, National Medical Center Hospital, and Kanagawa Central Adult Disease Hospital during the period from January 1965 to June 1975. Patients having primary bladder cancer, regardless of the number of tumors, as long as they were confined to the size of a collimating applicator, were consecutively selected for this treatment. A small number of T3 and T4 tumors were also included. The patients, 90 men and 27 women, ranged from 26 to 86 years of age; 2 patients were in their 30s, 11 in their 40s, 27 in their 50s, 32 in their 60s, 39 in their 70s, and 4 in their 80s.

The extent of the tumors was assessed by bimanual examination under anesthesia, cystoscopy, cystography, intravenous urography, and pelvic angiography. Extent and grade of tumors are presented in Table 1. The relationship between clinical and pathologic tumor extent for Ta, T1, and T2 is shown in Table 2. Random biopsies of apparently normal bladder mucosa were not performed.

B. LOCATION AND SIZE OF TUMORS IN THE BLADDER

Localization and the size of the tumors treated at the National Cancer Center Hospital are shown in Tables 3 and 4. Almost all of the tumors were on the ureteral orifice, posterior wall, and laterial walls, and size of the tumors was under 3.0 cm in diameter.

C. RESULTS
1. Survival Rate

As seen in Figure 4, 3-, 5-, and 10-year actuarial survival rates for all cases were 77.7, 67.5, and 52.8%, respectively. The 3-, 5-, and 10-year patient survival rates for Ta and T1 lesions were 91.0, 85.2, and 68.0%; for T2 lesions, 78.6, 64.3, and 41.6%; and for T3 lesions, 53.4, 26.7, and 26.7%, respectively.

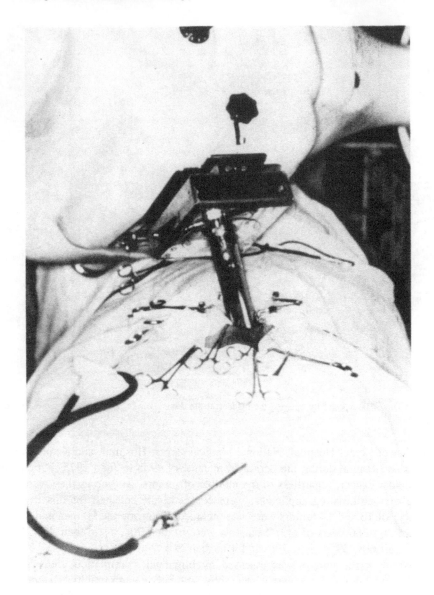

FIGURE 2.   Collimating electron beam applicator connected to the apparatus is introduced into the bladder to cover the tumor with a 1.5-cm margin.

2. Recurrences

Recurrence rates in Ta, T1, and T2 cases after treatment (Table 5) were 5.2% within 1 year and 11.1% within 2 years, 13.7% within 3 years, 17.3% within 4 years, 22.8% within 5 years, and 29.5% within 6 years. Local and heterotopic recurrence rates were extremely low. When the cases were classified into two groups, depending upon the number of tumors, recurrence in the solitary tumor group was 8.0%, while that in the multiple tumors group was 27.0% (Table 6). The recurrence rate increased in parallel with the grade of tumors (Table 7). Histopathologic grading followed AFIP classification. The lesion called "papilloma" was classified Grade 0 and was not included in this study. Five cases subsequently underwent total cystectomy because of multiple recurrences in the bladder after radiation therapy.

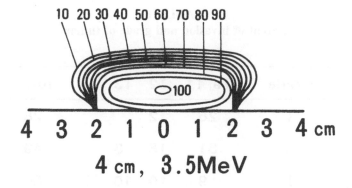

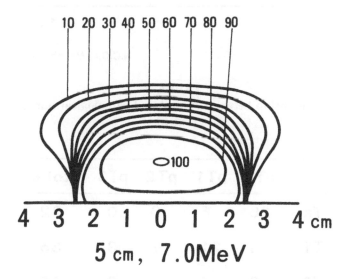

FIGURE 3. Depth-dose curves of 3.5- and 7.0-meV electrons.

D. COMPLICATIONS

Three patients complained of dull to colicky flank pain for several days after irradiation, presumably due to acute obstruction of the ureteral orifice that was included in the irradiation field. All of them recovered within 1 week, and no obstruction of the upper urinary tract was observed when examined by intravenous pyelography. No serious late complications were observed except in one patient who had a contracted bladder after 30 Gy of IORT and 31.5 Gy of external beam irradiation; 12 years later, urinary diversion was performed for this patient because of progressive bilateral hydronephrosis.

Hemorrhage and ulceration of the bladder mucosa are frequently encountered in patients treated with external and interstitial irradiation for uterine carcinoma. In our series, however, no such complications were observed. Tumors arising at the bladder neck or adjacent to the ureteral orifice were also treated with this method, but long-standing obstruction of the bladder neck or ureteral orifice did not occur in any case. One patient was treated with this method at two different sites in a single operative course, but had no complications up to 4 years later.

Radiation proctitis or other bowel damages were not experienced; probably because the dose distribution of electrons was restricted to the bladder wall, and the dose of additional external beam irradiation was under 40 Gy. Abdominal wall metastasis was not observed in our series, because according to the nature of this treatment, patients with a bladder full of tumors were not selected for treatment.

TABLE 1
Extent of invasion and grade of tumor

Grade	Ta, T1	T2	T3	T4	total
I	26	2			28
II	31	15	3		49
III	9	10	10	7	36
Unknown	1	1	2		4
					117

N.C.C.H. March, 1985.

TABLE 2
Relationship between clinical and pathological tumor extent

	pTa	pT1	pT2	pT3	total
Ta	26	6	0	0	32
T1	4	21	7	3	35
T2	0	4	16	8	28
					95

N.C.C.H. March, 1985.

E. INDICATIONS FOR IORT FOR BLADDER CANCER

According to the above-mentioned results, the best indication for treatment of bladder cancer with IORT is a solitary tumor at stage Ta, T1, or T2, less than 3.0 cm in diameter, histologic I, or Grade II. Concerning indications for this treatment for T3, T4, or Grade III lesions, it cannot be said positively that this treatment will be the best way to cure invasive cancer of the bladder, because there is an important problem with high metastatic rates to the lymph nodes with advanced cancer.[4,15,16] In the future, we have to try prospective studies on the indications for this treatment in invasive cancers.

IV. DISCUSSION

We have developed a new method for the treatment of superficial bladder cancer using single-fraction, high-dose electron irradiation.[10] As a principle, a solitary tumor was within the collimating electron beam applicator 6 cm in diameter. Some multiple-tumor cases, confined to the size of the applicator, were also treated.

TABLE 3
Site of tumors in the bladder

Site	No. of patients (%)	
Ureteral orifice	36	(43.9)
Posterior wall	18	(21.9)
Lateral walls	16	(19.5)
Vesical neck	7	(8.5)
Trigone	2	(2.4)
Dome	2	(2.4)
Anterior wall	1	(1.2)
Total	82	

N.C.C.H. March, 1985.

TABLE 4
Size of tumors

Size of tumors in diameter (cm)	No. of patients (%)	
Under 0.5	14	(17.1)
0.6–1.0	28	(34.1)
1.1–2.0	21	(25.6)
2.1–3.0	16	(19.5)
Unknown	3	(3.7)
Total	82	

N.C.C.H. March, 1985.

The following are the characteristic points of this treatment: (1) small, superficial tumors are selected; (2) relatively low energy electrons (4 to 6 meV) are used; electron dose can be equally distributed to the appropriate depth by proper selection of energy; in a deeper area than the beam range, the dose of the electron decreases as shown in Figure 3; when 3.5 meV is used, up to 1 cm depth can be covered with the 90% isodose line with nearly 0% dose at 2 cm, while 90% covers up to 2 cm with 0% dose at 4 cm if 7 meV is used; (3) high doses of electrons (25 to 30 Gy) can be given within a short time because of the high output; according to the nomogram proposed by Burns,[2] 30 Gy given in a single dose

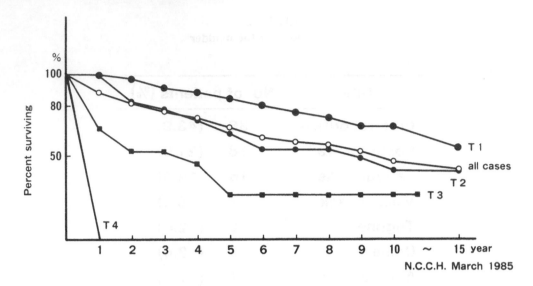

FIGURE 4.   Actuarial survival rate of bladder cancer cases after IORT.

TABLE 5
Posttherapeutic recurrences in stages Ta, T1, and T2

Follow-up period	No. of cases	Recurrent cases	%	Survival (%)
Within 1 year	95	5	5.2	100
2 years	90	10	11.1	92.7
3 years	80	11	13.7	88.5
4 years	69	12	17.3	84.3
5 years	57	13	22.8	80.0
6 years	44	13*	29.5	72.6

* Thirteen patients had one tumor recurrence during this period. Of them, Ta, T1 and T2 were 2, 4 and 7, respectively.

N.C.C.H. March, 1985.

is equivalent to 30 daily doses of 2 Gy; this dose, with an additional 30 to 40 Gy given by fractionated external irradiation, seems to be quite enough for the radical treatment of bladder cancer.

Normal vesical function was well preserved in most of the cases. No serious late effects were observed, such as ulcer formation in the bladder mucosa, hematuria, or dysuria. Only one patient had contracted bladder and underwent urinary diversion 12 years later because of progressive bilateral hydronephrosis.

One of the greatest merits of this method is the low recurrence rate after treatment. There are many reports suggesting that bladder cancer is a manifestation of generalized malignant diathesis of the urothelium.[6,8,14] This theory easily explains the high rate of recurrences in the bladder after therapy; that is, a new growth that was unrecognized but already persisting as a preneoplastic lesion in the urothelium. (We use the term "recurrence" in this text.) The reason for the extremely low recurrence rate after IORT should be explored.

TABLE 6
Recurrence rate in relation to multiplicity of tumors

	No. of cases	Recurrent cases	%
Solitary	88	7	8.0
Multiple	26	7	27.0
Unknown	3		
Total	117		

TABLE 7
Recurrence rate in relation to histological grade

Grade	No. of cases	Recurrent cases	%
I	28	1	3.6
II	49	3	6.1
III	36	9	25.0
Unknown	4	1	
Total	117	14	

Primary solitary small tumors were mainly selected for this therapy, and, presumably, to this was ascribed the low recurrence rate following IORT. As another possibility, we are considering the role of immunologic mechanisms in the process of tumor disappearance. Immediately after irradiation, the tumor and adjacent mucosa in the irradiation field show severe edema. As the edema subsides within 1 month, the shrinkage of the tumor occurs gradually. The tumor begins to look like a withered branch and finally fades away between 1 and 2 months. In some cases, the tumor persisted for more than 2 months, and transurethral resection was performed. Histology revealed no viable cancer cells. Cancer cells were heavily damaged by the radical high-dose irradiation. The immunocompetent cells sensitized by the antigenicity of the damaged cancer cells may attack the preneoplastic lesions as their target if present elsewhere in the bladder. Unfortunately, random biopsies were not performed in our series. At present, we cannot evaluate the effectiveness of additional external irradiation because there are not enough control cases; we have only five cases in all that were not given additional external irradiation. Studies are in progress on the immunologic processes in this type of treatment.

Cases with advanced tumors, that is, over T2 and high grade (Grade III), have shown poor results in the survival and recurrence rates. From these facts, this treatment is not adequate to cure invasive cancer of the bladder. Therefore, it is important that we should not fail to decide against using this treatment for invasive cancer.

V. SUMMARY

IORT using single-fraction, high-dose electron irradiation, was performed for 117 bladder cancer patients as a radical means of treatment for superficial bladder cancer. Additional fractionated external supervoltage irradiation covering the whole bladder was given in most of the cases. The 3-, 5-, and 10-year survival rates were 91.0, 85.2, and 68.0% for patients with T1 lesions, and 78.3, 64.3, and 41.6% for patients with T2 lesions, respectively. Heterotopic recurrence rates in the bladder were 5.3% within 1 year, 11.1% within 2 years, and 22.8% within 5 years. Normal vesical function was well preserved except in five patients who underwent total cystectomy because of multiple recurrences after radiotherapy; there was one patient who underwent urinary diversion because of a contracted bladder and progressive bilateral hydronephrosis. IORT was established as a reliable and superior method for the treatment of superficial bladder cancer because of its low recurrence rates and the good preservation of vesical functions after treatment.

REFERENCES

1. **Althausen, A. F., Prout, G. R., Jr., Daly, J. J.,** Non-invasive papillary carcinoma of the bladder associated with carcinoma in situ, *J. Urol.,* 116, 575, 1976.
2. **Burns, J. E.,** Nomogram for radiobiologically-equivalent fractionated doses, *Br. J. Radiol.,* 38, 545, 1965.
3. **Brosman, S. A.,** Experience with BCG in patients with superficial bladder carcinoma, *J. Urol.,* 128, 27, 1982.
4. **Drethler, S. P., Ragesdale, B. D., and Leadbetter, W. F.,** The value of pelvic lymphadenectomy in the surgical treatment of bladder cancer, *J. Urol.,* 109, 414, 1973.
5. **Greene, L. F., Hanash, K. A., and Farrow, G. M.,** Benign papilloma or papillary carcinoma of the bladder?, *J. Urol.,* 110, 205, 1973.
6. **Heney, N. M., Daly, J., Prout, G. R., Jr., Nieh, P. T., Heney, J. A., and Trebeck, N. E.,** Biopsy of apparently normal urothelium in patients with bladder carcinoma, *J. Urol.,* 120, 559, 1978.
7. **Koontz, W. W., Jr., Prout, G. R., Jr., Smith, W., Frable, W. J., and Minis, J. E.,** The use of intravesical thio-TEPA in the management of noninvasive carcinoma of the bladder, *J. Urol.,* 125, 307, 1981.
8. **Koss, L. G., Tiamson, E. M., and Robbins, M. A.,** Mapping cancerous and precancerous bladder changes. A study of the urothelium in ten surgically removed bladders, *JAMA,* 227, 281, 1974.
9. **Lamm, D. L., Thor, D. E., Winters, W. D., Stogdill, V. D., and Radwin, H. M.,** BCG immunotherapy of bladder cancer: inhibition of tumor recurrence and associated immuno responses, *Cancer,* 48, 82, 1981.
10. **Matsumoto, K., Kakizoe, T., Mikuriya, S., Tanaka, T., Kondo, I., and Umegaki, Y.,** Clinical evaluation of intraoperative radiotherapy for carcinoma of the urinary bladder, *Cancer,* 47, 509, 1981.
11. **Melicow, M. M.,** Histological study of vesical urothelium intervening between gross neoplasms in total cystectomy, *J. Urol.,* 68, 261, 1952.
12. **Pavon-Macaluso, M.,** Intravesical treatment of superficial (T1) urinary bladder tumors. A review of a 15-year experience, in *Diagnosis and Treatment of Superficial Urinary Bladder Tumors,* Montedison Lakemedel, Stockholm, 1978, 21.
13. **Pinsky, C. M., Camacho, F. J., Kere, D., Geller, N. L., Klein, F. A., Here, H. A., Whitmore, W. F., Jr., and Oettgen, H. F.,** Intravesical administration of Bacillus Calmette-Guerin in patients with recurrent superifical carcinoma of the urinary bladder: report of a prospective, randomized trial, *Cancer Treat. Rep.,* 69, 47, 1985.
14. **Schade, R. O. K. and Swinney, J.,** The association of urothelial atypism with neoplasia: its importance in treatment and prognosis, *J. Urol.,* 109, 619, 1973.
15. **Skinner, D. G., Tift, J. P., and Kaufman, J. J.,** High dose, short course preoperative radiation therapy and immediate single stage radical cystectomy with pelvic node dissection in the management of bladder cancer, *J. Urol.,* 127, 671, 1982.
16. **Smith, J. A., Jr. and Whitmore, W. F., Jr.,** Regional lymph node metastasis from bladder cancer, *J. Urol.,* 126, 591, 1981.
17. **Tortk, F. M. and Lum, B. L.,** The biology and treatment of superficial bladder cancer, *J. Clin. Oncol.,* 2, 505, 1984.
18. **Van Der Werf-Messing, B.,** Carcinoma of the bladder treated by suprapubic radium implants. The value of additional external irradiation, *Eur. J. Cancer,* 5, 277, 1969.
19. **Venema, R. J., Dean, A. L., Jr., Uson, A. C., Roberts, M., and Longo, F.,** Thiotepa bladder instillation; therapy and prophylaxis for superficial bladder tumors, *J. Urol.,* 101, 711, 1969.
20. **Whitmore, W. F., Jr.,** Management of bladder cancer, *Curr. Prob. Cancer,* 6, 1, 1979.

Chapter 20

INTRAOPERATIVE RADIATION THERAPY FOR BLADDER CANCER: A REVIEW OF TECHNIQUES ALLOWING IMPROVED TUMOR DOSES AND PROVIDING HIGH CURE RATES WITHOUT THE LOSS OF BLADDER FUNCTION

William U. Shipley

TABLE OF CONTENTS

I. INTRODUCTION

Bladder cancer is the eighth leading cause of death from cancer in this country. In 1986, approximately 41,000 new cases were recognized, and about 11,000 people died of bladder cancer. Despite some very encouraging results from both Europe and Japan, in the U.S. there has been very little exploration in the use of intraoperative radiation therapy (IORT) for the treatment of bladder cancer. The preferred method of treatment for patients with muscle-invading tumors in the U.S. has been radical cystectomy. For patients with superficial tumors, transurethral resection has been utilized, followed often by intravesicle installation of chemotherapy. Radiation therapy as the definitive treatment has largely been reserved for patients with invasive tumors who were older, medically inoperable, or who have unresected tumors. Radiation techniques requiring open surgical exploration have usually not been considered in these disadvantaged subgroups. However, when conventional definitive or full-dose radiation therapy has been used in "negatively" selected patients, permanent local control of the bladder tumor with the preservation of bladder function occurs in 25 to 50% of these patients (Table 1). Considerations of intraoperative techniques are then warranted, as they allow an improved radiation dose distribution throughout the tumor volume, and that will likely provide improved control and patient survival.

This review covers several recent reports (all retrospective) on the use of two operative radiation therapeutic approaches (IORT and interstitial implant) in the treatment of patients with primary bladder carcinoma. It will be shown that both techniques are effective in the treatment of selected patients with newly diagnosed solitary superficial tumors and that with muscle-invading tumors that are less than 5 cm, interstitial brachytherapy achieves excellent results. Finally, the suggestion is made that by combining external beam radiation therapy with an IORT boost using high-energy electrons, it is possible to cure patients with locally advanced tumors without losing bladder function.

II. IORT BY ELECTRON BEAMS

Matsumoto et al. reivewed the Japanese experience with IORT by combining the results of patients at the National Cancer Center Hospital, Tokyo, the National Medical Center Hospital, Tokyo, and the Kanagawa Central Adult Disease Hospital, Yokohama, from 1965 to 1968.[5] The tumors of 94 patients were clinically staged based on bimanual examination under anesthesia, cystoscopy, IVP, and often pelvic angiography as having Ta (32), T1 (34), or T2 (28) cancer. On *open* biopsy, the pathologic extent of the disease was very close to the original clinical staging — papillary noninvasive cancer was found in 30, carcinoma with invasion of lamina propria in 30, and carcinoma with superficial invasion of muscle in 23, and with deep invasion of muscle in 11. The tumor sizes (by largest diameter) in the 79 patients from the National Cancer Center Hospital were nearly all less than 3 cm; 50% were 1 cm or less, 27% were between 1.1 and 2.0 cm, and 19% were between 2.1 and 3.0 cm. Treatment was by open cystotomy and IORT, but without resection or fulguration. The IORT dose was 25 to 30 Gy by 3.5- to 7.5-meV electron beams delivered via cylinders of 4, 5, or 6 cm in internal diameter. In all but five patients, additional external beam irradiation was given postoperatively to the whole urinary bladder to a dose of 30 to 40 Gy in 15 to 20 d. The freedom from local recurrence rates were outstanding for these nonadvanced tumors; for stage Ta, 94%; for stage T1, 88%; and for stage T2, 82%. A total of 57 treated patients with stages Ta, T1, or T2 tumors had been followed for at least 5 years; of these, 81% were without evidence of recurrence or development of new bladder tumors. The actuarial 5-year survival rates for treated patients by clinical stage were: Ta and T1, 100%; T2, 62%; T3 (15) and T4 (7) patients, 7%. No local control rates were given for the few patients with locally advanced tumors. However, the depth dose of the 7.5-meV electron

TABLE 1
Full-dose External Beam Irradiation for Bladder Cancer

Series	Patient Number	Clinical Stage(s)	XRT dose (Gy)	Permanent local recurrence-free survival (%)
Miller[1]	428	A11	55—65	27
Parsons et al.[2]	15	T3, T4	<63	0
Timmer et al.[3]	76	T3, T4	60—65	41
Shipley et al.[4]	37	T2, T3	64—68	49

beam would very likely not have been penetrating enough to treat with full dose any stage T3 and T4 tumor that was thicker than 2 cm.

This 5-year 81% freedom from recurrence and/or the development of a new bladder tumor by IORT in Japan compares very favorably with the National Bladder Cancer Group experience with 259 patients with newly diagnosed stage Ta, T1, and T2 bladder cancers.[6] This was a surveillance study in which all patients were treated by transurethral resection (scored as "visibly complete" in 90% of the patients), often by prophylactic intravesical chemotherapy and only rarely by irradiation. The recurrence rate was 48% at 2 years and 61% at 5 years.

In the Japanese experience with 116 patients, there were very few complications reported, even though the IORT included the urethral orifice in 44%, and the bladder neck or trigone in 11%. Three patients had transient ureterovesicle junction obstruction, presumably due to edema. In one patient, bilateral hydronephrosis developed requiring urinary diversion. There was no reported hematuria or dysuria. Only 1 of 57 patients followed for greater than 5 years has developed clinically significant bladder contraction.[5] A recently reported study on canine bladder tolerance to IORT in foxhounds from the National Cancer Institute in Bethesda, MD, agreed with the earlier clinical experience from Japan, i.e., that relatively few acute or late harmful effects occurred.[7] In this study, anesthetized dogs were explored by laparotomy and a cystotomy incision that allowed the placement of a circular 5-cm treatment cylinder, and IORT to the bladder trigone and one ureteral orifice using 12-meV electrons. IORT doses of 0, 20, 25, 30, 35, and 40 Gy were given to each group of dogs which was then followed by serum creatinine, intravenous pyelogram, and cystometrics on a 3-monthly basis. There was no evidence of acute toxicity. With follow-up to 24 months, all dogs receiving 25 Gy or less had normal renal function, no abnormalities by repeat IVP, and no major loss of bladder volume or contractility by serial cystometrics. With IORT doses of 30, 35, and 40 Gy, some dogs developed hydronephrosis, but none had a major change in cystometric measurements. At autopsy, histologic changes revealed that the bladder epithelium remains intact without evidence of erosion or ulceration after all IORT does. Above 25 Gy, the ureteral orifice may be grossly stenosed by submucosal fibrosis. In general, these canine studies fully support the reported clinical tolerance to doses from 25 to 30 Gy by IORT given to part of the urinary bladder (usually <30%).

While our main emphasis at Massachusetts General Hospital using IORT has been in patients with colorectal or pancreatic carcinoma, we have treated three patients with locally advanced carcinoma of the urinary bladder, and one with ureteral cancer. In these instances, we have combined a course of 40 to 50 Gy of preoperative radiation therapy using conventional fractionation to the primary tumor and the regional lymph nodes, followed by an intraoperative electron beam boost using 15- to 23-meV electrons of from 18 to 22 Gy. There have been no local recurrences in these four patients. In the bladder-cancer patients,

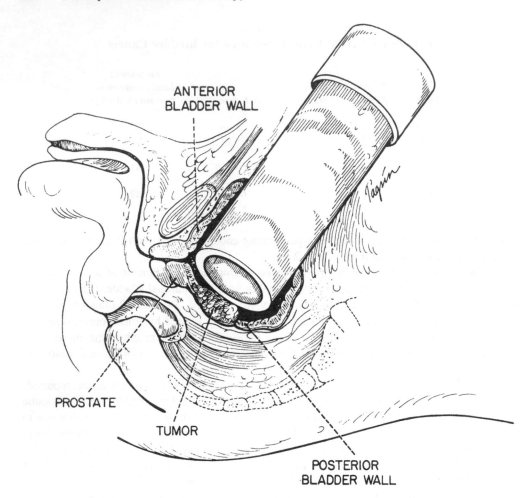

ANTERIOR
BLADDER WALL

PROSTATE

TUMOR

POSTERIOR
BLADDER WALL

FIGURE 1.   A sagittal schematic of intraoperative cylinder placement for delivery of IORT in the treatment of a patient with a locally advanced (stage T3b) bladder cancer. The bladder has been opened superiorly, and the treatment cylinder is angled laterally to avoid irradiating the right ureteral orifice and the rectum.

the tumor was clinical stage T4 in two, and in one, clinical stage T3b with a 6-cm mass obstructing the left ureteral orifice. The longest follow-up is available in the latter patient who is free of disease after 3.5 years. We have found that high-energy electron beams are necessary to cover adequately the extravesical extension of these tumors. The treatment cylinder is angled lateroinferiorly so that the anus and lower rectum and, in women, the lower vagina are not in the exit beam (Figure 1). We have had no difficulty with either bladder contracture or dysuria, including our most recent patient who had three doses of Cisplatin (70 mg/M^2) during her initial 50 Gy of preoperative irradiation.

III. BRACHYTHERAPY

The largest and most successful series of treating superficial bladder tumors with brachytherapy is from Rotterdam, where interstitial ^{226}Ra implants have been used over the last 25 years by van der Werf-Messing.[8-10] Patients were treated at the time of their first tumor, and only patients with solitary tumors less than 5 cm in diameter were selected. An open interstitial implantation of the radium needles was used. Intraoperatively, the radium needles are inserted into, and immediately adjacent to, the tumor with the bladder open at the time of a ventral cystotomy. The sutures attached to the needles are brought out through a separate track from the incision and are used to remove the needles following the delivery of 60 to 65 Gy. A total of 196 patients with T1 tumors have been treated with only 12% recurring in 5 years.[8] For 328 patients with stage T2 tumors, the recurrence rate within the bladder was 22% at 5 years.[9] Recently, they have modified their technique for treating patients with clinical stage T3 tumors less than 5 cm.[10] Preoperative radiation therapy (10.5 Gy in three 3.5-Gy fractions) is followed by a [226]Ra needle tumor implant for a dose of 35 Gy, and this is followed by a postoperative external beam radiation treatment of 30 Gy in 15 2-Gy fractions. In 41 treated patients, the overall 5-year survival is 57%. The local recurrence rate is only 8%. They report that bladder function has been satisfactory following this procedure, although they report that in two patients there were two deaths related to difficulties resulting from bilateral hydronephrosis due to severe radiation effects on the trigone in these two patients.

A second experience using radium needle implant from the Netherlands has recently been reported by Batterman et al.[11] They used a preoperative external beam radiation dose of either 10.5 Gy (three 3.5-Gy fractions) or 30 Gy in 15 fractions. This was followed by an open [226]Ra needle implant of from 45 to 60 Gy. They report, in 34 patients with T1 tumors, an 85% 5-year local control rate and a 72% 5-year survival rate. In 85 patients with clinical stage T2 tumors, they report a 74% local control rate at 5 years with a 5-year survival rate of 55%. They have 31 patients tumor free 5 to 10 years after treatment. These investigators commented on local failure in 3 of 5 patients who were implanted with tumors of 4 cm but < 5 cm in size. This group also reported some long hospital stays due to a delay in wound healing following removal of the radium needles; but no serious late reactions were observed in the bladder or intestines.

Recently, two institutions have reported their experience using after-loading ^{192}Ir interstitial implants for patients with only moderately invasive bladder tumors. The first is reported by Pierquin's group in Creteil, France.[12] They have used a single-plane, after-loading ^{192}Ir implant combined with complete gross tumor removal and an external iliac lymph node dissection. In 55 patients with pathologic stage T1 (31), T2 (14), or T3 (10) tumors, they report 84% are free of bladder recurrences or reoccurrences and a 67% NED survival at 5 years. With careful attention to the Paris system of dosimetry,[13] they use a dose of 60 Gy when the tumor margins are microscopically positive or no segmental cystectomy was done, and a dose of 45 Gy when the margins are negative. Their target volume includes 1 to 2 cm of healthy tissue around the incision and the full thickness of the bladder wall. The implanted plastic tubes are not loaded with active ^{192}Ir sources until seventh postoperative day to allow for initial healing of the cystotomy incision. Among the 55 patients, only 4 bladder complications were observed — 2 vesicocutaneous fistulae that closed with conservative management, 1 bladder neck stricture, and 1 contracted bladder. These results seem very good for tumors with limited muscle invasion. However, they are not clearly better than segmental cystectomy alone in carefully selected patients or segmental cystectomy followed by postoperative irradiation. The limitation of this elegant technique is that only thicknesses of 1 cm can be irradiated, thus precluding treatment of patients with clinical stage T3b tumors. Also precluded are patients with tumors invading the bladder neck because the plastic tubing is difficult to place within the trigone.

Finally, a group from the University of Pennsylvania has reported a pilot study of 14 patients combining preoperative external beam irradiation with an after-loading ^{192}Ir implant in patients who are not candidates for a segmental cystectomy.[14] For tumors less than 3 cm, 10 to 15 Gy external beam radiation was followed by ^{192}Ir interstitial implant, delivering 60 to 77 Gy. For tumors from 3 to 5 cm, 40 Gy of external beam radiation was followed by an additional 30 to 40 Gy by ^{192}Ir implant; 3 patients had T1 tumors and 11 had T2 tumors. While the median follow-up of this series is only 22 months, the actuarial local control rate at 2 years is 80%, and the survival rate is 68%. To date, only two complications have been noted: one vesicocutaneous fistula and one contracted bladder.

IV. SUMMARY

Based on extensive experience from Tokyo and Rotterdam, newly diagnosed Ta and T1 tumors can be controlled with a very high probability (90%) by high-dose IORT combined with a lower dose of external beam radiation to the entire bladder. For tumors of less than 4 or 5 cm that deeply invade the muscle, brachytherapy combined with 40 Gy of pelvic external beam radiation therapy seems to be both well tolerated and locally effective. For tumors that allow a limited partial cystectomy, "adjuvant" local radiation therapy by after-loading ^{192}Ir implant around the cystotomy incision may allow extension of the indications for segmental cystectomy and assure local control without the loss of bladder function. However, postoperative external beam irradiation in this setting will likely achieve the same goal. Finally, for locally advanced tumors deeply involving the trigone in patients in whom radical cystectomy is not possible or desired, combined electron beam IORT and 50 Gy external beam irradiation of the whole pelvis seems, based on limited experience, well tolerated and may achieve a higher probability of local control than is possible with conventional external beam therapy alone.

ACKNOWLEDGMENTS

I would like to thank Ms. Anne Macualay for her assistance in preparation of the manuscript and Ms. Edith Tagrin for her medical drawing.

REFERENCES

1. **Miller, L. S.,** Bladder cancer: superiority of preoperative irradiation therapy and cystectomy in clinical stages B2 and C, *Cancer*, 39, 973, 1977.
2. **Parsons, J. J., Thar, T. L., Bova, F. A., et al.,** An evaluation of split-course irradiation for pelvic malignancies, *Int. J. Radiat. Oncol. Biol. Phys.*, 6, 175, 1981.
3. **Timmer, P. R., Hartlief, H. A., and Hoojikaas, J. A.,** Bladder cancer: pattern of recurrence in 142 patients, *Int. J. Radiat. Oncol. Biol. Phys.*, 11, 899, 1985.
4. **Shipley, W. U., Rose, M. A., Perrone, T. L. et al.,** Full-dose irradiation for patients with invasive bladder carcinoma: clinical and histologic factors prognostic of improved survival, *J. Urol.*, 134, 679, 1985.
5. **Matsumoto, L., Kakizoe, T., Mikuriya, S. et al.,** Clinical evaluation of intraoperative radiotherapy for carcinoma of the urinary bladder, *Cancer*, 47, 509, 1981.
6. **Cutler, S. J., Heney, N. M., and Friedell, G. H.,** Longitudinal study of patients with bladder cancer: factors associated with disease recurrence and progression, in *Bladder Cancer: AUA Mongraphs*, Vol. 3, Bonney, W. W. and Prout, G. R., Jrs., Eds., William & Wilkins, Baltimore, 1982, 35.
7. **Kinsella, T., Sindelar, W., DeLuca, A. et al.,** Tolerance of the canine bladder to intraoperative radiation therapy: an experimental study, *Int. J. Radiat. Oncol. Biol. Phys.*, 11, 187, 1985.
8. **van der Werf-Messing, B. and Hop, W. L. P.,** Carcinoma of the urinary bladder (T1NXMO) treated either by Radium implant or by transurethral resection only, *Int. J. Radiat. Oncol. Biol. Phys.*, 7, 299, 1981.
9. **van der Werf-Messing, B., Menon, R. S., and Hop, W. L.,** Cancer of the urinary bladder T2, T3 (NXMO) treated by interstitial Radium implant: second report, *Int. J. Radiat. Oncol. Biol. Phys.*, 7, 481, 1983.
10. **van der Werf-Messing, B., Menon, R. S., and Hop, W. C.,** Carcinoma of the urinary bladder T3NXMO treated by combination Radium implant and external beam radiation: second report, *Int. J. Radiat. Oncol. Biol. Phys.*, 9, 177, 1983.

11. **Batterman, J. J. and Tierie, A. H.,** Results of implantation for T1 and T2 bladder tumors, *Int. J. Radiat. Oncol. Biol. Phys.,* 11, 188, 1985.
12. **Maseron, J. J., Marinello, G., Pierquin, B. et al.,** Treatment of bladder tumors by Iridium-192 implantation: the Creteil technique, *Radiat. Ther. Oncol.,* 4, 111, 1985.
13. **Dutrieux, A., Marinello, G., and Wambersie, A.,** *Dosimetrie et Encurietherapie,* Masson, Paris, 1982.
14. **Straus, K. L., Littman, P., Wein, A. J. et al.,** Interstitial Iridium-192 treatment for invasive bladder carcinoma, *Int. J. Radiat. Oncol. Biol. Phys.,* 11, 189, 1985.

Chapter 21

INTRAOPERATIVE RADIATION THERAPY FOR PROSTATIC CANCER

Masaji Takahashi

TABLE OF CONTENTS

I. INTRODUCTION

Since the advent of high-energy radiation therapy equipment in the 1960s, external beam radiation therapy has played a major role in the management of prostatic cancer[1] in addition to hormonal therapy and radical or transurethral prostatectomy. In most reports, a dose of 60 to 76 Gy was delivered to the prostatic lesions with conventional fractionation;[2-6] better results in survival and local control were achieved in patients selected to receive higher doses depending on tumor size or stage.[7-9] It was, however, noticed that prostate irradiation of 65 to 72 Gy with or without pelvic irradiation of 45 to 50 Gy produced an overall complication rate of 24%,[6] with 5 to 12% incidence of bladder and bowel injuries,[10] the most common problems with external beam irradiation.

In recent years, interstitial radiation therapy has been applied using ^{125}I seeds[11] and [198]Au colloid and grains[12,13] by directly infiltrating tumors and tumor beds. Also, a 160-meV proton beam has been used to deliver a boost dose to a carefully defined prostatic tumor volume.[14] By employing these treatment techniques, increased doses could be delivered to the prostatic lesion without increasing treatment-related morbidity. With the same purposes as those of brachytherapy and proton beam irradiation, intraoperative radiation therapy (IORT) with electron beams has been performed for the treatment of prostatic cancer at Kyoto University Hospital since 1972.[15,16] In this report, we offer a review of the procedure and the preliminary results of IORT for carcinoma of the prostate.

II. TECHNIQUES

A. OPERATIVE PROCEDURE FOR IORT

In an operating room, the patient is placed in the exaggerated lithotomy position, and an inverted U-shaped incision is made in the perineum. The dissection is continued upwards to achieve direct exposure of the prostatic tumor and to separate the posterior surface of the tumor from the rectum. Then, as shown in Figure 1, the perineal wound is temporarily closed and draped, and the patient is moved to a radiation therapy room under general anesthesia.

The radiotherapist should be present during surgery so that the choice of optimal energy of electron beam and radiation field (treatment cone) can be correctly made by measuring the three-dimensional size of the tumor.

In the radiation therapy room, the patient is placed again in the exaggerated lithotomy position, and the perineum is reopened for electron beam irradiation (Figure 2). A Young's tractor is passed per urethra into the bladder. By pulling the handle of the tractor strongly toward the patient's head, the prostatic tumor can be pushed toward the perineum because the pubis acts as a fulcrum. Then, as illustrated in Figure 3, the tumor is positioned within a sterile treatment cone which is inserted through the perineal incision. At each treatment time, it should be confirmed by digital rectal examination that the rectum is outside the treatment cone and the path of the electron beam. Figure 4 shows IORT with a betatron electron beam for a patient with prostatic cancer.

After IORT has been completed, the perineum is closed while the patient is still in the radiation therapy room.

B. RADIATION CONDITIONS
1. Electron Energy and Field Size

The selection of an optimal energy of electron beam is made depending on the depth of the lesion so that the whole tumor volume can be surrounded with the 90% isodose curve, and in addition, the normal tissues behind the tumor should be exposed to as minimal a dose as is possible. Accordingly, energies selected may be 12 to 18 meV.

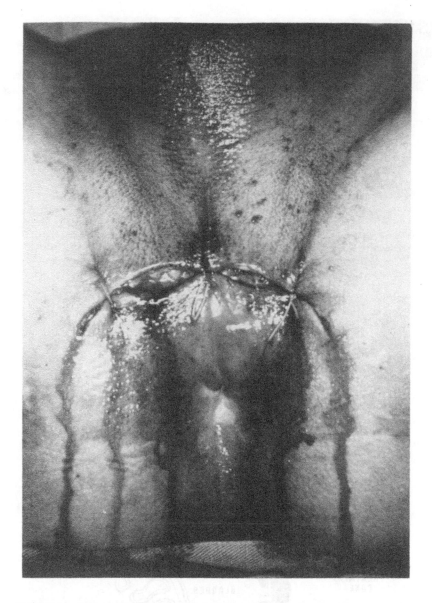

FIGURE 1. A perineal inverted U-shaped incision is temporarily closed in an operating room before a patient is moved to a radiation therapy room.

A treatment cone is selected out of those with circular ends 3 to 5 cm in diameter, or with elliptical ends of 3 × 4 or 4 × 5 cm dimensions.

Energies actually selected in our early series were 10, 12, and 14 meV. The selection was made based on the concept that 80% of the maximum dose should be delivered to the deep surface of the tumor.[16] Recently, a 90% dose level has been used for energy selection, and the treatment cones with an elliptical end for the radiation field.

2. Radiation Dose

IORT for prostatic cancer comprises two treatment modalities; one is to perform IORT alone, and the other as a boost in conjunction with external beam radiation therapy. In the light of our clinical results, single intraoperative doses required for achieving local control are at least 33 to 35 Gy by IORT alone, or 25 Gy as a boost in conjunction with external

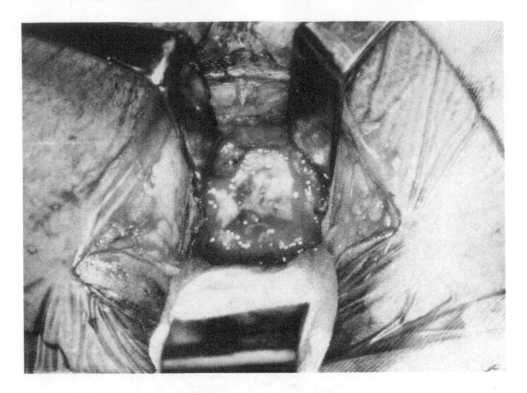

FIGURE 2.   The perineum is reopened in a radiation therapy room. The prostatic tumor is directly visualized.

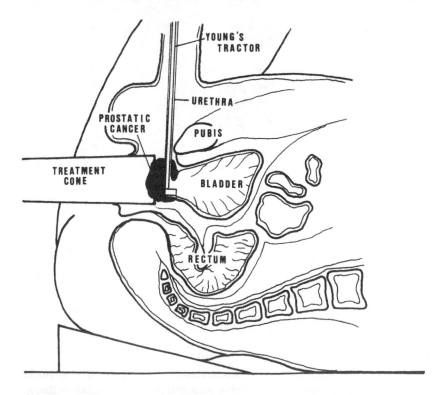

FIGURE 3.   Diagrammatic representation of IORT for prostatic cancer by the perineal approach. With a patient placed in the exaggerated lithotomy position, a treatment cone is inserted via perineum toward the tumor which is pushed forward to the cone by the Young's tractor. Note the pubis as a fulcrum.[16]

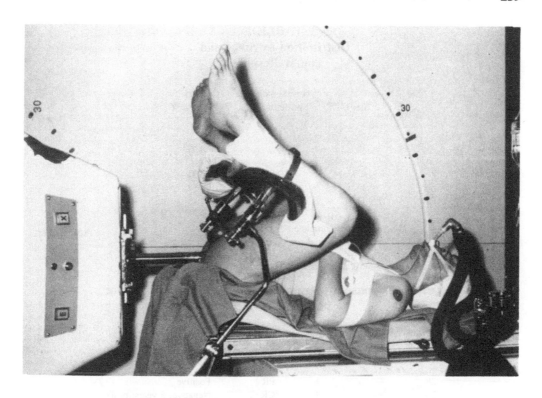

FIGURE 4.   IORT for a patient with prostatic cancer using a betatron.

beam radiation therapy, where 50 Gy is delivered to the whole pelvis in conventional fractionation of 1.8 to 2.0 Gy/d, five treatments per week. As for the sequence of IORT and external beam radiation therapy, IORT is recommended first. If not, there is some risk of delayed healing of the perineal incision.

III. CLINICAL RESULTS

A. PATIENTS

Between June 1972 and January 1985, 18 patients with histologically proven adeno-carcinoma of the prostate were treated by IORT with curative intent for stage A_2, B, and C diseases and with palliative intent for stage D. The patients were staged according to the American Urological System.[17]

Of 18 patients, 8 had not received any previous treatment, and the remaining 10 had persistent disease that showed poor response to hormonal manipulation or had relapsed following transurethral prostatectomy. In these ten patients, staging was also performed in the same manner as in the first eight patients. The stage distribution was comprised of one stage A_2, five stage B_2, ten stage C, and one stage D_1 and one stage D_2.

B. TUMOR RESPONSE

After treatment, all the patients have received follow-up examinations at regular intervals by radiotherapists and urologists. The evaluation of the response of prostatic tumors was made based on serial rectal examination, retrograde urography, CT scan, or perineal needle biopsy. Tumor response was graded as complete regression (CR), partial regression (PR), and no response (NR): CR was defined as clinical disappearance of the tumor, PR as regression greater than or equal to 50% in the size of prostatic nodule, and NR as less than 50% decrease or no change. In prostatic cancer, tumor regressions are slow, and, furthermore,

TABLE 1
Distribution by Stage and Tumor Response

Stage	Number of patients	Clinical response
A_2	1	CR[a]
B_2	5	CR in 4, PR[b] in 1
C	10	CR in 10
D_1	1	CR
D_2	1	CR

[a] CR: complete response.
[b] PR: partial response.

TABLE 2
Tumor Responses by Tumor Dose Given by IORT with or without External Beam

Dose (Gy)		Number of patients	Clinical response	Histological examination
IORT	EBRT[a]			
28	—	1	PR	Positive
30	—	1	CR	Negative, 5 years; positive at the 6th year
33	—	2	CR in 2	Negative in one, s/o[b] positive in one
34	—	1	CR	Negative
35	—	1	CR	Negative
20	50	1	CR	s/o positive
25	50	11	CR in 11	Negative in 11

[a] EBRT: external beam radiation therapy.
[b] s/o: suspicious of.

the clinical evaluation of response was complicated because of diffuse induration throughout the treated tissues. The final decision regarding a clinical response was therefore made 3 months after treatment.

Table 1 shows the stage distribution and the incidence of clinical responses according to stage. Of 18 patients, 17 achieved CR, and the remaining one with stage B_2 disease, PR.

Early in this series, various single doses of 28 to 35 Gy with electron beams were delivered to the prostatic lesion with curative intent. More recently, IORT has been applied as a boost dose in conjunction with external beam radiation therapy using 10-millielectronvolt peak (meVp) X-rays, where an intraoperative dose of 20 or 25 Gy limited to the prostatic lesion and a total dose of 50 Gy in conventional fractionation to the whole pelvis were delivered.

Table 2 shows a correlation between radiation doses and tumor responses. In the patient who failed to achieve CR, a single dose of 28 Gy had been delivered to the prostatic lesion by IORT alone. A needle biopsy performed during follow-up showed carcinoma cells with moderate degeneration, and this was compatible with the clinical response, PR. The patient who achieved CR by a single exposure to 30 Gy maintained negative histologic proof of recurrence of cancer for 5 years following the treatment. At the sixth year, however, a biopsy showed local recurrence of disease in the primary site. In one of two patients who

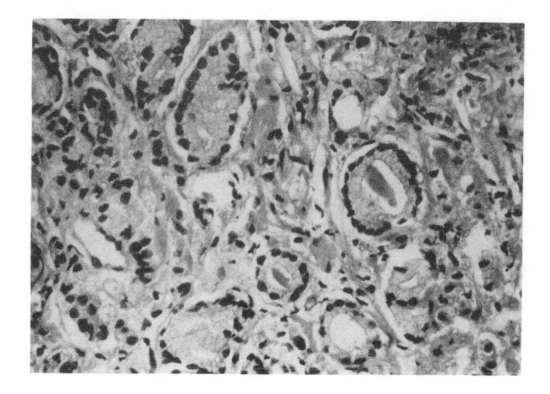

A

FIGURE 5. Histological specimens of prostatic cancer (A) before and (B) 1 year after a single intraoperative radiation dose of 33 Gy. Well-differentiated tubular adenocarcinoma is replaced by fibrous tissue.

received 33 Gy intraoperatively and achieved CR, abnormal cells with marked degeneration were noted and were suspected of being residual carcinoma cells. This patient has, however, maintained CR for 20 months since the treatment was performed. In the remaining three patients who received single doses of 33 to 35 Gy, it was confirmed by both serial rectal examination and needle biopsy that they achieved CR and remained local recurrence-free during the follow-up period of 1 to 7 years.

All of the 12 patients treated by a combination of intraoperative electrons and external beam photons achieved CR. Biopsies showed no evidence of malignant residuals in all but one who received an intraoperative dose of 20 Gy. Since then, he has been treated by hormonal therapy and has maintained CR for better than 4 years.

Figure 5 shows histological specimens that reveal well-differentiated tubular adenocarcinoma previous to the treatment (A) and no evidence of malignancy 1 year after a single exposure to 33 Gy.

C. SURVIVAL

The cumulative survival curve is shown in Figure 6. Four patients died: one with stage C disease of acute hepatitis at the tenth month after treatment, and the remaining three with stage B_2, C, and D_2 lesions of generalized disease. Except for the patient with stage B_2 disease who received 28 Gy by IORT alone, the other three patients had local tumor control at the time of death. Calculation of survival rates using the Kaplan-Meier method yields 79.9 and 59.9% for 5 and 10 years, respectively.

D. MORBIDITY

Table 3 summarizes acute and chronic complications related to IORT alone or as a boost

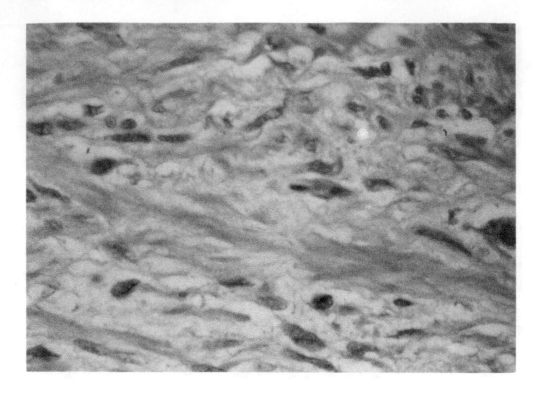

FIGURE 5B.

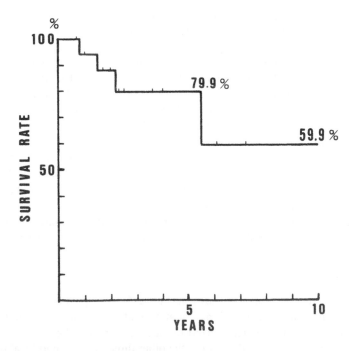

FIGURE 6.   Survival curve by the Kaplan-Meier method.

in conjunction with external beam radiation therapy in 18 patients with prostatic cancer. Hematuria occurred in every patient immediately after treatment and lasted 1 to 4 weeks.

TABLE 3
Summary of Major Complications

Complication	Treatment mode	Incidence
Hematuria		
Lasted 2—4 weeks	28—35 Gy/ IORT alone	6/6
Lasted 1—2 weeks	20—25 Gy/IORT plus 50 Gy/ EBRT[a]	12/12
Contracted bladder	60 Gy/ EBRT 3 years after 28 Gy/ IORT	1/1
	Others	0/17
Urethral stricture	All	0/18
Rectal injury	All	0/18

[a] EBRT: external beam radiation therapy.

The duration of hematuria appeared to be related to the intraoperative dose rather than the external beam irradiation; that is, it lasted 2 to 4 weeks in patients treated intraoperatively with 28 to 35 Gy, and 1 to 2 weeks in those treated with 20 or 25 Gy. The occurrence of hematuria was attributed not only to IORT, but also to manipulation of the Young's tractor which was inserted into the urinary bladder. After bleeding for a limited period, all of the patients had resolution and no recurrence of the symptom.

Pollakiuria, which was persistent after the treatment, developed in two patients who received external irradiation in addition to IORT. One patient, who received external irradiation with 60 Gy 3 years after IORT with 27 Gy, developed a contracted bladder. As this patient had no symptoms of radiation-induced cystitis until external irradiation was delivered, this suggested that his severe complication might be caused by the additional external beam dose of 60 Gy. In another patient treated with an external beam dose of 50 Gy following IORT with 25 Gy, pollakiuria resolved within 6 months, and no recurrence of same was observed. Diarrhea or soft stool occurred only in patients who received external irradiation, and the incidence and severity of the symptoms were the same as those related to usual external beam radiation therapy. None of the patients developed any chronic symptom of rectal injury and/or urethral stricture.

There was a problem with delayed wound healing of the perineal incision in two patients treated by IORT following external irradiation. In the remaining 16 patients who underwent IORT alone or previous to external irradiation, delayed wound healing or complications secondary to infection did not occur.

On the whole, the complications of IORT for prostatic cancer appeared quite acceptable.

E. TECHNIQUE CONSIDERATIONS

As for different operative procedures to place the treatment cone to the prostatic tumor, the retropubic and the transsacral approaches in addition to the perineal route may also be used. Of these routes, the perineal approach was employed in our study because it is technically easier and less invasive. During this procedure, the posterior surface of the prostatic tumor was separated from the rectum by blunt finger dissection. When the tumor was pushed toward to the treatment cone with a Young's tractor, the rectum remained apart from the tumor (Figure 3). In addition, it was confirmed by digital rectal examination at each treatment time that the rectum was outside the treatment cone and the path of electron beam. These careful manipulations were responsible for none of the patients suffering acute and/or chronic injuries of the rectum (Table 3). The uretha tolerated treatment well. Although it was fully exposed to radiation, none of the patients had symptoms secondary to urethral strictures induced by radiation.

One of the physical advantages of electron beams can be found in the low incidence of bladder injuries (Table 3). Although a contracted bladder occurred in one patient who received external beam irradiation with 60 Gy independent of IORT with 28 Gy at an interval of 3 years, this patient had no symptoms related to IORT until external beam irradiation was delivered. None of the remaining 17 patients developed any chronic bladder symptoms. These results indicated that with electrons of appropriate energy there is a rapid fall-off of radiation dose in the urinary bladder behind the prostatic tumor.

The first problem met on performing IORT was to decide an optimal single dose of electrons. As a result of delivering various single doses of 28 to 35 Gy to the prostatic tumor by IORT alone, it became clear that at least 33 Gy was required for achieving local control.

Data collected from previous publications show that the incidence of pelvic lymph node metastases with prostatic cancer ranges from 7 to 36% in stage B and 38 to 69% in stage C.[2,4,11,18] This strongly suggests that pelvic lymph nodes should be treated with an adequate dose of external beam irradiation. Thus, IORT was applied as a boost in conjunction with external beam irradiation of 50 Gy to the whole pelvis, and accordingly, the single intra-operative boost dose was decreased to 25 Gy. In all 11 patients who received 25 Gy intraoperatively in conjunction with an external dose of 50 Gy, local control was achieved with no histological evidence of malignancy at the time of analysis (Table 2).

It has been previously reported that local control was achieved in 70 to 88% of patients with stage C disease treated by external beam radiation therapy,[6,9] while postirradiation morbidity was seen with a wide spectrum of clinical syndromes.[10] Although interstitial implantation led to better results in local control,[11-13] this dropped with increase in tumor volume,[11] where a good distribution of dose could not be obtained. A better homogeneity of dose distribution can be provided by IORT with electron beams rather than interstitial implantation. Our preliminary results compare favorably with those previously reported.

IV. CONCLUSIONS

Single intraoperative doses of 33 to 35 Gy alone or 25 Gy in conjunction with external beam dose of 50 Gy are considered to be optimal, because local control can be achieved with these dose levels and maintained without serious acute or chronic complication. In conclusion, a high possiblity of local control with minimal morbidity may be expected with IORT in patients with stage B and C carcinoma of the prostate.

REFERENCES

1. **Bagshaw, M. A., Kaplan, H. S., and Sagerman, R. H.,** Linear accelerator supervoltage radiotherapy. VII. Carcinoma of the prostate, *Radiology*, 85, 121, 1965.
2. **Bagshaw, M. A., Ray, G. R., Pistenma, D. A., Castellino, R. A., and Meares, E. M.,** External beam radiotherapy of primary carcinoma of the prostate, *Cancer*, 36, 723, 1975.
3. **Lipsett, J. A., Cosgrove, M. D., Green, N., Casagrande, J. T., Melbye, R. W., and George, E. W.,** Factors influencing prognosis in radiotherapeutic management of carcinoma of the prostate, *Int. J. Radiat. Oncol. Biol. Phys.*, 1, 1049, 1976.
4. **Perez, C. A., Baner, W., Garza, R., and Royce, R. K.,** Radiation therapy in the definitive treatment of localized carcinoma of the prostate, *Cancer*, 40, 1425, 1977.
5. **del Regato, J. A.,** Long-term curative results of radiotherapy of patients with inoperable prostatic carcinoma, *Radiology*, 131, 291, 1979.
6. **Kurup, P., Kramer, T. S., Lee, M. S., and Phillips, R.,** External beam irradiation of prostatic cancer, *Cancer*, 53, 37, 1984.
7. **Neglia, W. J., Hussey, D. H., and Johnson, D. H.,** Megavoltage radiation therapy for carcinoma of the prostate, *Int. J. Radiat. Oncol. Biol. Phys.*, 2, 873, 1977.

8. **Harisiadis, L., Veenema, R. J., Senyszyn, J. J., Puchner, P. J., Tretter, P., Romans, N. A., Chan, C. H., Lattimer, J. K., and Tennenbaum, M.,** Carcinoma of the prostate. Treatment with external radiotherapy, *Cancer,* 41, 2131, 1978.

9. **Perez, C. A.,** Presidential address of the 24th annual meeting of the American Society of Therapeutic Radiologist: carcinoma of the prostate, a vexing biological and clinical enigma, *Int. J. Radiat. Oncol. Biol. Phys.,* 9, 1427, 1983.

10. **Pilepich, M. V., Krall, J., George, F. W., Asbell, S. O., Plenk, H. D., Johnson, R. J., Stetz, J., Zinninger, M., and Walz, B. J.,** Treatment-related morbidity in phase III RTOG studies of extended-field irradiation for carcinoma of the prostate, *Int. J. Radiat. Oncol. Biol. Phys.,* 10, 1861, 1984.

11. **Hilaris, B. S., Kim, J. H., and Tokita, N.,** Low energy radionuclides for permanent interstitial implantation, *Am. J. Roentgenol. Radiat. Ther. Nucl. Med.,* 126, 171, 1976.

12. **Flocks, R. H., O'Donghue, E. P. N., Milleman, L. A., and Culp, D. A.,** Surgery of prostatic carcinoma, *Cancer,* 36, 705, 1975.

13. **Chan, R. C. and Gutierriz, A. E.,** Carcinoma of the prostate. Its treatment by a combination of radioactive gold-grain implant and external irradiation, *Cancer,* 37, 2749, 1976.

14. **Duttenhaver, J. R., Shipley, W. U., Perrone, T., Verhey, L. J., Goitein, M., Munzenrider, J. E., Prout, G. R., Parkhurst, E. C., and Suit, H. D.,** Protons or megavoltage X-rays as boost therapy for patients irradiated for localized prostatic carcinoma, *Cancer,* 51, 1599, 1983.

15. **Abe, M. and Takahashi, M.,** Intraoperative radiotherapy: the Japanese experience, *Int. J. Radiat. Oncol. Biol. Phys.,* 7, 863, 1981.

16. **Takahashi, M., Okada, M., Shibamoto, Y., Abe, M., and Yoshida, O.,** Intraoperative radiotherapy in the definitive treatment of localized carcinoma of the prostate, *Int. J. Radiat. Oncol. Biol. Phys.,* 11, 147, 1985.

17. **Murphy, G. P.,** Prostatic cancer: progress and change, *Cancer,* 28, 104, 1978.

18. **Pistenma, D. A., Ray, G. R., and Bagshaw, M. A.,** The role of megavoltage radiation therapy in the treatment of prostatic carcinoma, *Semin. Oncol.,* 3, 115, 1976.

Chapter 22

INTRAOPERATIVE ELECTRON BEAM RADIATION THERAPY FOR GYNECOLOGICAL MALIGNANCIES

Alfred L. Goldson, Gregorio Delgado, Ebrahim Ashayeri, and Edmund S. Petrilli

TABLE OF CONTENTS

I. INTRODUCTION

The incidence and mortality of invasive cancer of the cervix has been steadily decreasing in North America since the turn of the century. In the U.S., however, it is still an important female cancer among socioeconomically disadvantaged population groups such as blacks, Puerto Ricans, Mexicans, and poor whites.[1] It is the number one cancer in most developing countries. The human impact of cervical cancer is much greater than statistics indicate, since cervical cancer occurs at a much younger age than other gynecologic cancers and has a higher incidence with multiparous women.

Current conventional treatment of cervical cancer is limited to the pelvis. Standard radiotherapeutic treatment consists of a combination of external beam radiation therapy to the pelvis with intracavitary brachytherapy applications. The average external fields usually measure 15×15 cm and do not extend above the aortic bifurcation. Standard surgical procedures, such as radical hysterectomy, lymphadenectomy, and exenterations, are also limited to the pelvis.

However, there is a group of patients for whom conventional irradiation alone has limitations, e.g., those patients with large metastatic pelvic lymph nodes outside the usual pelvic radiation field (para-aortic nodes) or large central tumors with parametrial involvement.[2,3]

A number of recent studies have shown that the incidence of para-aortic lymph node metastases in patients with cancer of the cervix is much higher than expected (Table 1). Early attempts to treat the para-aortic nodes with external radiation therapy have resulted in high complication rates (Table 2). This is not surprising in view of the high doses delivered to the treatment field. External beam radiation therapy after retroperitoneal exploration of the lymph nodes has not appeared to improve survival. Most authors feel that the risk-benefit ratio does not justify routine para-aortic irradiation with external beam techniques.[11]

In an attempt to circumvent the morbidity and mortality associated with conventional external beam irradiation, we initiated a pilot study using intraoperative electron beam irradiation of the para-aortic nodes and large metastatic lymph nodes of the pelvis.[12,13]

Intraoperative radiation therapy (IORT) or "direct view irradiation" is a surgical-radiotherapist team approach to unresectable or partially resectable malignant neoplasms of the various body cavities and subcutaneous soft tissues. An external beam of radiation, preferably electrons because of the sharp and rapid fall-off in depth dose, is delivered during surgery with the tumor exposed.

This direct visualization has several advantages: the technique permits accurate beam direction, precise limitation of the radiation field to the tumor, and the ability to physically retract or block with lead shields sensitive organs such as the skin, small intestines, ureters, and nerves in the treatment volume. The IORT boost dose can be preceeded by or followed by conventional fractionated external beam irradiation. The theoretical advantages are a high radiation tumor dose without a concomitant increase in treatment morbidity and mortality.

IORT is not a new idea. Like other recently revived techniques, such as hyperthermia and radiation sensitizers, IORT was used in the pioneering days of radiation therapy by European[14-16] and American[17-19] radiotherapists. However, the difficulty in combining an operating room and a radiation therapy suite, as well as the small field and the low penetration of the beam from orthovoltage therapy units, restricted its usefulness, and no significant clinical series were accumulated.

The current revival of IORT is credited to the work of Abe[20,21] at Kyoto University in Japan and our own work at Howard University Hospital in Washington, D.C.[22-25]

II. PRECLINICAL RADIATION BIOLOGY

Preclinical animal studies conducted at several institutions in the U.S. provided fun-

TABLE 1
Frequency of Paraaortic Metastases in Cervix Cancer

Author	Method	Stage	Para-aortic metastases Number	Percent
Piver[4]	Lymphangio		7 of 17	31
Averette[5]	Exploration		27 of 70	39
Buchsbaum[2]	Exploration	II-IV	9 of 34	27
Delgado[6,7]	Exploration	II-IV	13 of 31	42

TABLE 2
Complication Rates after External Radiotherapy of the Para-aortic Area in Cancer of the Cervix

Author	Dose	Time (weeks)	Severe complications Number	Percent
Nelson[8]	60	6	4/94	4
Lepanto[9]	50	5	5/26	19
Piver[4]	60	6	12/21	57
Wharton[3]	55	6	10/24	42
Delgado[10]	45	6	6/13	46

damental data on normal tissue tolerances to single high doses of intraoperative electron beams. At Howard University Hospital, dogs were irradiated by Goldson[26] to the retroperitoneum, including the aorta and vena cava, with single electron beam doses of 20, 30, and 40 Gy. After 16 months, the animals were sacrificed. Grossly, the aorta and vena cava appeared normal; microscopically, there was some degree of intimal thickening of the vessels, but the overall integrity of the great vessels was maintained. In contrast, the small intestines tolerated intraoperative electron beam treatment poorly, with progressive ulcerations and gangrenous bowel developing when single doses exceeded 20 Gy. Radiobiological studies carried out at the National Cancer Institute by Sindelar[27] and Tepper[28] demonstrated that dog aortas subjected to single doses of electron beam irradiation up to 50 Gy maintained structural integrity. Microscopically, there was subintimal and medial fibrosis in the aortic wall at doses above 30 Gy. The changes noted seemed to be dose related, but there was no significant narrowing of the vessels.

The tolerance of the great vessels to single high-dose IORT electrons is significant because these structures are routinely irradiated in the treatment of the para-aortic nodes.

The tolerance of the kidneys and ureters to single high-dose IORT had to be established to further understand the radiation biology of the retroperitoneum. High-dose IORT electrons to the kidney illustrated a renal sensitivity, resulting in parenchymal atrophy and hyalinization necrosis with doses as low as 20 Gy.[29] Clinically, this can be avoided by surgical dissection of the ureters and retracting them out of the treatment portal.

It is often wise to mobilize and fix the ureters outside the treatment portal to avoid their incarceration in the subsequent fibrotic reaction which often takes place within the irradiated area of the retroperitoneum.

Additional canine studies indicated the maximum tolerance doses were 15 Gy for the colon, 25 Gy for the small intestine, and 30 Gy for the bladder.[29]

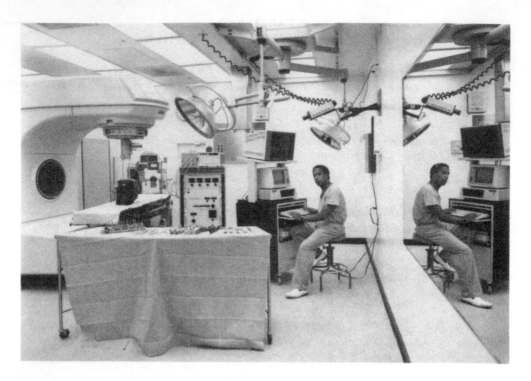

FIGURE 1.   Dedicated in 1976, the Howard University Intraoperative Radiotherapy Suite is a complete surgical facility equipped with a Clinac-18 accelerator and a Clini-Therm® hyperthermia unit.

III. IORT FACILITIES AND EQUIPMENT AT HOWARD UNIVERSITY HOSPITAL

A. IORT EQUIPMENT

At Howard University Hospital, IORT was inaugurated in November 1976 with a dedicated facility (Figure 1). At that time the Howard facility was the only one worldwide where the surgery and irradiation were initiated and completed in the same suite. The dedicated IORT suite houses a Varian® Clinac-18 linear accelerator and measures 25 × 25 feet.

Modification of the suite included equipotential grounding of all electrical equipment, including the accelerator, conductive flooring, separate air circulation, surgical lights, isolation transformers, and a nitrous oxide, oxygen, and suction column. An isolation panel was installed for electrical outlets and to supply adequate power for future intraoperative hyperthermia techniques.

An electron-producing accelerator offers the preferred characteristics for IORT. The electron beam delivers its effective dose in a few centimeters of tissue with a rapid fall-off of dose beyond this critical distance. The effective dose range in centimeters of tissue is determined by the energy of the electron beam, i.e., 6, 9, 12, or 18 meV. By applying this physical property to the known thickness of the involved nodes, the lowest possible effective energy can be selected to give a homogenous dose distribution throughout the tumor-bearing volume, while minimizing the dose to the great vessels and the spinal cord. A homogenous tumor dose in a single exposure is calculated at the 90% isodose curve and is delivered at approximately 5 Gy/min, facilitating a short IORT treatment time. The loss of "skin sparing" is no disadvantage for IORT — the skin is physically retracted out of the way of the electron beam. The bremsstrahlung (photon) contamination is less than 5% at all energies.

Specially designed IORT treatment collimators (or beam shapers) were fabricated for this unique treatment procedure. The electron beam collimator consists of an outer anodized

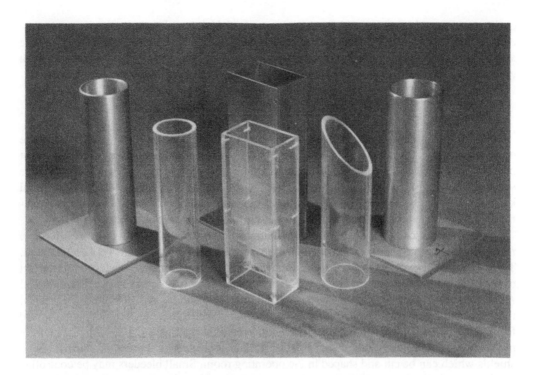

FIGURE 2.   Specially designed anticrush telescoping collimators were designed for the IORT procedure. Various shapes and bevels are available for each clinical setting.

or hard-coated aluminum collimator and a telescoping inner Lucite® collimator, both 30 cm long and with $1/4$-in.-thick walls (Figure 2). Both collimators overlap by 10 cm. The lower Lucite® collimator provides clear visualization of the tumor volume and confirms that the normal tissues have not drifted into the treatment field. The Lucite® collimator also acts as a secondary retraction device in that it provides a physical barrier between surrounding normal tissue and the treatment field, and the telescoping effect of the Lucite® collimator is an additional inherent safety factor. The inner Lucite® portion of the collimator can telescope into the aluminum section for a distance of 20 cm. These characteristics prevent any undue static pressure against vital structures that the collimator may rest upon during the IORT. The treatment collimators come in various dimensions and shapes, e.g., round, rectangular, and square. Certain collimators are designed with a beveled edge to facilitate insertion under the costal arch and against the pelvic sidewalls for certain clinical situations. The aluminum portion of the collimator is autoclaved, and the Lucite® portion is gas sterilized prior to each procedure. Both segments are numbered and stored in the cabinets in the IORT suite.

B. SURGICAL EQUIPMENT

Conventional surgical instruments are used to carry out the dissection of the retroperitoneum and the pelvis. The standard metal retractors, Metzambaum scissors, tissue and hemostatic forceps, and the like are used during the surgical procedure as well as during the IORT phase of the operation.

C. ANESTHESIA EQUIPMENT

Standard anesthesia procedures are followed during surgery and IORT. However, during the short interval during which radiation is administered to the tumor, the anesthesia team, as well as the rest of the surgical team, must leave the room. Therefore, a second multichannel oscilloscope capable of remotely monitoring arterial blood pressure, respirations, electro-cardiogram, and pulse rate was installed in the surgical suite, where it can be used by the anesthesia team during the short interval or IORT. Beyond this, no extraordinary anesthesia equipment is required.

IV. BASIC PROCEDURE TECHNIQUES

A surgical-radiotherapeutic team approach is the cornerstone of a successful outcome of the procedure. Preoperative consultation between the team members provides for the best positioning of the patient on the operating table and the optimum surgical incision site. The surgeon's clear understanding of the capabilities of the IORT technique and the physical knowledge of the size and flexibility of the IORT collimators provide him with the funda-mental data needed to offer the radiotherapist the best exposure to perform the IORT.

In all anatomical locations, be it the cranium, thorax, abdomen, pelvis, or soft tissues, maximal surgical resection of the tumor and its regional nodes should always be attempted. This provides for a major reduction in tumor cell burden and increases the potential effect of the IORT as well as the postoperative conventional fractionated irradiation that follows. Along with the appropriate resections and anastomoses, additional dissection of normal tissues in the immediately adjacent areas may be indicated so that they too may be removed from the IORT field, thereby minimizing toxic effects of treatment. Tissues that cannot be physically retracted out of the beam may be further protected by the use of sterilized lead shields which can be cut and shaped in the operating room. Small bleeders may be controlled by the use of metal clips without the fear of them inducing significant radiation scatter or shielding of micrometastases, which may lie in their immediate vicinity. If at all possible, any anastomosis should be performed after the IORT procedure in order to reduce any unnecessary stress upon the anastomosis as a result of the insertion of the collimator.

The IORT aspects of the procedure are conducted in the following manner. After surgical resection or exposure, the limits of the unresected primary tumor, or the tumor bed, or regional nodes are determined and measured in all three dimensions. Upon determining the surface area of the region to be irradiated, the appropriate size and shape collimator is selected so as to encompass the tumor with a 1- to 2-cm margin. The selection of the appropriate electron beam energy is determined by the anterior-posterior thickness of the target volume. Technically, the electron energy is selected so that the 90% isodose line of that specific energy falls at least 1 cm deeper than the most posterior aspect of the target volume. Depending on the clinical presentation, either microscopic or gross disease, a single dose of electrons from 15 to 25 Gy is selected. The appropriate treatment collimator is placed down over the target volume, care being taken to retract normal tissues out of the way. Lap towels and metal retractors are also used to maintain the normal tissues in a safe position. The patient is then positioned under the collimator of the treatment gantry to which the aluminum portion of the treatment collimator has been attached. The operating table is then adjusted so as to dock the aluminum segment to the Lucite® portion of the treatment collimator. Before leaving the treatment room, the anesthesiologist checks the patient's vital signs and the surgeon assesses the status of hemostasis. After confirmation of the patient's stability, all members of the team leave the IORT suite. The anesthesiologist monitors the patient's vital signs via a second oscilloscope mounted inside the treatment control area. The dose rate for most linear accelerators currently in use for this technique is approximately 5 Gy/min, resulting in treatment times usually lasting from 2 to 6 min, depending on the IORT dose prescribed. If during the delivery of the IORT dose any abnormalities are noted in the patient's vital signs, the accelerator can be turned off by the anesthesiologist by simply opening the door, thus allowing immediate entry into the room to assist the patient. Unlike interstitial implantation of radioisotopes, the patient is never radioactive. Table 3 outlines the Howard-Georgetown pilot study protocol.

TABLE 3
Treatment Protocol for Radiation Therapy

Intraoperative irradiation
  Para-aortic area[a]

Negative nodes	15 Gy	9—12 meV
Positive nodes		
A. Microscopic metastasis (surgically removed)	20 Gy	9—12 meV
B. Grossly positive (biopsy only)	25 Gy	9—12 meV
Pelvis area: lymph nodes		
A. Microscope metastasis	15 Gy	9—12 meV
B. Grossly positive nodes	25 Gy	9—12 meV
Parametria	25 Gy	9—12 meV

External irradiation ^{60}Co or X-ray

Para-aortic nodes (unresectable)	25 Gy
Pelvis	45—50 Gy

Intracavitary applications:^{137}Cs

Pelvis	2 applications (48 h each)

Administered to all patients having treatment for primary cancer.

V. PATIENTS AND METHODS

A total of 19 patients received IORT for advanced cervical cancer after a staging laparotomy; 16 of the patients had primary cancer, and 3 had recurrent cancer. Only patients with stage II, III, IV, or recurrent cancer were selected for the study.

All patients underwent a clinical staging procedure that included physical examination, chest X-ray, intravenous pyelogram, cystoscopy, barium enema, proctoscopy, lymphangiogram, and a computed tomography scan when clinically indicated. When the lymphangiogram revealed positive lymph nodes, needle biopsies of the para-aortic nodes were attempted.

All 16 patients with primary cancer received IORT to the para-aortic area, and some patients received additional IORT to the parametrium and pelvic sidewalls.

Three patients had pelvic and leg pain due to the recurrence of cervical carcinoma in the pelvic sidewall, which was confirmed histologically by surgery. These three patients had been treated for stage II (one patient) and III (two patients) cervical carcinoma with external irradiation and intracavitary radium 2 years before. Intraoperative irradition was given to the sites of recurrence for palliation.

After clinical staging, the patients were taken to the IORT facility for surgery.

VI. INTRAOPERATIVE IRRADIATION OF PARA-AORTIC AREA

After a complete exploration of the abdomen, a para-aortic lymphadenectomy or para-aortic node biopsy was performed as follows. The peritoneum was opened at the level of the bifurcation of the aorta and extended cephalad for 5 cm. The mesentery of the small bowel was retracted, and the aorta and the vena cava were visualized. After the right ureter and the ovarian blood vessels were identified and retracted laterally, the fatty tissue containing the lymph nodes anterior and lateral to the vena cava was carefully dissected and removed. After this, a similar dissection was performed on the left side anterior and lateral to the aorta. The dissections were performed about 5 to 8 cm above the bifurcation of the aorta. Metallic clips were placed at the highest area of dissection.[6,13] When the lymph nodes were large and fixed to the vena cava, only biopsies were performed.

The peritoneum parallel and lateral to the descending colon was opened and pulled medially for better exposure in some cases. After the aorta was exposed, the lymph nodes suggesting metastatic tumor were biopsied and the area marked with Hemoclips®.

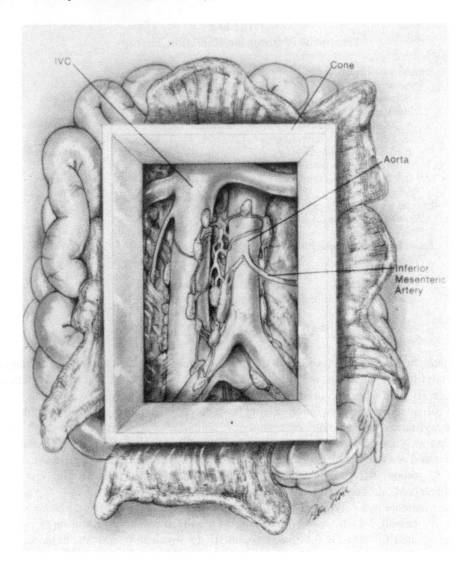

FIGURE 3.   The small intestines and ureters are retracted away and the IORT collimator is seen covering the para-aortic lymph node area.

The patient was then positioned under the linear accelerator, the clear Lucite® section of the treatment collimator was connected to the anodized aluminum portion of the collimator that had been attached to the collimator head of the accelerator (10 × 4 cm) (Figure 3). A maximum dose of 25 Gy was delivered in 5 min with an electron beam of 9 to 12 meV. During this time, the patient was alone in the operating room and was monitored by a television screen and by a continuous trace of pulse, respiration, and blood pressure. After completion of the IORT, the applicator was removed.

VII. INTRAOPERATIVE PELVIC RADIATION TECHNIQUE

After the para-aortic nodes were treated, the bowels were packed upwards and the pelvis was carefully explored. On the left side, the retroperitoneal spaces were entered on top of the psoas muscle; the sigmoid colon was retracted medially, bringing it up from its retro-peritoneal insertion (Figure 4). The ureter was identified and retracted medially. The blood

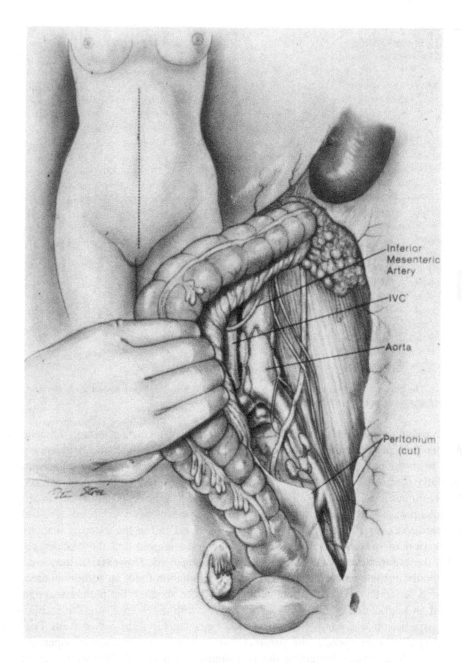

FIGURE 4. The retroperitoneal space above the psoas muscle is entered, and the rectosigmoid is retracted medially so as not to be included in the radiation field.

vessels were identified, including the common, external, and internal iliac arteries and veins. With blunt dissection, the pararectal space was entered medial to the internal iliac artery. The rectum and the rectosigmoid were then retracted medially. The avascular space lateral to the bladder was then identified and bluntly dissected medial to the pelvic blood vessels, and the paravesical space was identified. The bladder was then retracted medially. With two fingers, one in the pararectal space and the other in the paravesical space, all tissues, the rectosigmoid, and the bladder were retracted medially so as not to include these structures in the IORT field (Figure 5).

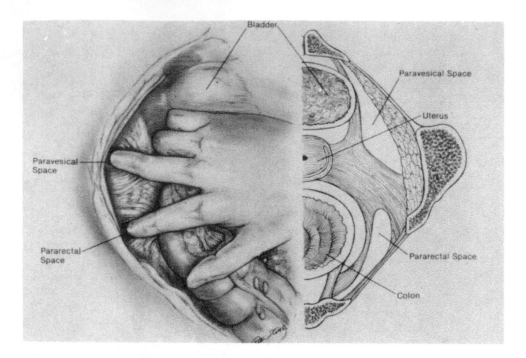

FIGURE 5.   The pararectal and paravesicle space and space of Retzius are opened, and the abdominal viscera retracted medially so as not to be included in the radiation field.

Large pelvic nodes were removed for confirmation of metastatic tumor. Dissection of the bladder was performed from the suprapubic space (of Retzius); the bladder was then detached from the pubic area, bladder pillars were transected, and the bladder was dropped and medially retracted. At this time, the remainder of the abdominal viscera was retracted and the treatment applicator (6 × 10 or 6 × 15 cm) was introduced after ascertaining that the previous para-aortic intraoperative field of irradiation was not overlapped. The field size was selected to cover all the pelvic nodes from the distal end of the external iliac artery to the bifurcation of the aorta (Figure 6). With the rectosigmoid and the bladder retracted medially, the parametria were included in the radiation field. However, if they were very bulky and only a small part could be included in the radiation field, an additional area might be irradiated separately. After the applicator(s) had been secured, the patient was again left alone, and an application of 25 Gy IORT was given with the 9- to 23-meV electron beam.

After irradiation was completed, dissection began in the right pelvic wall. The retroperitoneal spaces were opened, the pararectal and paravesical spaces were opened as described, and all structures including the rectosigmoid and the bladder were retracted. In some cases, the cecum was also retracted upwards. Again, the lymph nodes, the pelvic wall, and the parametria were placed within an appropriately sized field to cover the pelvic nodes but not to overlap the field from the paraaortic IORT marked earlier by metallic clips. After all the structures were separated and retracted, the patient was again put under the linear accelerator and given IORT monitored from the control room. The peritoneum and then the abdominal wall were closed by retention sutures.

VIII. EXTERNAL BEAM RADIATION THERAPY

At 10 days postIORT, the patients were given pelvic external beam radiation therapy with a Clinac-18 accelerator; 2 weeks after this was concluded, they had intracavitary cesium

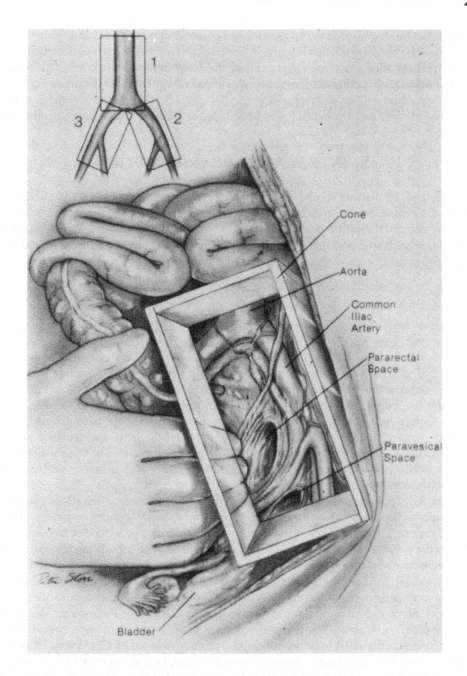

FIGURE 6. A view (upper left) of the three fields covering the lymphatics, the parametria, and pelvic and para-aortic area (lower right). The applicator is placed so the parametria and lymph nodes will be irradiated after the retroperitoneal spaces are opened and the rectum, sigmoid, and bladder retracted so as not to be included in the radiation field.

applications. In two patients whose para-aortic nodes were grossly positive with metastasis, 25 Gy of fractionated external beam radiation was directed toward the area of disease defined at the time of surgery with surgical markers. The radiation portals covered the upper border of the pelvic field with adequate gap and a matchline superior to the interspace between T12 and L1.

A minimum total dose of 45 Gy was delivered homogeneously to the pelvis in daily dose increments of 1.8 to 2.0 Gy (midplane calculation). Four or five fractions were given per week for 4 to 5 weeks. Standard anterior and posterior opposing field arrangements were used unless the clinical situation suggested the need for four-field or rotational techniques.[3]

External radiation portals designed to match the extent of the disease covered the external iliac, hypogastric, and obturator lymph nodes. Treatment was based on the following boundaries: (1) superior — the interspace between L4 and L5, (2) inferior — upper third of obturator foramen, and (3) lateral — at least 1 cm beyond the lateral bony margin of the pelvis at its widest point.

IX. INTRACAVITARY IRRADIATION

A total of 14 patients received intracavitary cesium treatment by a fixed afterloading Fletcher-Suit intracavitary applicator. Intracavitary treatment began approximately 2 weeks after completion of external beam pelvic and/or para-aortic irradiation. The second intracavitary treatment was performed 1 to 2 weeks after the first treatment; 2000 to 3000 mg-h were delivered in each 48-h application. The dose to point A ranged from 45 to 65 Gy.

X. RESULTS

Table 4 shows the cancer stage and cell type for the 19 patients in the study and the status of their para-aortic nodes. Of the 19 patients, 16 had primary cancer and 3 had recurrent disease; 16 patients had squamous cell carcinoma and 3 had adenocarcinoma. Two patients had grossly positive nodes, nine patients had microscopically positive nodes, and eight had negative nodes. Table 5 shows the therapy the patients received. When this mode of therapy first began, only the para-aortic area was treated with IORT. All 16 patients with primary cancer received IORT to the para-aortic areas; 11 of these patients had positive para-aortic nodes; 5 did not. Six of the former and two of the latter also received IORT to the pelvic nodes, iliac nodes, parametrium, and/or pelvic sidewalls. The three patients with recurrent pelvic sidewall disease after IORT of their primary cervical cancer received IORT to the pelvic area only.

After IORT, 16 patients were given external beam irradiation to the pelvis. The three other patients had external beam irradiation and intracavitary cesium treatment of their cervical cancer 2 years before. Those patients with recurrent pelvic sidewall disease had IORT to the pelvic sites only. In addition, the two patients with grossly positive para-aortic nodes were treated with an additional 25 Gy external beam therapy to the para-aortic area. After external irradiation, 14 patients had intracavitary applications: 12 double, 2 single. Of the remaining patients, two refused intracavitary applications; the three other patients with tumor recurrence had received intracavitary applications as part of their primary treatment. The 11 patients with positive para-aortic nodes are dead, 1 from other causes than cancer. The survival range was 10 to 36 months with a median survival of 17 months. Of the five patients primarily treated with negative para-aortic nodes, two are alive and free of disease. Two patients died of disease and the other from unrelated causes. The median survival for this group was 33.3 months with a range of 17 to 71 months (Table 6).

The three patients with recurrent disease died from cancer after therapy. In two of these patients, reexploration was done to rule out recurrence. In one patient, the irradiated lymph nodes were negative, and in the other patient, the irradiated pelvic mass recurrence was also negative. In both cases, the therapy was IORT alone.

XI. TREATMENT-RELATED TOXICITY

The composite of treatment-related complications are noted in Table 7. Two patients died of arterial hemorrhage related to pelvic necrosis and disruption of the hypogastric artery.

TABLE 4

Patients with Advanced Cervical Cancer Receiving Intraoperative Irradiation by Cancer Stage, Cell Type, and Status of Para-aortic Nodes

| | Number of patients | | | | |
| | Cell type | | Para-aortic node status[a] | | |
Stage	Squamous	Adenocarcinoma	Positive	Negative	Total
II	3	2	2	3	5
III-IV	10	1	9	2	11
Recurrent[b]	3	0	0	3	3
Total	16	3	11	8	19

[a] Three patients had therapy to site of recurrence only. Five patients with paraaortic nodes had 15 Gy to the para-aortic area as per Table 2.

[b] Patients had prior radiation therapy for cervical cancer, treatment given to recurrence in the pelvic sidewall.

TABLE 5

Patients with Advanced Cervical Cancer Receiving Intraoperative Irradiation, External and/or Intracavitary Radiation Therapy and Para-aortic Node Status

| | Para-aortic nodes (number of patients) | | |
	Positive	Negative	Total
Radiation therapy			
Total number of patients	11	8	19
Intraoperative irradiation			
Para-aortic nodes	11	5	16
Pelvic nodes/iliac nodes/parametria	6	2	8
Pelvic sidewall[a]	0	3	3
External irradiation			
Before intraoperative irradiation	0	3	3
After intraoperative irradiation	10	6	16
Intracavitary application[b]			
Single	2	0	2
Double	5	7	12

[a] Three patients with pelvic wall recurrence after radiation therapy for cervical cancer had only pelvic intraoperative irradiation.

[b] The three patients with recurrence had received prior treatment with intracavitary radium. Two other patients refused intracavitary cesium.

TABLE 6

Present Status of Patients with Advanced Cervical Cancer Receiving Intraoperative Irradiation

	Median survival (months)	Range (months)
+ Para-aortic nodes (11)[a]	17	10—36
− Para-aortic nodes (5)[b]	33	17—71

[a] Dead, one from causes other than cancer.

[b] Two N.E.D.

TABLE 7
Treatment-Related Complications

Complication	No. of incidents[a]
Arterial hemorrhage	2[b]
Pelvic abscess	1[b]
Radiation neuritis	2
Ureteral obstruction	1
Vena cava laceration	2
Leg edema	3
Prolonged ileus	2

[a] The first five complications listed occurred in only four patients.

[b] Three patients had fatal treatment complications. One was free of disease, one had a small volume of residual disease, and one was clinically free of disease without post-mortem confirmation.

When arterial embolization failed to control the bleeding in the first patient, laparotomy was performed. Extensive pelvic necrosis was present, and the completely disrupted right hypogastric artery was ligated near the defect, close to the common iliac artery. Necrosis of the sigmoid colon required resection and colostomy, and microscopic tumor was found in the specimen on pathologic examination. The patient later experienced a fatal recurrent hemorrhage. The second patient required ileocystostomy 8 months after IORT for left ureteral obstruction caused by extensive pelvic fibrosis. In 3 months, the patient suffered a vaginal hemorrhage that was incompletely controlled by arterial embolization; the bleeding persisted. She refused further treatment and died. Autopsy revealed rupture of the left hypogastric artery 5 mm below the common iliac bifurcation in an area adjacent to a necrotic lymph node. No tumor was present.

Two instances of neurologic injury occurred: one patient manifested a unilateral femoral nerve deficity, the other had severe pelvic pain and weakness of the legs. Neurologic evaluation resulted in a differential diagnosis of radiation neuritis vs. tumor involvement of the lumbar plexus. On exploration, no tumor was found, although extensive pelvic fibrosis was present. The left ureter was damaged in one patient during the difficult dissection and required reanastomosis. Persistent postoperative leakage occurred from a drain placed near the ureteral repair, even though a nephrostomy had been previously placed prior to reexploration. After 8 months, the patient died of sepsis related to a left pelvic abscess. She was still clinically free of cancer. A post-mortem examination was not obtained.

Two vena cava injuries and three instances of prolonged ileus were surgical complications unrelated to IORT per se.

Of note is the fact that the major complications observed were located primarily in the pelvis, where the IORT dose was combined with external beam irradiation and intracavitary irradiation (Figure 7).

Obviously, the additive radiation effect of all three modalities proved more toxic than anticipated.

The only treatment complications noted in the abdomen and the para-aortic region were vena cava lacerations and prolonged ileus which were surgically related.

XII. DISCUSSION

Conventional radiation therapy to the para-aortic lymph nodes has its limitations; it does not necessarily enhance survival, and it frequently results in complications in the gastroin-

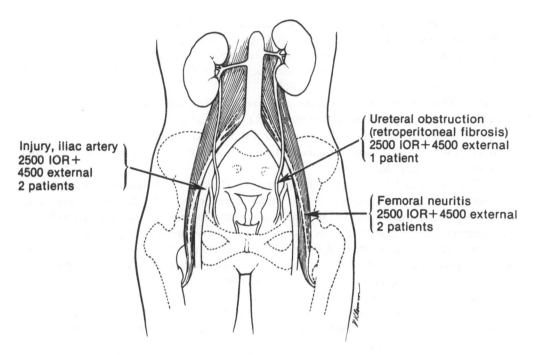

FIGURE 7. The major treatment-related complications were located in the pelvis, where IORT was combined with external beam irradiation and intracavitary ^{137}Cs irradiation.

testinal tract. The use of intraoperative electron beam irradiation permits irradiation of affected areas without including sensitive organs. With dissection of the retroperitoneal spaces in the para-aortic area, the intestines are retracted from the radiation field. The peritoneum lateral to the sigmoid is entered, and the paravesical, pararectal, and suprapubic spaces are identified; the dissection is then developed so that the sigmoid, rectum, and bladder can be retracted away from the radiation field separately on each pelvic sidewall. Thus, the pelvic organs are not irradiated intraoperatively, and external beam irradiation and intracavitary cesium therapy can be added to the treatment regimen. In this way, the areas of frequent failure, such as the pelvic lymph nodes and parametria, get additional radiation without affecting the rectosigmoid or bladder.

The original study design was directed solely toward the use of IORT electrons for the para-aortic lymph node chain. This was later modified to expand the application of IORT to the parametria and pelvic sidewall.

Analysis of the toxicities of treatment indicates a cluster of events in the pelvis when compared to the para-aortic region. When single-dose IORT was given to the para-aortic nodes alone there were no radiation-related complications. However, the combination of IORT electrons, external beam irradiation, and intracavitary irradiation to the pelvis proved to have a greater radiobiologic effect than anticipated. The preclinical animal studies were accurate for single-dose electrons to the structures of the retroperitoneum, but these data could not be extrapolated to the pelvic tissues.

Animal data have demonstrated aortic and vena caval tolerances of 30 to 40 Gy in a single dose. Two patients in our study died from hypogastric arterial disruption and hemorrhage related to vascular necrosis as a result of the combined treatment. This complication could be avoided by decreasing the amount of IORT given to the pelvic area when it is combined with additional external beam radiation therapy. One of these two patients was free of cancer; the other had a small amount of residual disease.

Atherosclerotic blood vessels in older patients with cervical cancer may be more sensitive to injury than normal tissues. The patients who had vascular and neurologic complications in this report received IORT doses of 15 to 25 Gy to these structures and additional doses of approximately 80 to 100 Gy derived from subsequent external beam and intracavitary therapy. Patients with histories of atherosclerotic vascular disease may represent a subset of patients at risk for late sequelae from IORT.

After a femoral nerve deficit was observed in one patient, thin lead shields have routinely been placed over the psoas muscles during IORT to protect the femoral nerve. Since then, no similar problems have occurred. The case of severe lumbar plexus neuropathy and ureteral obstruction were complications of radiation therapy from fibrosis of the pelvic sidewall, and each required surgical intervention.

Although the full biologic effects of single high-dose IORT treatment are not well understood, they appear to exceed those of similar doses delivered by standard fractionation.

Intraoperative irradiation used in conjunction with conventional fractionated irradiation has demonstrated a capacity to reduce large tumor volumes in this study. However, it did not appreciably alter the pattern of failure because all the patients who died of disease had persistent pelvic cancer with or without distant metastases. Unfortunately, only three patients had autopsy and/or laparotomy to determine the tumoricidal effects of IORT electrons on the para-aortic nodes. The rationale for investigating IORT in gynecology is to improve tumor control relative to treatment complications. The results of this study suggest that although it appears to assist in the local control of large tumors, a favorable effect on survival has not been demonstrated.

The substantial treatment-related morbidity that occurred clearly indicates the need for further basic investigation to determine the appropriate dose guidelines prior to future clinical studies.

REFERENCES

1. End Results in Cancer, Rep. No. 4, National Institute, U.S. Department of Health, Education and Welfare, 1972, 104.
2. **Buchsbaum, H. J.,** Paraaortic lymph node involvement in cervical carcinoma, *Am. J. Obstet. Gynecol.,* 113, 942, 1972.
3. **Wharton, J. T., Jones, H. W., III, Day, T. G., Jr. et al.,** Preirradiation celiotomy and extended field irradiation for invasive carcinoma of the cervix, *Obstet. Gynecol.,* 49, 333, 1977.
4. **Piver, M. S. and Barlow, J. J.,** Paraaortic lymphadenectomy, aortic node biopsy, and aortic lymphangiography in staging patients with advanced cervical cancer, *Cancer,* 32, 367, 1973.
5. **Averette, H. E., Dudan, R. C., and Ford, J. H.,** Exploratory celiotomy for surgical staging of cervical cancer, *Am. J. Obstet. Gynecol.,* 13, 1090, 1972.
6. **Delgado, G., Smith, J. P., and Ballantyne, A. J.,** Scalene node biopsy in carcinoma of the cervix: pelvic and paraaortic lymphadenectomy, *Cancer,* 35, 784, 1975.
7. **Delgado, G., Chun, B. K., Caglar, H., et al.,** Paraaortic lymphadenectomy in gynecologic malignancies confined to the pelvis, *Obstet. Gynecol.,* 50, 418, 1977.
8. **Nelson, J. H., Jr., Macassaet, M. A., Therese, L. et al.,** The incidence and significance of paraaortic lymph node metastases in late invasive carcinoma of the cervix, *Am. J. Obstet. Gynecol.,* 118, 749, 1974.
9. **Lepanto, P., Littman, P., Mikuta, J. et al.,** Treatment of paraaortic nodes in carcinoma of the cervix, *Cancer,* 35, 1510, 1975.
10. **Delgado, G., Caglar, H., and Walker, P.,** Survival and complications in cervical cancer treated by pelvic and extended field radiation after paraaortic lymphadenectomy, *Am. J. Roentgenol.,* 130, 141, 1978.
11. **Chism, S., Park, R., and Keys, H.,** Prospects for Paraaortic irradiation in treatment of cancer of the cervix, *Cancer,* 35, 1505, 1975.
12. **Goldson, A. L., Delgado, G., and Hill, L. T.,** Intraoperative radiation of the paraaortic nodes in cancer of the uterine cervix, *Obstet. Gynecol.,* 52, 713, 1978.
13. **Delgado, G., Goldson, A. L., Ashayeri, E., Hill, L. T., Petrilli, E. S., and Hatch, K. D.,** Intraoperative radiation in the treatment of advanced cervical cancer, *Obstet. Gynecol.,* 63, 246, 1984.

14. **Finsterer, H.,** Zur therapic inoperable magen and darmkarzinome mit freilegung and nachfolgen der rontgenbestrachlung, *Strahlentherapie,* 6, 205, 1915.

15. **Henschke, U. and Henschke, G.,** Zur technik der opertion-strahlung, *Strahlentherapie,* 74, 223, 1944.

16. **Fuchs, G. and Ueberal, R.,** Die intraoperative roentgentherapie des blasen Karzinoms, *Strahlentherapie,* 135, 280, 1969.

17. **Pack, G. and Livingston, E., Eds,** Palliative irradiation of gastric cancer, in *Treatment of Cancer and Allied Diseases,* Vol. 2, Hoeber, New York, 1940, 1100.

18. **Eloesser, L.,** The treatment of some abdominal cancers by irradiation through the open abdomen combined with cautery excision, *Ann. Surg.,* 106, 645, 1937.

19. **Beck, C.,** On external roentgen treatment of internal structures (eventration treatment), *N.Y. State J. Med.,* 90, 621, 1919.

20. **Abe, M., Takahashi, M., Yabumoto, E. et al.,** Clinical experiences with intraoperative radiotherapy of locally advanced cancers, *Cancer,* 45, 40, 1980.

21. **Abe, M. and Takahashi, M.,** Intraoperative radiotherapy: the Japanese experience, *Int. J. Radiat. Oncol. Biol. Phys.,* 7, 863, 1981.

22. **Goldson, A. L.,** Preliminary clinical experience with intraoperative radiotherapy, *J. Natl. Med. Assoc.,* 70, 493, 1978.

23. **Goldson, A. L.,** Past, present and future prospects of intraoperative radiotherapy (IORT), *Semin. Oncol.,* 8, 59, 1981.

24. **Goldson, A. L., Ashayeri, E., Jacobs, M., Nibhanupudy, J. R., Manning, J., and Streeter, O. E., Jr.,** Intraoperative Radiotherapy, Proc. Varian's Fourth European Clinac User's Meet., Malta, 1984, 99.

25. **Goldson, A. L., Streeter, O. E., Jr., Ashayeri, E., Collier-Manning, J., Barber, J., and Fan, K.,** Intraoperative radiotherapy for intracranial malignancies: a pilot study, *Cancer,* 54, (Suppl. 12), 2807, 1984.

26. **Goldson, A. L.,** Radiobiology of intraoperative electron beam therapy, in *Proc. of the Symp. on Electron Beam Therapy,* Chu, F. and Laughlin, J. S., Eds., Memorial Sloan-Kettering, New York, 1979, 139.

27. **Sindelar, W. F., Tepper, J., Travis, E. L. et al.,** Tolerance of retroperitoneal structures to intraoperative radiation, *Ann. Surg.,* 196, 601, 1982.

28. **Tepper, J., Sindelar, W., Travis, E. et al.,** Tolerance of canine anastomeses to intraoperative radiation therapy, *Int. J. Radiat. Oncol. Biol. Phys.,* 9, 1983.

29. **Gunderson, L. L., Tepper, J., Biggs, P. J., Goldson, A. L., Martin, J. K., McCullough, E. C., Rich, T. A., Sindelar, W. F., and Wood, W. C.,** Intraoperative ± external beam irradiation, *Curr. Prob. Cancer,* VII(11), 1983.

Chapter 23

INTRAOPERATIVE RADIATION THERAPY FOR COLORECTAL CANCER

Leonard L. Gunderson, J. Kirk Martin, Robert W. Beart, and Jennifer Fieck

TABLE OF CONTENTS

I. INTRODUCTION

External beam irradiation has been combined with surgical resection, chemotherapy, and/or immunotherapy for locally advanced colorectal cancer. When radiation is combined with surgery for residual disease after resection,[1-7] or for initially unresectable disease,[1-3,6-10] although local control and survival can be obtained in some patients, the risk of local recurrence is too high at 30 to 50%. No improvements in survival or local control were seen in a Mayo Clinic series that combined immunotherapy with irradiation.[6]

Both Massachusetts General Hospital (MGH)[11-13] and Mayo Clinic[13,14] have initiated pilot studies which add a boost dose with intraoperative irradiation therapy (IORT) using an electron beam in addition to the previous combinations of external beam irradiation and resection. This is an attempt to decrease local recurrence and improve survival with an acceptable risk of complications when compared to results achieved with external beam techniques.

The intent of this chapter is to discuss the indications for and results of aggressive combined techniques that include IORT. Results obtained with only external beam techniques ± resection will be discussed to demonstrate the need for higher doses of irradiation. Technical considerations and the results with IORT will be presented, and the potential for the future will be discussed.

II. EXTERNAL BEAM IRRADIATION ± RESECTION

A. PRIMARY IRRADIATION

The marked palliative and occasional curative value of radiation therapy for locally advanced colorectal lesions is evident in the literature. Good or excellent palliation is obtained in approximately 75% of patients with recurrence, but only an infrequent cure.[1,3,6,7,15] Although radiation therapy results seem to be better in patients with inoperable (surgical or medical) and/or residual carcinoma, there is need for improvement. Wang and Schulz obtained cures in 12.5% (2/16) of the inoperable group and 22% (2/19) of the group with partial resection.[1]

Cummings et al. presented a series from the Princess Margaret Hospital[16] in which a group of 123 patients had been treated with radical external beam irradiation without resection from 1970 to 1977 (preferred dose of 45 to 50 Gy in 2.5-Gy fractions, 5d/week — equivalent to approximately 55 to 60 Gy delivered in 1.8-Gy fractions). In the 67 patients who presented with tumor fixation, local control was achieved in only 6/67 (9%), and 5-year actuarial survival was only 2%.

In a recent Mayo Clinic series, 44 patients with locally advanced rectal cancer (7 unresectable, 7 resected but residual, 30 locally recurrent) received 50-Gy split-course pelvic irradiation with or without adjuvant immunotherapy.[6] In patients in whom the site of initial tumor progression could be evaluated, 28 of 31 (90.3%) experienced local progression within the radiation field, and in 17 (55%), it was the only site of disease.

B. RESECTION PLUS IRRADIATION (PRE- OR POSTOPERATIVE)

In the residual disease analyses from MGH[5] and Albert Einstein (AE),[2,4] the incidence of local failure (LF) after subtotal resection and external beam irradiation varied by the amount of residual disease — 50 to 52% (AE, 9/18; MGH, 12/23) if there was a gross residual vs. 15 to 30% (AE, 2/13; MGH, 9/30) if there was only microscopic residual. In the MGH analysis, a possible dose-response correlation was seen in the group with microscopic residual with an 11% LF risk (1/9) if the boost was ≥60 Gy and 33% (7/21) if the boost dose was ≤55 Gy. In patients with gross residual, a dose-response correlation could not be discerned.

In patients with disease that is unresectable for cure due to tumor fixation to an unresectable structure, a number of institutions have given preoperative radiotherapy in an attempt to shrink the lesion, allow resection, and possibly improve local control and survival.[3,6-10] Although 50 to 75% of such patients may have the disease resected after 45 to 50 Gy given over 5 to 6 weeks, the incidence of local recurrence in the resected group ranged from 35 to 45% in series from Tufts,[9] MGH,[10] and Oregon.[8] In the MGH analysis, patients whose disease was not resected after preoperative irradiation were all dead within 3 years. Long-term survival was seen in approximately 30% of those whose tumors were resected.

III. INTRAOPERATIVE AND EXTERNAL BEAM IRRADIATION ± RESECTION

In the U.S. IORT trials, some of the most favorable results have been obtained in patients who present with colorectal lesions that are unresectable for cure, have residual disease after resection, or have recurrent but localized disease. While this site was not emphasized in the Japanese trials,[17,18] some of the results have been encouraging. In a recent report of combined results from many institutions, 5 of 14 colon cancer patients were alive.[18] Of the eight colon patients described by Abe et al. (included in the combined analysis), one was alive and free of disease at 9 years and 8 months following treatment and one at 10 years, despite retroperitoneal invasion and unresected nodal disease in both.[17]

A total of 67 colorectal cancer patients have received IORT plus external beam irradiation during the tenure of the primary author (Gunderson) at either MGH or Mayo Clinic. Close interaction is necessary between the surgical and radiotherapy teams during both surgical exploration or resection as well as during IORT. Surgical and radiotherapy techniques utilized in both institutions have been discussed previously.[11-14] In the published MGH series, 32 patients had a minimum follow-up of 20 months.[12] All received 45 to 50 Gy in 1.8-Gy fractions, with multiple field external beam techniques and resection when feasible. In addition, all had an IORT electron beam boost of 10 to 15 Gy to the remaining tumor or tumor bed. In the Mayo Clinic series, 33 of 35 patients had surgical debulking of disease before or after similar external beam treatment. The IORT doses vary from 10 to 20 Gy depending on the amount of disease remaining after attempts at resection.[14]

The techniques employed in the IORT series allow the safe delivery of much higher effective doses of radiation than can be delivered with only external beam techniques. With external beam irradiation, the presence of dose-limiting organs, such as the small bowel, restricts doses to 45 to 50 Gy given in 25 to 28 fractions in many patients.[3,7,19,20] Even when the small bowel can be excluded, doses within boost fields are usually not carried beyond a combined dose of 60 to 70 Gy. The biologic effectiveness of single-dose irradiation is considered equivalent to two to three times that quantity of fractionated external beam treatment.[21] In view of that, the effective dose in the IORT field, when added to the 45 to 50 Gy delivered in 25 to 28 fractions with external beam techniques, is 65 to 80 Gy for an IORT dose of 10 Gy, 75 to 95 Gy with a 15-Gy boost, and 85 to 110 Gy with a 20-Gy IORT dose.

A. SURVIVAL

In the MGH group of 32 patients treated with IORT combined with external beam irradiation,[12] survival has been higher than that seen in previous series of MGH patients treated with external beam techniques with or without resection.[7,10] In the seven patients with residual disease who received IORT, although five of seven had gross residual disease after resection, survival paralleled that of patients treated with external beam therapy for microscopic residual disease.[12] In ongoing IORT trials at MGH,[13] survival in the group of patients who present with recurrence is stable at approximately 30% between 3 and 4 years

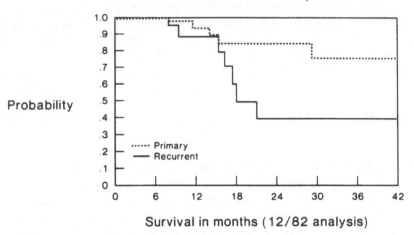

FIGURE 1. Survival results at MGH for locally advanced rectal cancer patients treated with external beam X-ray therapy and IORT electron boost with or without resection, primary (N = 24) vs. recurrent disease (N = 17) presentation (analysis performed December 1982). (From Gunderson, L. L. et al., *Curr. Prob. Cancer*, 7, 55, 1983. With permission.)

(Figure 1), in contrast to an expected long-term survival of 5 to 10% when treated with standard techniques.[1,3,7] The poorer survival in the recurrent vs. primary disease presentation is due to a higher incidence of both local and systemic failure in the group of patients with recurrent disease. In the residual disease and recurrent disease patients, survival improvements with IORT plus external irradiation may be due in part to case selection, since patients who were found to have metastasis prior to or at the time of exploration did not receive the IORT boost, and their survival is not reflected in the survival curves. The marked improvement in local control that can be achieved with the aggressive IORT approaches, however, could also be responsible for the improvement in survival.

The results from the group of 16 IORT patients from MGH with initially unresectable disease[12] are the most intriguing, since patients were selected in similar fashion to a previous group of patients treated with only preoperative irradiation and resection.[10] Survival curves revealed a statistical advantage for the group who received the IORT boost that does not appear to be due to a difference in case selection (Figure 2). More patients in the IORT group had surgical transection of tumor in spite of preoperative irradiation and resection (4/16 vs 1/14). Gross disease persisted beyond the muscularis propria in 75% of the specimens in both groups.

In the Mayo Clinic IORT series of 35 patients survival results parallel those achieved at MGH (Figure 3); 25 of 35 (66%) are alive with 19 (54%) free of disease (Table 1). Of the 12 who expired, 3 had no evidence of disease progression. Disease progression has occurred in only 2/9 (22%) who received high-dose preoperative irradiation (50 Gy in 28 fractions) vs. 10/24 (42%) when resection preceded the high dose irradiation.

B. FAILURE PATTERNS
1. Local Control

In published MGH trials, local control appears to be improved in both those patients with residual disease and those with initially unresectable disease who received an IORT boost[12] vs. those who received only external beam irradiation[5,10] (Table 2). Most local regrowths in the MGH IORT series have appeared in patients who presented with recurrence or those who had gross residual disease after partial resection.

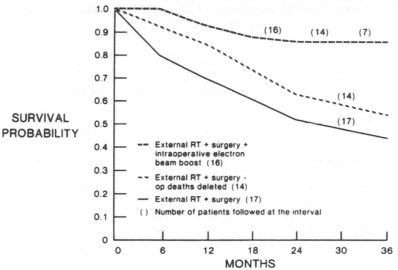

FIGURE 2.   Comparison of crude survival for combination of resection and external beam irradiation vs. resection plus external beam and intraoperative irradiation for patients with disease that is unresectable for cure due to disease fixation (Curve 1 vs 3 — p <.01 to .025 dependent on method of calculation; Curve 1 vs. 2 — p <.05 to 0.1) (From Gunderson, L. L., Cohen, A. M., Dosoretz, D. E., Shipley, W. U., Hedberg, S. E., Wood, W. C., Rodkey, G. V., and Suit, H. D., *Int. J. Radiat. Oncol. Biol. Phys.*, 9, 1601, 1983. With permission.)

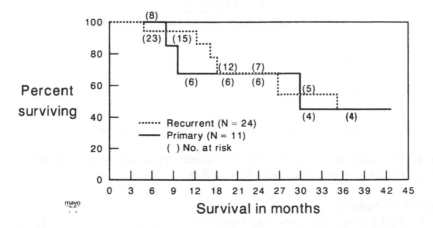

FIGURE 3.   Kaplan-Meier survival curve of 35 patients with locally advanced colorectal cancer treated with external beam and intraoperative irradiation at Mayo Clinic (analysis performed March 1985).

In the Mayo Clinic series, the single central failure (CF — within IORT field) and three of four LFs (in external beam field) have occurred in patients who presented with recurrent disease. The fourth LF occurred within an area of inital tumor fixation that was resected with negative but narrow margins and received 50 Gy in 28 fractions external beam therapy,

TABLE 1

Survival and Disease Status, Colorectal IORT Plus External Beam Therapy, Mayo Clinic

Disease category (number of patients)	Alive		Dead	
	NED[a]	Failure	NED[a]	DOD[a]
	No (%)	No. (%)	No. (%)	No. (%)
Primary (11)				
Resected, residual (9)	5(56)	0	1(11)	3(33)
Unresectable for cure				
Resected after XRT[a] (2)	2	0	0	0
Recurrent (24)				
Resected, residual (17)	9(53)	3(18)	1(6)	4(24)
Unresectable for cure (7)	4(57)	0	1(14)	2(29)[b]
Resected after XRT[a] (5)	3	0	0	2[b]
Never resected (2)	1	0	1	0
Total 35	19(54)	4(11)	3(9)	9(26)

Note: Analysis performed March 1985.

[a] NED = no evidence of disease; DOD = died of disease; XRT = X-ray therapy.
[b] One patient received only 25.2 Gy preoperative due to a previous course of external beam irradiation.

TABLE 2

Local Failure vs. Treatment Method for Locally Advanced Primary Colorectal Cancer, MGH[5,10,12]

	Method of irradiation		
	External beam alone		External beam & IORT[a]
	Number at risk	Percent local failure	
Partial resection			0/7
Microscopic residual	30	30%	
Gross residual	23	52%	
Resected after preoperative irradiation	27	43%	0/16

[a] Five of seven patients with partial resection of tumor had gross residual cancer.

but no IORT. Although 23 of 33 evaluable patients presented with recurrent disease, the total local failure rate thus far is only 12% (4/33)

2. Distant Metastases

In the IORT series from both MGH and Mayo Clinic, systemic failure has been more common in patients when surgery preceded high-dose preoperative irradition. In the MGH series,[12] in patients who presented with primary disease, the comparative systemic failure incidence was 3/6 (50%) vs. 2/16 (12.5%) — systemic failure was a possibility, but not proven in a third patient — maximum 3/16 (19%). That trend is also seen in the Mayo Clinic series in Table 3 (DM or PS in 10/24 or 42% when surgery preceded irradiation vs. 2/9 or 22%). Whether the lower incidence is due to a different treatment sequence (i.e., preoperative irradiation may alter implantability of cells spread at time of resection) or is due to a difference in case selection cannot be ascertained, as choice of treatment sequence was not controlled in either series.

TABLE 3
Colorectal Disease Category Versus Failure, Mayo Clinic, IORT Plus
External Beam Therapy

Disease category	Number of patients	No. of failures (percent)	Patterns of failure (any component)			
			CF	LF	DM	PS
Resected, residual	24	10(42)				
Primary	8[a]	3	0	1[b]	3	0
Recurrent	16[a]	7	1[c]	2[c]	5	2[c]
Unresectable-resected after XRT	7	2(29)	0	0	0	0
Primary	2	0	0	0	0	0
Recurrent	5	2	0	1[d]	2	0
Recurrent-unresectable after XRT	2	0	0	0	0	0
Totals	33(35)[a]	12(36)	1(3)	4(12)	10(30)	2(6)

Note: CF = central failure; LF = local failure; DM = distant metastasis; PS = peritoneal
seeding. Analysis performed March 1985.

[a] 33 of 35 patients evaluable for patterns of failure — deleted are two patients who died of
intercurrent disease with no evidence of cancer at 1 and 3 months.
[b] LF in area of initial tumor fixation to posterior abdominal wall that was resected and
received 50.4 Gy in 28 fractions with external beam irradiation but no IORT.
[c] One patient had CF, LF, and PS (received only 10 Gy by IORT boost).
[d] Received only 25.2 Gy in 14 fractions by external beam irradiation as had been treated
previously with external beam irradiation.

C. MORBIDITY

A significant increase in soft tissue complications has not been encountered in the MGH
series of patients who received an IORT boost in comparison to patients with similar disease
extent treated with external beam irradiation alone.[22] Some problems with delayed wound
healing have been encountered in IORT patients that developed an infection in the pelvis
or a perineal wound after preoperative irradiation and abdominoperineal resection.[12-14,22]
Neither the magnitude nor the incidence of such problems was increased when compared
with patients treated with only preoperative irradiation and resection at MGH[10,22] or at other
institutions. The healing problems are presumably related to the advanced stage of the tumor
growth or regrowth (10 of the initial 32 MGH patients and 24 of the 35 Mayo Clinic patients
presented with recurrence), the difficulty of the surgical resection or reresection, and the
aggressive radiation therapy.

Problems with delayed pelvic pain have occurred in both the MGH and Mayo Clinic
series, but have been reversible in most patients. It is uncertain whether this finding is a
result of radiation fibrosis, neuropathy, or a combination. The exact incidence and severity
is being evaluated as a function of disease presentation, extent of surgery, and combined
dose of IORT and external beam irradiation. Motor deficits have been rare in contrast to a
recent report from the National Cancer Institute.[23]

IV. CONCLUSIONS AND FUTURE POSSIBILITIES

The long-term results of an aggressive treatment approach for locally advanced colorectal
malignancies (initially unresectable, residual after resection, and local recurrence) are dependent on the metastatic potential of the tumor at the treated site. Distant failures in the

MGH and Mayo Clinic series were most common in patients who presented with recurrent disease or had partial resection of primary disease prior to moderate-dose external beam irradiation. With both primary and recurrent disease, it may be preferable to deliver the external irradiation prior to an attempted resection and IORT boost (deliver 45 to 50 Gy in 25 to 28 fractions; restage approximately 4 weeks later, do partial or gross total removal, and give IORT boost if feasible). Theoretical advantages of this sequence include: (1) potential alteration in implantability of cells that may be disseminated at the time of partial surgical resection (spread of cells probably more likely in patients with gross transection of tumor); (2) can delete patients found to have metastases at the restaging workup or at laparotomy and spare them the potential risks of an IORT boost; and (3) the interval between external and intraoperative irradiation is less apt to be prolonged. If the resection and IORT boost are the initial phase of treatment and the patient develops postoperative complications, the interval to the start of external irradiation may be prolonged to the degree that the combined IORT plus external doses do not have an additive antitumor effect, but only an additive effect on normal structures (i.e., added risk but no potential gain).

While the aggressive local treatment approaches outlined in this chapter appear to be appropriate, treatment of the liver and/or peritoneal cavity with intraperitoneal chemotherapy or radiocolloids, infusion chemotherapy, external beam radiation, or combinations may be necessary in the subsets of patients whose tumors have high metastatic potential. If either infusion chemotherapy of the liver[24,25] or intraperitoneal chemotherapy decrease the incidence of liver metastases in ongoing trials with colon cancer, it would be worthwhile to consider the same approach with locally advanced rectal cancer.

The potential for improvements in local control ± survival with radiation therapy is considerable when used both externally and as an intraoperative boost in colorectal lesions which are initially unresectable (later resection whenever feasible) or have resection but residual disease. Even with locally recurrent lesions, the aggressive multimodality approaches have resulted in long-term survival of 30 to 40% vs. an expected 5 to 10% result with conventional techniques. Randomized trials will be needed to compare standard treatment to treatment which includes an IORT boost to see if previous observed differences are true advantages or are merely due to differences in case selection.

V. ACKNOWLEDGMENTS

The authors appreciate the effort of Julie Boland and the Mayo Clinic Typing Service for assistance in the preparation of this manuscript. L. L. Gunderson and J. K. Martin were supported in part by the National Cancer Institute, Contract CM-27528.

REFERENCES

1. **Wang, C. C. and Schulz, M. D.,** The role of radiation therapy in the management of carcinoma of the sigmoid, rectosigmoid, and rectum, *Radiology,* 79, 1, 1962.
2. **Turner, S. S., Vieira, E. F., Ager, P. J., Alpert, S., Efrow, G., Ragins, H., Weil, P., and Ghossein, N. A.,** Elective postoperative radiotherapy for locally advanced colorectal cancer, *Cancer,* 40, 105, 1977.
3. **Gunderson, L. L., Cohen, A. M., and Welch, C. W.,** Residual, inoperable, or recurrent colorectal cancer: surgical radiotherapy interaction, *Am. J. Surg.,* 139, 518, 1980.
4. **Ghossein, N. A., Samala, E. C., Alpert, S., Bosworth, J. L., and Turner, S. S.,** Results of postoperative radiotherapy in patients who had incomplete resection of a colorectal cancer, *Dis. Colon Rectum,* 24, 252, 1981.
5. **Allee, P. E., Tepper, J. E., Gunderson, L. L., and Munzenrider, J. E.,** Postoperative radiation therapy for incompletely resected colorectal carcinoma. *Int. J. Radiat. Oncol. Biol. Phys.,* in press.

6. **O'Connell, M. J., Childs, D. S., Moertel, C. G. et al.,** A prospective controlled evaluation of combined pelvic radiotherapy and methanol extraction residue of BCG (MER) for locally unresectable or recurrent rectal carcinoma, *Int. J. Radiat. Oncol. Biol. Phys.,* 8, 1115, 1982.

7. **Gunderson, L. L., Rich, T. A., Tepper, J. E., Dosoretz, D. E., Russell, A. H., and Hoskins, R. B.,** Large bowel cancer: utility of radiation therapy, in *Gastrointestinal Malignancy,* DeCosse, J. J. and Sherlock, P., Eds., Martinus Nijhoff, Boston, 1984, 189.

8. **Stevens, K. R., Allen, C. V., and Fletcher, W. S.,** Preoperative radiotherapy for adenocarcinoma of the rectosigmoid, *Cancer,* 37, 2866, 1976.

9. **Emami, B., Pilepich, M., Willett, C., Munzenrider, J. E., and Miller, H. H.,** Management of unresectable colorectal carcinoma (preoperative radiotherapy and surgery), *Int. J. Radiat. Oncol. Biol. Phys.,* 8, 1295, 1982.

10. **Dosoretz, D. E., Gunderson, L. L., Hoskins, B., Hedberg, S. E., Shipley, W. U., Blitzer, P. H., and Cohen, A. M.,** Preoperative irradiation for localized carcinoma of the rectum and rectosigmoid: patterns of failure, survival, and future treatment strategies, *Cancer,* 52, 818, 1983.

11. **Gunderson, L. L., Shipley, W. U., Suit, H. D., Epp, E. R., Nardi, G., Wood, W., Cohen, A., Nelson, J., Battit, G., Biggs, P. J., Russell, A., Rockett, A., and Clark, D.,** Intraoperative irradiation: a pilot study combining external beam irradiation with "boost" dose intraoperative electrons, *Cancer,* 49, 2259, 1982.

12. **Gunderson, L. L., Cohen, A. M., Dosoretz, D. E., Shipley, W. U., Hedberg, S. E., Wood, W. C., Rodkey, G. V., and Suit, H. D.,** Residual, unresectable, or recurrent colorectal cancer: external beam irradiation and intraoperative electron beam boost ± resection, *Int. J. Radiat. Oncol. Biol. Phys.,* 9, 1597, 1983.

13. **Gunderson, L. L., Tepper, J. E., Biggs, P. J., Goldson, A., Martin, J. K., McCullough, E. C., Rich, T. A., Shipley, W. U., Sindelar, W. F., and Wood, W. C.,** Intraoperative ± external beam irradiation, *Curr. Prob. Cancer,* 7, 1, 1983.

14. **Gunderson, L. L., Martin, J. K., Earle, J. D., Byer, D., Voss, M., Fieck, J., Kvols, L., Rorie, D., Martinez, A., Nagorney, D. M., O'Connell, M. J., and Weber, F.,** Intraoperative and external beam irradiation ± resection: Mayo pilot experience, *Mayo Clin. Proc.,* 59, 691, 1984.

15. **Gunderson, L. L., Tepper, J. E., Dosoretz, D. E., Kopelson, G., Hoskins, R. B., Rich, T. A., and Russell, A. H.,** Patterns of failure after treatment of gastrointestinal cancer, *Cancer Treat. Symp.,* 2, 181, 1983.

16. **Cummings, B. J., Rider, W. D., Harwood, A. R., Keane, T. J., and Thomas, G. M.,** External beam radiation therapy for adenocarcinoma of the rectum, *Dis. Colon Rectum,* 26, 30, 1983.

17. **Abe, M., Takahasi, M., Yabumoto, E., Adachi, H., Yoshii, M., and Mori, K.,** Clinical experience with intraoperative radiotherapy of locally advanced cancers, *Cancer,* 45, 40, 1980.

18. **Abe, M. and Takahashi, M.,** Intraoperative radiotherapy: the Japanese experience, *Int. J. Radiat. Oncol. Biol. Phys.,* 5, 863, 1981.

19. **Gunderson, L. L., Meyer, J. E., Sheedy, P., and Munzenrider, J. E.,** Radiation oncology. XVIII, in *Alimentary Tract Radiology,* 3rd ed., Margulis, A. R. and Burhenne, H. J., Eds., C. V. Mosby, St. Louis, 1983, 2409.

20. **Gunderson, L. L., Russell, A. H., Llewellyn, H. T., Doppke, K. P., and Tepper, J. E.,** Treatment planning for colorectal cancer: radiation and surgical techniques and value of small bowel films, *Int. J. Radiat. Oncol. Biol. Phys.,* 11, 1379, 1985.

21. **Suit, H. D.,** Radiation biology: a basis for radiotherapy, in *Textbook of Radiotherapy,* 2nd ed., Fletcher, G. H., Ed., Lea & Febiger, Philadelphia, 1973, 75.

22. **Tepper, J. E., Gunderson, L. L., Orlow, E., Cohen, A. M., Hedberg, S. E., Shipley, W. U., Blitzer, P. H., and Rich, T.,** Complications of intraoperative radiation therapy, *Int. J. Radiat. Oncol. Biol. Phys.,* 10, 1831, 1984.

23. **Sindelar, W. F., Kinsella, T. J., Hoekstra, P. et al.,** Treatment complications in intraoperative radiotherapy, *Int. J. Radiat. Oncol. Biol. Phys.,* 11, 117, 1985.

24. **Taylor, I., Rowling, J. and West, C.,** Adjuvant cytotoxic liver perfusion for colorectal cancer, *Br. J. Surg.,* 66, 833, 1979.

25. **Taylor, I., Machin, D., Mullee, M., Trotter, G., Cooke, T., and West, C.,** A randomized controlled trial of adjuvant portal vein cytotoxic perfusion in colorectal cancer, *Br. J. Surg.,* 72, 359, 1985.

Chapter 24

INTRAOPERATIVE RADIATION THERAPY OF SOFT TISSUE SARCOMAS

Joel E. Tepper, William C. Wood, and Herman D. Suit

TABLE OF CONTENTS

I. INTRODUCTION

There has been substantial interest shown in the use of electron beams intraoperatively for the treatment of soft tissue sarcomas, primarily retroperitoneal sarcomas, at the Massachusetts General Hosptial (MGH) and the National Cancer Institute (NCI). Because of the rarity of this tumor, however, experience has been limited. In addition to the interest in the treatment of retroperitoneal sarcomas, there has been some experience from a number of Japanese centers in the treatment of extremity sarcomas where intraoperative radiation therapy (IORT) has been used after surgical resection.

II. RESULTS OF CLINICAL TRIALS

Abe et al.[1] have reported results from 28 patients who were treated at 7 Japanese institutions. At the time of the report, 21 of the 28 patients were alive, with 5 of the 21 patients having survived for greater than 5 years. The major advantage of this approach over external beam irradiation is the ability to keep overlying skin out of the radiation field. The radiation was given in a single dose of 30 to 40 Gy. Field size ranged from a 3-cm circle to large rectangular fields of 12 cm. There was no component of treatment given by fractionated external beam techniques. A substantial number of these patients had residual disease at the time of the delivery of IORT. Local control was obtained in 73% (11/15) of the patients. This percentage is quite good considering that many patients were treated for recurrent disease and with gross residual after surgery.

There is also a trial on the use of IORT for retroperitoneal soft tissue sarcomas at NCI. Previous trials at the NCI of surgical resection plus high-dose postoperative external beam radiation (>50 Gy) had shown a high level of toxicity.[2]

In their recent phase III trial, patients were randomized to IORT or no IORT after maximum surgical resection. The IORT dose was generally 20 Gy and was combined with the hypoxic cell sensitizer misonidazole. Patients randomized to IORT received an additional postoperative external beam dose of 30 to 40 Gy given with conventional fractionation. In the control arm, the surgical resection was followed by postoperative radiation therapy to doses of 44 to 55 Gy. Preliminary evaluation shows a 5-year survival of approximately 45%, with no obvious difference between the two treatment groups either in survival or disease-free survival. There is also no clear difference in local recurrence rates, although the local failure was slightly less in the patients treated with IORT.[3]

The complications of therapy were generally acceptable. One major concern was that five patients in the IORT group developed significant neuropathy with pain and paresthesia that has persisted over a substantial length of time. All of these patients had tumors that were close to the nerves producing the neuropathy and received the full radiation dose. It is not clear that the toxicity was strictly related to the IORT and not to a combination of the treatment modalities, including surgical resection, external beam irradiation, and misonidazole. One patient developed a sacral osteonecrosis and one had a vertebral body fracture, although it is not clear that this was caused by IORT. The patients have acutely tolerated these radiation treatments very well despite the fact that the field sizes were extremely large and often encompassed an entire hemiabdomen and required adjoining fields. For this abuttment, the group at the NCI has used an applicator which they call the "squircle", which has one half of the applicator rectangular and the other portion circular. This allows for ease in field matching without having to block with lead at one end of the field.

Gunderson et al.[4] of the Mayo Clinic had treated seven patients as of April 1984. Of these seven, five were alive, three without evidence of disease. Four of the seven patients had recurrent disease which was partially resected; two had primary and unresectable sarcoma; and one patient had a primary sarcoma which was partially resected. The follow-up in this series is still short, but it indicates some ability to control even recurrent sarcomas with IORT.

At the MGH, 20 patients with sarcoma of soft tissues have had IORT as a component of their treatment. In most patients, IORT was judged to be the only reasonable option to deliver a high radiation dose. As has been true with other tumor categories at the MGH, IORT has been used as a supplement to the other therapeutic modalities. Thus, in all the patients, IORT has been combined with high-dose external beam radiation therapy and surgical resection if feasible. For the retroperitoneal tumors, which constitute the majority of the sarcomas treated with IORT, we have delivered 40 to 50 Gy preoperatively. We favor the preoperative approach for a number of reasons. First, a high-dose preoperative regimen sterilizes a large percentage of tumor cells. As the resection of these tumors is virtually always marginal, the preoperative treatment decreases the likelihood of tumor seeding in the peritoneal cavity at resection and minimizes the importance of a "microscopic" tumor cut-through. Second, there is often some decrease in the size of the mass and some pseudoencapsulation of the tumor which facilitates the surgical resection. Occasionally, an unresectable tumor becomes resectable. Third, and perhaps most important, the external beam radiation can be delivered both more effectively and with better patient tolerance when delivered preoperatively. In most of the patients the primary retroperitoneal sarcoma is large (10 cm). Irradiation of the tumor bed postresection means that the stomach and the small and large intestine may have moved into the region where the tumor was previously located. In addition, there may be some normal tissues, such as the small bowel, which were previously adherent to the tumor, but following preoperative radiation treatments may have been freed from the tumor and not require resection. If treated preoperatively, adherent small bowel may not be in the radiation field. When using preoperative irradiation, the very large tumor mass acts to push much of the normal tissue outside of the treatment volume. Thus, it is usually quite feasible to give daily doses of 1.8 Gy with excellent tolerance. This usually cannot be done postoperatively.

We have generally treated patients with one fraction per day through AP-PA portals, as the tumor usually extends from the retroperitoneal surface to the anterior abdominal wall. Hence, normal tissue sparing may not be obtained with lateral fields. At times, we have found oblique fields helpful to minimize the dose to normal structures such as the spinal cord and kidney. Patients are given approximately 4 weeks rest after the external beam irradiation (40 to 50 Gy) prior to the surgical resection. IORT as a single dose of 15 Gy is given to the tumor bed if there is no gross residual tumor; 20 Gy is delivered if gross residual is present.

The anatomic sites of sarcoma among the 20 patients who received IORT at the MGH through July 1, 1986 were as follows: extremities, 5; chest cavity, 2; and retroperitoneum, 13. As of August 1986, 8 of the 20 patients have died and 10 developed tumor recurrence. Two patients have developed failure within the radiation field; in both patients, the tumor was unresectable at the time of IORT. Nine patients have developed distant metastatic disease (one patient had both local and distant disease recurrence). One patient with distant metastatic disease had resection of the metastases and is now without evidence of tumor.

In the patients treated to date, the actuarial survival rate is 60% at 3 years and 39% at 5 years, with actuarial disease-free survival of 38 and 37% at 3 and 5 years, respectively. The actuarial local control rate at 5 years is 80%, despite the very large size of these tumors. This compares to a 5-year local control rate of 54% in a historical series of retroperitoneal sarcomas treated with surgery and external beam irradiation from MGH.[5] Complications have generally been minor and easily solved. One patient had difficulty in wound healing, but that patient was also on Adriamycin® chemotherapy. One patient developed a late bowel obstruction which required surgical resection. One of the patients with a chest sarcoma developed postoperative pneumonitis (which was thought not to be related to the IORT) and subsequently died of this complication.

III. SUMMARY

Despite the fact that there is not at present a large amount of information available, there is reason for encouragment in the treatment of soft tissue sarcomas with IORT. Japanese data indicate a high local control rate in a group of patients with recurrent and residual disease after surgical resection. The data from the MGH and the NCI indicate that IORT at a dose of 15 to 25 Gy can be tolerated in large areas of the retroperitoneum and can be combined with substantial surgical resections. The NCI phase III trial does not allow conclusions regarding the efficacy of IORT compared to external beam therapy and surgical resection. The MGH data are showing a lower local failure rate than a historical trial of surgical resection and external beam irradiation for retroperitoneal sarcomas. As is true in other sites, the major advantage of IORT is likely to be in combination with surgical resection and external beam radiation therapy. Because of the relative rarity of these tumors, it is very likely that formal randomized studies will require a multiple-institution collaborative effort.

REFERENCES

1. **Abe, M. and Takahashi, M.,** Intraoperative radiotherapy: the Japanese experience, *Int. J. Radiat. Oncol. Biol. Phys.,* 7, 863, 1981.
2. **Glen, J., Sindelar, W. F., Kinsella, T., Glatstein, E., Tepper, J. E., Costa, J., and Baker, A.,** Results of multimodality therapy of resectable soft-tissue sarcomas of the retroperitoneum, *Surgery,* 97, 316, 1985.
3. **Kinsella, T., Sindelar, W., Glatstein, E., and Rosenberg, S.,** Preliminary results of a prospective randomized trial of intraoperative (IORT) and low dose external beam radiotherapy vs high dose external beam radiotherapy as adjunctive therapy in resectable soft tissue sarcomas of the retroperitoneum, *Int. J. Radiat. Oncol. Biol. Phys.,* 12, 183, 1986.
4. **Gunderson, L., Martin, J. K., Earle, J., Byer, D. E., Voss, M., Fieck, J. M., Kvols, L. K., Rorie, D., Martinez, A., Nagorney, D. M., O'Connell, M. J., and Weber, F. C.,** Intraoperative and external beam irradiation with or without resection: Mayo pilot experience, *Mayo Clin. Proc.,* 59, 691, 1984.
5. **Tepper, J. E., Suit, H., Wood, W. C., Proppe, K. H., Harmon, D., and McNulty, P.,** Radiation therapy of retroperitoneal soft tissue sarcomas, *Int. J. Radiat. Oncol. Biol. Phys.,* 10, 825, 1984.

Chapter 25

INTRAOPERATIVE RADIATION THERAPY AT THE MASSACHUSETTS GENERAL HOSPITAL

Joel E. Tepper, William U. Shipley, William C. Wood, Andrew L. Warshaw, and George L. Nardi

TABLE OF CONTENTS

I. INTRODUCTION

The Massachusetts General Hospital (MGH) was the second institution in the U.S. to begin using intraoperative radiation therapy (IORT), with treatments beginning in 1978. Throughout this time there has been a standard philosophy of using IORT as a boost radiation dose, supplemented in all cases by high-dose external beam radiation therapy and, in situations where it was feasible, by surgical resection. Never did we think it advisable to use IORT as the sole primary treatment. There are inherent radiobiological limitations to the use of IORT because there is no opportunity for hypoxic cells to reoxygenate between radiation fractions, and because there will be a substantial number of cells in a relatively radioresistant phase of the cell cycle when single dose radiation is employed. The major advantage of IORT is to avoid giving radiation doses that are beyond those tolerated by normal tissues. As most normal tissues (such as the small bowel, colon, or stomach) will tolerate doses in the range of 45 Gy, it seemed advisable to take full advantage of the reoxygenation of cells, and redistribution of cells in the cell cycle that can be obtained with external beam fractionated radiation, as well as the wide field coverage best accomplished by this modality.

At MGH, we have had to transport patients from the operating room to the radiation therapy department for IORT. Because of this logistic limitation we have been limited to using IORT on one patient per week. Because of this, we have made a conscious effort to treat only a few defined anatomic sites so that worthwhile information could be obtained rather than having a smattering of cases available at a wide variety of sites.

II. TECHNIQUE

We have used IORT solely with high-energy electrons. We utilize a Varian® Clinac-35 linear accelerator for all treatments. A thorough physics evaluation and workup of the Clinac-35 has been described by Biggs et al.[1] Modifications have included the addition of a special collimation system on the head of the linear accelerator to try to maximize the quality of the electron dose distribution.

We have available a large collection of Lucite® applicators, including circular applicators with internal diameters ranging from 4 to 9 cm. We also found it helpful to have beveled edges available on a number of applicators, the most useful bevels being those of 15 and 30°. These have been necessary for obtaining a good approximation of the end of the treatment applicator on the tumor volume. We also used elliptical applicators of various sizes and found them to be quite helpful. Although rectangular applicators are also available, we have found these less useful as it can be difficult to place a large rectangle (with squared off corners) inside an abdominal incision. As is true for many other institutions, we have used a sliding applicator system, so that the Lucite® applicator extends into an aluminum tube attached to the accelerator head. In our system there is a hole in the side of the applicator into which instruments can be inserted. This hole does not affect the electron dosimetry significantly and allows one to insert suction devices or light sources and to manipulate the area inside the applicator. It is also useful for insertion of a side-mounted perioscope through which the entire field can be visualized after the treatment applicator is in the final position.

We have found it essential for a thorough physics evaluation to be made of the IORT equipment. The physics evaluation has included a determination of the applicator ratio (given dose per monitor unit) for each applicator and for each electron energy. Measurements have also been made of the surface dose so that there is no underdosing of the most superficial tissues. For energies greater than 9 meV, the surface dose is not a problem, since our tumor doses are quoted at the 90% isodose line; and the surface dose at higher energies is generally 90% or greater. We also made in-depth determinations of the dose fall-off, and the full beam profiles and isodose curves have been documented. One must be aware that the effective field width (distance between 90% isodose lines across the field) is less than the actual applicator size, and this must be taken into consideration when prescribing the radiation dose, in addition to the flatness and symmetry of the beam at various depths and energies.

The general technique for tumors, such as locally advanced rectal carcinoma, has been to deliver high-dose preoperative radiation therapy to approximately 50 Gy, which is completed approximately 4 weeks prior to the surgery.[2] The patient is then taken to the operating room with the intent of doing a surgical resection whenever feasible. For most tumors (not including pancreatic adenocarcinoma) we have encouraged the surgeons to perform a resection, even if it is thought that there will be some gross residual disease left. This is done because we believe the likelihood of local control with radiation therapy will be maximized if the bulk of the tumor is resected. As patients have received high-dose preoperative irradiation, the risk of tumor seeding from the surgical procedure should be small. Patients with pancreatic carcinoma have generally had low-dose preoperative radiation therapy. We have not thought it feasible to combine high-dose external beam radiation therapy plus pancreaticoduodenectomy with IORT.

After the completion of the resection, but before anastomoses are performed, the patient is evaluated for IORT. Areas of known gross or microscopic residual disease or areas at very high risk for microscopic residual are determined both from adherence noted during the surgical resection and by a review of the pathological specimen. Often biopsies for frozen section evaluation are taken from circumferential margins or other areas that are thought to be at high risk for residual tumor. For rectal carcinoma, these are typically located on the sacrum or on the pelvic sidewall. The surgeon and the radiation therapist then define the exact applicator size and the approach that is most appropriate. For most abdominal tumors a direct anterior abdominal approach is used. However, after an abdominal-perineal resection, a perineal approach is sometimes most appropriate to irradiate a distally located tumor. When selecting the appropriate applicator, we are very careful in excluding normal structures not at risk for tumor involvement from the radiation field. For pelvic tumors, the normal tissues of greatest concern are the ureters and small bowel — which has a tendency to move down into the radiation field. One must also be certain that the rectum is adequately removed from the field (after low anterior resection) and that bladder irradiation is minimized (for anterior pelvic tumors). For tumors in the upper abdomen, one must consider the radiosensitivity of small bowel, stomach, kidney, ureters, and spinal cord. Previous radiobiologic studies have shown that ureters and bile ducts are relatively sensitive to high single doses, and these structures may need to be mobilized to avoid irradiation. If it is thought that a ureter is involved with tumor, we then irradiate the ureter with the understanding that late fibrosis or stricture will likely occur. Occasionally, strips of lead are cut and inserted into the radiation field to protect normal tissues which are not easily moved out of the field. A determination is made of the depth of the tissue at risk for gross or microsopic tumor residual so that the appropriate electron energy can be chosen.

The patient is then prepared for transportation to the radiation therapy department. After hemostasis has been obtained, the abdomen is closed with stay sutures and is covered with a plastic adhesive sterile drape. Additional sterile drapes are placed over the patient, and he is then transferred to a Surgi-Lift® stretcher and switched to portable anesthesia equipment. The radiation therapy department room has previously been prepared so that it can act effectively as an operating room. Full surgical supplies are made available and portable operating room lights are supplied. The patient is transferred to the radiation therapy treatment couch and returned to standard anesthesia equipment. The patient is then redraped and the wound is reexposed. The previously selected applicator is placed over the treatment area. As mentioned earlier, often times a suction catheter is placed at the base of the wound to avoid any accumulation of blood that would decrease the depth of electron penetration during

TABLE 1
Patients Treated with IORT at
the MGH

Pancreas	72
Rectum	54
Soft tissue sarcoma	20
Colon	9
Cervix	7
Bladder	3
Stomach	3
Other	7
Total	175

irradiation. After the treatment applicator is attached to the machine, the radiation is delivered over approximately 3 to 5 min. We think it is important that the IORT field be observed both immediately prior to and immediately after the treatment. Even though it is unlikely that one would be able to correct an error in the IORT delivery after the fact, it is important to know if any errors have occurred. If only wound closure is required, the surgery is usually completed in the radiation therapy department. However, if more extensive surgery, such as anastomoses, are required, the patient is transferred back to the operating room for completion of the procedure.

III. RESULTS

The overall group of patients treated at MGH with IORT are shown in Table 1. The largest group of patients are those with locally advanced adenocarcinomas of the rectum and pancreas. The rectal tumors were those which we thought to be unresectable with curative intent because of adherence or fixation of the tumor to the sacrum, pelvic sidewall, or anterior structures. There have been a number of previous studies evaluating the use of high-dose preoperative radiation therapy to a dose of 45 to 50 Gy, followed by surgical resection. In data from MGH, Tufts, and the University of Oregon, it has been shown that 50 to 75% of patients are able to have a potentially curative resection after the high dose preoperative radiation therapy, but the local failure rate has remained 35 to 45%, despite the preoperative treatment. In addition, data from MGH have shown that in patients who have a surgical resection with residual disease, local failure occurs in approximately 40% of the patients, despite the delivery of high dose postoperative radiation. Rectal carcinoma was also thought to be an excellent model for the use of IORT because it has a propensity to remain localized and is a disease in which a substantial cohort of patients have local failure alone.

The protocol used at MGH has been to treat these patients preoperatively with a dose of 50.4 Gy delivered in 28 fractions through a 4-field box technique. With this approach we hope to decrease the tumor bulk to allow a potentially curative resection to be performed. The preoperative radiation therapy is also intended to sterilize areas of microscopic extension of the disease in regions where there may be no clinical fixation and to have treatment of regional nodal disease which will not be resected. The patients have approximately 4 weeks rest after the completion of the external beam therapy, at which time either a low anterior resection or an abdominal-perineal resection is performed, depending on the level of the tumor. At the time of resection the tumor is carefully evaluated for areas at high risk for residual disease, either gross residual or positive or close surgical margins. In patients in whom there was found to be no areas thought to be at especially high risk, no IORT was delivered. In the other patients, we gave IORT doses in the range of 10 to 20 Gy, generally using 15 Gy for microscopic residual and 20 Gy for gross residual cancer.[3]

TABLE 2
IORT for Locally Advanced Rectal Cancer —
MGH

	Primary	Recurrent
Number of patients	31	22
Local control rate (actuarial)		
24 months	90%	46%
48 months	85%	30%
Actuarial survival rate (48 months)	52%	25%
Local failure alone	3	5
Local and distant failure	0	7
Distant failure alone	13	5
No evidence of disease	15	5

An analysis has been performed as of April 1986; 31 patients had primary locally advanced disease, and 22 patients had local recurrences after previous surgical resection, with their recurrence being locally unresectable. We have analyzed our results both in terms of whether the tumor was primary or recurrent at presentation, and to the extent of surgical resection which was performed (Table 2). Of the 31 patients with primary locally advanced disease, 18 patients had grossly complete surgical resections, with only one patient having local recurrence; and 12 patients have had partial surgical resection with only two having local recurrence. Of the 22 patients with locally recurrent/locally advanced disease, 9 had complete surgical resection with 2 local recurrences; 8 patients had partial resection with 6 local recurrences; and 5 patients have had unresected disease, of whom 4 have had local recurrence. Thus, the failure has been substantially higher with the locally recurrent disease, no doubt partially related to the amount of surgical resection which could be performed. Overall, patients with primary locally advanced disease had a median survival of 49 months compared to a median survival of 31 months in the patients with locally advanced/locally recurrent tumors. In comparing the results to our previous series with high-dose preoperative radiation therapy alone at MGH, there appears to be a distinct advantage in terms of local control and in terms of survival for the patients with primary tumors.

We have thought it very important when evaluating a treatment regimen such as IORT to evaluate the complications very carefully, too. For this additional therapeutic regimen to be worthwhile, the increase in local control should be accomplished without a substantial increase in complications. We have done a careful evaluation of the complication rate after IORT in the rectal carcinoma patients and have compared this to patients who have been treated with high-dose preoperative radiation therapy alone for locally advanced disease and a second group of patients treated with surgery alone at MGH for nonlocally advanced disease (Table 3).[4] These results show no increase in the complication rates in the patients with primary locally advanced disease with the addition of IORT. There is a modest increase in the complication rate with high-dose preoperative radiation therapy, surgical resection, and IORT compared to surgery alone for patients with nonlocally advanced tumors. However, in the locally advanced disease patients, the surgical procedure is much more difficult because of the locally advanced nature of the tumor (regardless of the use of radiation) and is at least a partial contributor to the complication rate. In the patients with locally recurrent disease, we have seen a substantially higher complication rate. This has included a syndrome of pelvic pain in three patients; in one this has persisted. The exact etiology of the pain syndrome is not clear, but it seems likely that it is related to fibrosis and secondary nerve entrapment. There has also been greater difficulty with soft tissue healing after combined external beam, IORT, and resection in the patients with locally recurrent disease.

TABLE 3
Complications After Radiation Therapy of Rectal Cancer — MGH

	Surgery alone (nonadvanced tumors)	External beam radiotherapy & surgery (locally advanced tumors)	External beam radiotherapy & surgery & IORT (locally advanced primary tumors)	External beam radiotherapy & surgery & IORT (locally advanced recurrent tumors)
Total complications	13	10	6	9
Total patients with complications	13	8	5	8
Total patients	80	23	24	17
Percent patients with complications	16%	35%	21%	47%

IV. PANCREAS

Most of the institutions using IORT in the U.S. and Japan have had a significant experience in the treatment of adenocarcinoma of the pancreas. Many of the initial studies used IORT alone and did not combine it with either external beam radiation or surgical resection. As discussed earlier, we feel strongly that IORT be used as a boost modality. Although early in our series, we used IORT in combination with a Whipple resection (pancreaticoduodenectomy), the morbidity from this combination was high, and we have discontinued this approach. Thus, all but four of our patients have had radiation therapy alone without concomitant surgical resection. The patients whose tumors were thought to be amenable to surgical resection have been treated with Whipple resection, generally followed by high-dose external beam radiation therapy, but without IORT.

Treatment protocol development at MGH has been an evolutionary process since the initiation of our studies. All patients have a standard presurgical evaluation which includes abdominal CT scan. Most patients also have angiography to assess their tumor for resectability and have recently had a laparoscopy to screen for the presence of metastastic disease. Approximately 40% of the patients without any evidence of metastases during the rest of the workup were shown to have liver metastases or peritoneal seeding at laparoscopy.[5] At present, patients receive 10 Gy in five fractions preoperatively through anterior and posterior portals. There is then immediate surgical exploration and definition of the tumor extent. As mentioned earlier, if surgical resection is performed, no IORT is delivered. We are not using IORT for patients with evidence of metastatic disease. Although the initial IORT dose was 15 Gy, at present a dose of 20 Gy is given to the tumor mass with high-energy electrons. Virtually all patients have both a gastric and biliary bypass performed. Postoperatively, the patients receive 39.6 Gy delivered in 22 fractions through a 4-field approach to cover the primary pancreatic tumor mass and the regional lymphatics.[6-8] No attempt has been made to formally cover the tail of the pancreas for lesions of the pancreatic head, although there is some risk of tumor in the distal pancreas and in distal pancreatic and splenic hilar lymph nodes. The external beam irradiation is given in conjunction with 3 days of 5-fluorouracil chemotherapy.

As of April 1986, a total of 66 patients have been treated with a median survival of 13.5 months. We have observed good pain palliation, and in a previous analysis it was shown that approximately 50% of the patients have had complete sustained relief of pain from the use of IORT and external beam irradiation. The 13.5-month survival is superior to the results that have been reported with other local treatment regimens without IORT. We also performed a study to evaluate the utility of misonidazole, an hypoxic cell radiosensitizer, in conjunction with IORT. The treatment is exactly as described earlier, except

TABLE 4
IORT for Locally Advanced Pancreatic Cancer — MGH

Number of patients	66
(4 with resection)	
Patients without resection	62
Median survival	13.5 months
Actuarial survival rate (12 months)	59%
Actuarial local control rate (12 months)	70%
Local failure rate	40% (25/62)
Distant metastases	61% (38/62)
No evidence of disease	27% (17/62)

that in addition to the IORT, patients received 3.5 gm/M^2 of misonidazole intravenously approximately 30 min prior to irradiation. In an analysis of 41 patients who have been treated with misonidazole, compared to an earlier group of patients treated without the sensitizer, we have not seen any substantial difference in terms of either local control or long-term survival. At present, the sensitizer is not being used at MGH.

Local failure has remained a substantial problem in this group of patients, despite the high dose of radiation. Of 62 patients treated without surgical resection, 25 have had local failure. Distant metastases were seen in 38 patients. Of the 62 patients, 17 had no evidence of disease at the time of last analysis (Table 4).

Although this approach seems to improve the median survival and produces good palliation, it is clear that the long-term curability will be low.

V. MISCELLANEOUS

Despite the fact that we have emphasized locally advanced rectal and pancreatic carcinoma, we have treated a few patients with other tumors. As of the April 1986 analysis, there have been 13 patients treated for gastrointestinal sites other than the rectum for reasons of local tumor adherence or fixation. Seven patients have been treated for carcinoma of the cervix.[9] In addition, 20 patients have been treated for soft tissue sarcomas, the majority of these being sarcomas of the retroperitoneum.[10] A more detailed discussion of the retroperitoneal tumors is in the chapter on sarcomas.

VI. SUMMARY

To date, we have treated approximately 175 patients with IORT at MGH. We have been consistent in our use of IORT as a boost, always combining it with high-dose external beam radiation therapy and, where appropriate, with surgical resection. We have been very encouraged with the results in locally advanced primary rectal carcinomas and believe there has been a decrease in the local failure rate and an improvement in long-term survival. We think we have benefited patients with locally advanced nonmetastatic adenocarcinoma of the pancreas, but the long-term survival and long-term local control have not been as good as we would have hoped. We plan to proceed with investigation of additional sites in the future, including carcinoma of the urinary bladder and para-aortic lymph nodes for carcinoma of the cervix; we will continue with the basic philosophy described above.

REFERENCES

1. **Biggs, P. J., Epp, E. R., Ling, C. C. et al.,** Dosimetry, field shaping and other considerations for intraoperative electron therapy, *Int. J. Radiat. Oncol. Biol. Phys.,* 7, 875, 1981.
2. **Gunderson, L. L., Cohen, A. M., Dosoretz, D. E. et al.,** Residual, unresectable or recurrent colorectal cancer: external beam irradiation and intraoperative electron beam boost, *Int. J. Radiat. Oncol. Biol. Phys.,* 9, 1597, 1983.
3. **Tepper, J., Cohen, A. M., Wood, W. C. et al.,** Intraoperative electron beam radiotherapy in the treatment of unresectable rectal cancer, *Arch. Surg.,* 121, 421, 1986.
4. **Tepper, J., Gunderson, L. L., Orlow, E. et al.,** Complications of intraoperative radiation therapy, *Int. J. Radiat. Oncol. Biol. Phys.,* 10, 1831, 1984.
5. **Warshaw, A. L., Tepper, J. E., and Shipley, W. U.,** A unique role of laporoscopy in staging and planning for pancreatic cancer, *Am. J. Surg.,* 151, 76, 1986.
6. **Wood, W., Shipley, W. U., Gunderson, L. L. et al.,** Intraoperative irradiation for unresectable pancreatic carcinoma, *Cancer,* 49, 1272, 1982.
7. **Shipley, W. U., Wood, W. C., Tepper, J. E. et al.,** Intraoperative electron beam irradiation for patients with unresectable pancreatic carcinoma, *Ann. Surg.,* 200, 289, 1984.
8. **Shipley, W. U., Tepper, J., Warshaw, A., and Orlow, E.,** Intraoperative radiation therapy for patients with pancreatic cancer, *World J. Surg.,* 8, 929, 1984.
9. **Dosoretz, D., Tepper, J., Shimm, D. et al.,** Intraoperative electron beam irradiation in the management of gynecologic malignancies, *Appl. Radiol.,* 13, 61, 1984.
10. **Tepper, J., Suit, H. D., Wood, W. et al.,** Radiation therapy of retroperitoneal soft tissue sarcoma, *Int. J. Radiat. Oncol. Biol. Phys.,* 10, 825, 1984.

Chapter 26

MAYO CLINIC EXPERIENCE WITH INTRAOPERATIVE AND EXTERNAL BEAM IRRADIATION WITH OR WITHOUT RESECTION

Leonard L. Gunderson, J. Kirk Martin, David M. Nagorney, Jennifer Fieck, Alvaro Martinez, and John D. Earle

TABLE OF CONTENTS

I. INTRODUCTION

The intent of this chapter is to present the experience of a Mayo Clinic multidisciplinary program which combines intraoperative irradiation (IORT) with external beam irradiation and, when feasible, surgical resection. Existing facilities in the radiation oncology department were renovated to provide a temporary facility for IORT. The renovation included construction of an operating room (Curie OR) adjacent to a Varian® Clinac-18 linear accelerator which provided electron energies ranging from 6 to 18 meV. The intent of the temporary facility was to allow the Mayo Clinic to quickly mount an IORT treatment program utilizing existing space and equipment. Between April 1981 and October 1985, 136 patients had been treated for locally advanced malignancies in the abdomen and pelvis, and the results from the initial 115 patients are reported. The future direction of IORT within our institution is also discussed.

II. MATERIALS AND METHODS

A. PATIENT SELECTION AND WORKUP

Patient selection for Mayo Clinic IORT studies is based upon the presence of a locally advanced malignancy (primary or recurrent) and the absence of disseminated disease. Lesions can be unresectable for cure on the basis of tumor fixation, or residual disease may remain after a subtotal resection. The IORT approach must permit direct irradiation of unresected or residual tumor within single or abutting IORT fields with a minimum or total lack of intervening normal tissues or organs.

While the approach of preselecting patients for IORT varies by institution, our method has involved (1) definition of tumor size, location, and extent preoperatively with noninvasive imaging techniques, or (2) exploring patients first in regular operating rooms at Methodist or St. Mary's Hospitals, then performing IORT in appropriate patients as a second procedure. While the latter approach achieves the best patient selection, it does necessitate a second operation with all the inherent risks. Patients have not been excluded solely because of age — the range in age has been from 2 to 79 years.

Routine preoperative evaluation has included a chest film, serum chemistries, hematology and coagulation profiles, and CT scans. Liver scans or ultrasound, CT-guided thin-needle biopsies, peritoneoscopy, and other procedures have been performed on a more selective basis.

Before the IORT procedure, baseline studies are obtained of structures or organs that may be included in the IORT field whenever this is feasible (i.e., a baseline upper gastrointestinal series in patients with pancreatic cancer, a baseline excretory urogram in patients with colorectal lesions involving or adjacent to the ureter). Serial follow-up studies can then be used to evaluate structural changes that may occur as a result of the aggressive combined modality approach.

B. OPERATIVE FACTORS

Prophylactic antibiotic coverage with a cephalosporin has been used in the immediate perioperative period in all patients, and nutritional support may be an important consideration in some. Since many patients with pancreatic malignancies will have lost 10% or more of their body weight from their malignancy, preoperative hyperalimentation or placement of a feeding tube jejunostomy at the time of IORT has been utilized selectively.

1. Facility and General Approaches

Currently, most operating rooms across the country are widely separated from radiation facilities. The cost and space required to encorporate a modern linear accelerator within an operating room as a dedicated IORT facility precluded their use in most initial IORT pilot trials. Consequently, most institutions using IORT have elected to transport the patient from the regular operating room to the radiation therapy area and back to the operating room, and their required procedures have been described in detail.[1-7] This approach has potential shortcomings, including maintenance of sterility, insurance of patient safety, and duration of anesthesia; however, it has been successfully used by most Japanese investigators[2] in addition to Massachusetts General Hospital (MGH),[1,5,8-10] National Cancer Institute (NCI),[6] and others.

Our institution attempted to avoid some of these problems by converting an existing area in the radiation therapy department into a standard operating room (Curie OR) with adjoining facilities for scrub sinks. The room was modified to provide for anesthetic gas evacuation, suction, and positive pressure ventilation. A standard operating table and lights are used. Patients are explored, the tumor is exposed, and the IORT applicator is selected. The patient is then moved with the aid of a Surgi-Lift® down a short, isolated corridor to the linear accelerator room for applicator placement and treatment. Because fluid buildup over a tumor or tumor bed could alter the thickness of a treatment volume and create a risk of underdosage at depth, constant suction is maintained alongside the applicator during treatment of all sites. During the IORT treatment, the patient is automatically ventilated. Blood pressure, heart rate, and electrocardiogram are monitored continuously by closed circuit television. Following IORT, the patient is returned to the Curie OR where additional procedures are performed, as indicated, and wounds are closed. The patient is then moved to the Methodist Hospital recovery room. The operating team and instruments as well as anesthesia and blood bank support are provided from the Methodist Hospital.

When major resections are contemplated, they are usually performed in the regular operating rooms in either of the two hospitals staffed by Mayo Clinic physicians. Decisions regarding indications for and the technique of IORT are made at that exploration by the surgeon and radiation oncologist, and the patient is reexplored in the Curie OR within 1 to 10 d.

2. Technical Aspects

In patients who have been through a recent major operation before IORT, the timing of the reoperation is of importance. Pragmatically, an "early" reoperation in 1 to 7 d has been found to be technically the safest, but patients have been reexplored as late as 10 d. Between 1 and 4 weeks, adequate exposure can be difficult to achieve because of inflammatory changes and adhesions associated with dense induration. Such changes usually resolve and allow reoperations after 4 to 6 weeks. An additional reason for early reoperation is to minimize changes in appearance of the operative areas of resection and to maximize adequate coverage of the area at high risk. Even in patients with unresected pancreas lesions, problems with mobilization of the stomach and reexposure of the tumor have been increased if the interval is 8 to 10 d instead of earlier.

Other limiting factors influencing adequate exposure are prior procedures, particularly the presence of a double bypass (biliary and gastric) with jejunum in patients with pancreatic cancer.[11] The jejunal loop extends directly across the gastrocolic omentum at the site where entry into the lesser sac is necessary to treat head lesions and can prevent the use of IORT. The biliary bypass does not usually present a problem as it either lies above the pancreas (choledochoduodenostomy) or lateral to it (cholecystojejunostomy).

The choice of incision varies with the disease site. Bilateral subcostal incisions give excellent exposure for upper abdominal malignancies (pancreas, bile duct), but midline or long oblique incisions can also be utilized. In pelvic malignancies (colorectal or sarcomas), a lower midline incision is chosen. If the area to be treated is very low, usually below the tip of the coccyx, a perineal approach is used. When the first operation proceeds IORT by only a few days and the entire external beam component of irradiation has already been delivered, the perineal incision can be temporarily packed open until IORT and can be closed with drainage at that procedure. If a longer interval exists between resection and IORT, the perineal incision should be closed after the initial resection and reopened for IORT. When the latter approach is utilized, the pelvic floor should be reconstructed to displace small bowel away from the area at risk.

Radio-opaque clips are placed to define tumor extent and thereby aid the precise delivery of IORT and external beam irradiation (if the latter was not completed preoperatively). We prefer a single small vascular clip to mark superior, inferior, lateral, and medial margins of unresected or residual disease or areas of adherence. The sparse placement of small Hemoclips® produces only minimal interference with subsequent CT examinations. Titanium clips produce less CT artifact, but sometimes they cannot be identified on lateral simulator films due to their decreased density.

C. RADIATION FACTORS (INTRAOPERATIVE AND EXTERNAL BEAM)

The intent of treatment in all patients has been to use IORT electrons for a "boost" dose in conjunction with external beam photons.[1,5,7] The external beam component of treatment usually includes potential nodal drainage sites. Patients receive 45 to 50 Gy in 1.7- to 1.8-Gy fractions over 5 to 6 weeks either before or after the IORT boost. This is delivered by 6- or 10-meV photon beams from isocentric linear accelerators. Multiple-field portals and field shaping are employed to limit the doses to normal tissue.

With lesions that are initially unresectable for cure due to disease fixation but in whom later resection may be feasible (colorectal lesions, sarcomas, etc.), the radiotherapy preference is to deliver 45 to 50 Gy preoperatively in an attempt to convert the lesion to one that is potentially resectable and to alter implantability of cells that may be spread at the time of resection.[12,13] Resection is undertaken 3 to 5 weeks later in the regular operating room, and the IORT boost is delivered to the remaining tumor or tumor bed at the time of reexploration in the Curie OR in 1 to 10 d.

With unresectable pancreatic lesions, high-dose preoperative irradiation has not been used as standard treatment, since the intent has not been to attempt later resection. In this group, a single preoperative dose of 5 Gy has been delivered with a 4-field technique to gross tumor plus at least a 2-cm margin on the day prior to the IORT boost in 21 patients. This was an attempt to alter potential implantability of cells.[14,15] Postoperatively, 45 Gy external beam therapy was given over 5 weeks with 1.8-Gy fractions starting 3 to 6 weeks after IORT in conjunction with bolus IV-5FU 500 mg/M^2 on 3 consecutive days, weeks one and five. If patients did not receive a 5-Gy preoperative dose, they had 50.4 Gy in 28 fractions in 5.5 weeks given postoperatively with a field reduction after 45 Gy.

The dose used in the IORT boost is calculated at the 90% isodose line, and has varied from 10 to 20 Gy, and is dependent on the amount of disease: microscopic residual (m) — 10 Gy, gross or macroscopic residual (g) ≤2 cm — 15 Gy, unresected or gross residual >2 cm — 17.5 to 20 Gy. This dose variability has been shown to be appropriate in initial MGH and Mayo Clinic analyses, but may have to be modified as longer follow-up is achieved and both local control and normal tissue tolerance can be evaluated. In patients with recurrent lesions, we have changed our minimum IORT dose to 15 Gy, even when all gross tumor is resected. The biologic effectiveness of single-dose irradiation is considered equivalent to two or three times that radiation quantity of fractionated external beam treatment.[16] In view of that, the effective dose within the IORT boost when added to the 45 to 50 Gy delivered in 25 to 28 fractions with external beam techniques is 65 to 80 Gy, with a 10-Gy IORT boost, 75 to 95 Gy with a 15-Gy IORT boost, and 85 to 110 Gy with a 20-Gy IORT boost.

The choice of electron beam energy and applicator size is based on the thickness and volume of unresected or residual tumor.[1-7] Our institution has a wide variety of methyl

TABLE 1
Patient Group — Curie OR (April 1981 to March 1985)

Primary tumor site	Explored	Treated	Reason for no treatment			Technical	Other
			Metastases				
			Liver	PS[a]	Both		
Pancreatic	79	52	12	7	3	1	4[b]
Colorectal	40	35	2	0	1	2	0
Biliary duct	11	8	1	2	0	0	0
Gastric	1	1	—	—	—	—	—
Sarcoma	9	9	—	—	—	—	—
Gynecologic	4	3	0	0	0	0	1
Pediatric, ret- roperitoneal	5(6)	5(6)	—	—	—	—	—
Genitourinary	2	2	—	—	—	—	—
Total	151	115	15	9	4	3	5

[a] PS = peritoneal seeding.
[b] Malignancy could not be confirmed (3); too large (1).

methacrylate applicators available so that the tumor volume can be encompassed with approximately a 1-cm margin (7-cm tumor = 9 cm applicator). The Clinac-18 linear accelerator has electron energies ranging from 6 to 18 meV. For the unresected pancreas lesions, 18-meV electron energy has routinely been selected (90% depth dose at 5 to 5.5. cm). When a majority of tumor has been resected, as found in most of our colorectal and sarcoma cases and at other sites, the energy has varied from 9 to 15 meV, depending on the degree of beam obliquity relative to the resected surface (a true vertical docking would be most desirable, but is rarely feasible in pelvic cases).

The physics and technical aspects of using IORT boosts have been presented in previous publications[1,17] and are detailed elsewhere in this book. We prefer to use an electron beam rather than orthovoltage beam for the IORT boost because of its inherent advantages in dose distribution and the relative lack of differential absorption in normal tissues.

III. RESULTS

A. TOTAL PATIENT GROUP

As of our March 1985 analysis, a total of 151 patients had been explored in the Curie OR, and 115 had received an IORT electron boost (Table 1). In 28 of the 36 patients who were not treated, the boost was withheld because of either hemotogenous or peritoneal spread of disease. The main disease sites are gastrointestinal (pancreas, colorectum, and bile duct) and soft tissue sarcomas. In addition, three patients with gynecologic malignancy, two with genitourinary primaries, and six patients with retroperitoneal pediatric malignancies have been treated (one of the six is included with the sarcoma subset).

TABLE 2
Patient Group — Disease Category and Site, Gastrointestinal
(April 1981 to March 1985)

Disease category	Number patients	Pancreas	Colorectum	Biliary duct	Stomach
Primary, resected-residual	11	2	9	0	0
Primary, unresectable	59	49	2[a]	8	0
Recurrent, resected-residual	18	0	18	0	0
Recurrent, unresectable	8	1	6[b]	0	1
Total	96	52	35	8	1

[a] Resected after 50 Gy — res (m), res (g).

[b] 1 patient had disease recurrence after 40 Gy, had additional 25 Gy in 14 fractions, then resection and IORT 20 Gy; 2 patients had 50 Gy in 28 fractions preoperatively, but remained unresectable; another 45 Gy in 25 fractions preoperatively, but unresectable; 2 patients had partial resection after 45 to 50 Gy.

TABLE 3
Survival and Disease Status By Site, Upper Gastrointestinal

Status (number of patients)	Pancreas (P)[a]	Bile duct (B)	Interval (months)
Alive (22)			
No disease progression (19)	11[b]	5	(P) range 2—24 (3>12)
			(B) range 1—22$^{1/2}$ (2>12)
With disease (3)	3	0	(P) 1, 7, 29$^{1/2}$
Dead (39)[a]			
No disease progression (3)[c]	1	1	(P) 7$^{1/2}$[d], (B) 4, (G) 5[c]
Disease progression (29)	27	2	(P) range 3.5—19.5 (11 ≥12)
			(B) 37
Uncertain (7)	7	0	(P) range 1—11 (B) 6$^{1/2}$
Total 60[c]	49(52)[b]	8	

Note: Analysis performed March 1985.

[a] Two patients had resection but residual tumor (dead at 5$^{1/2}$ and 6 months).

[b] Three additional patients had not completed external beam therapy.

[c] Single gastric (G) cancer patient dead without evidence of disease at 5 months (aspiration pneumonia).

[d] No residual disease at autopsy.

B. GASTROINTESTINAL MALIGNANCIES

As discussed previously, only patients with locally advanced disease have been included in the Mayo Clinic studies (Table 2). All patients with biliary duct cancer and most with pancreatic cancer presented with unresectable primary lesions (8/8 and 49/52, respectively). In our colorectal group, 24 of 35 patients presented at the time of a localized recurrence and only 11 had primary disease.

1. Survival and Disease Status

Survival and disease status for patients with upper gastrointestinal lesions is shown in Table 3. Five of eight biliary duct cancer patients are alive without evidence of disease progression with two of five alive over 1 year (15 and 22.5 months). Of the remaining three patients, one died of sepsis at 4 months, one died at 37 months of a pulmonary embolus,

TABLE 4
Incidence and Patterns of Failure, Gastrointestinal

Site	Number of patients evaluable	Number of patients failing			
		CF No.-%	LF No.-%	DM No.-%	PS No.-%
Pancreas	30/42[a]	2-5	3-7	21-50	12-29
Colorectum	12/33[b]	1-3	4-12	10-30	2-6
Bile duct	1/6[c]	1-17	1-17	—	—
Total	43/81	4-5	8-10	31-38	14-17

Note: CF = central failure in IORT field, LF = local failure in external beam field, DM = distant metastasis, PS = peritoneal seeding. Analysis performed March 1985.

[a] Ten additional patients with failure patterns unevaluable — (have not completed treatment (three), uncertain status (five), localized PS at IORT (one), other (one).

[b] Two additional patients died of intercurrent disease at 1 and 3 months.

[c] Patterns of failure unevaluable in two additional patients as they died at four and $6^{1}/_{2}$ months with no evidence of disease progression. The patient with CF, LF died of a pulmonary embolus at 37 months and persistent local tumor was found at autopsy.

and local residual tumor was confirmed at atuopsy, and the third died at 6.5 months of uncertain cause with persistent tumor, but no evidence of disease progression. In the pancreas group, 11 of 49 patients who had completed both the IORT and external beam irradiation were alive and without evidence of disease progression, with only 3/11 alive more than 12 months (13, 15.5, and 24 months); 1 patient died of intercurrent disease at 7.5 months and was free of disease at autopsy, 27 died of disease, and 7 died with cause and tumor status uncertain.

2. Failure Patterns

Only 4 of 81 patients (5%) evaluable for patterns of failure had evidence of tumor progression within the IORT boost field (Table 4). Three of these four patients had unresected disease, and the fourth was a patient with partial resection of a recurrent lesion. An additional four patients (total 8/81 or 10%) had progression in the external beam field. Both blood-borne and peritoneal progression have been common in patients who presented with pancreatic malignancies with a majority of blood-borne metastases occurring in the liver (liver only — 13/21, liver and lung — 1, lung only — 5, other — 2).

C. MISCELLANEOUS SITES (SARCOMA, GYNECOLOGIC, GENITOURINARY, PEDIATRIC)

Of our 115 patients, 19 presented with tumors at nongastrointestinal sites. Disease extent is listed in Table 5, and survival and disease status in Table 6. Of the 19 patients, 12 are alive without evidence of disease progression with 6/12 at risk at least 1 year. As seen in Table 7, central or local failure has occurred in only 1/19 (5%) patients, but blood-borne spread has been proven in 6/19 (32%). Peritoneal spread has not been identified as a pattern of disease progression in this group of patients.

IV. CONCLUSIONS AND FUTURE POSSIBILITIES

A. GASTROINTESTINAL CANCERS

As noted in the chapter on colorectal cancer, the long-term results of an aggressive local

TABLE 5
Patient Group Miscellaneous Tumors (Sarcoma, Gynecologic [Gyn], Pediatric, Genitourinary [GU] Tumors)

Disease category	Number of patients	Sarcoma	Gyn	Pediatric retroperitoneal	GU
Primary, resected-residual	3	1	0	2	0
Primary, unresectable	6	2[a]	1[a]	2[a]	1
Recurrent, resected-residual	7	6	0	1	0
Recurrent, unresectable	3[b]	0	2[b]	0	1[a]
Total	19	9[c]	3	5	2

[a] Five patients had disease resected after 50 Gy: two had gross residual disease in tumor bed, one — pelvis, one — retroperitoneal; one — nonexistent margins; two had gross residual disease in iliac and para-aortic lymph nodes, one primary uterine cervix cancer and one recurrent ureter cancer.

[b] Unresectable after 45 and 50 Gy preoperatively.

[c] Adult — eight, pediatric (retroperitoneal sarcoma) — one.

TABLE 6
Survival and Disease Status By Site — Sarcoma, Gynecologic (GYN), Pediatric (Ped), Genitourinary (GU) Tumors

Status	Sarcoma	Gyn	Ped	GU	Survival by disease site[a] (months)
Alive (13)					
NED[b] (12)	5	2	5	0	(S) 2, 4, 16, $20^1/_2$, 33 (Gyn), 18, 26 (Ped) 5, 5, $6^1/_2$, $8^1/_2$, 22
With disease (1)	1	0	0	0	(S) $32^1/_2$
Dead (6)					
With disease (6)	3	1	0	2	(S) 3, 9, $37^1/_2$ (Gyn), 9 (GU), $12^1/_2$, $14^1/_2$
Total 19	9	3	5	2	

[a] S: sarcoma; Gyn: gynecologic; Ped: pediatric; GU: genitourinary.

[b] NED — no evidence of disease.

TABLE 7
Incidence and Patterns of Failure, Miscellaneous Tumors

Disease site	Number of failures	Patterns[a]
Sarcoma	4/9	DM (4)
Gynecologic	1/3	DM
Pediatric retroperitoneal	0/5	
Genitourinary	2/2	DM, LF + CF

[a] DM = distant metastasis; LF = local failure, CF = central failure.

approach for locally advanced gastrointestinal malignancies (initially unresectable, residual after resection, and locally recurrent) are dependent on the metastatic potential of the tumor at the treated site. With locally advanced biliary and colorectal cancer, if local control is achieved, there is a good chance that this may result in long-term survival, since systemic failure is less common than with gastric, pancreatic,[18] and gall bladder primaries. In the latter tumors, abdominal failure occurs frequently with resectable as well as unresectable lesions. Although the aggressive local treatment approaches outlined in this book may still be appropriate with cancers of the latter sites, treatment of the liver and/or peritoneal cavity may be indicated in an attempt to increase survival (intraperitoneal chemotherapy or radiocolloids, infusion chemotherapy, external beam irradiation, or combination thereof). We have nearly completed case accession to a phase II tolerance study which combines upper or total abdominal irradiation (wide-field XRT) and infusion 5FU with aggressive treatment of the tumor lymph node region with external beam therapy and IORT approaches.[18] In a small group of patients who received wide-field irradiation and chemotherapy with both intraperitoneal and infusion of 5FU there were problems with excess toxicity, and we have no plans to utilize both intraperitoneal chemotherapy and wide-field irradiation in future trials. In a subsequent trial, external beam irradiation will be limited to a tumor lymph node field, and abdominal prophylaxis will be with intraperitoneal chemotherapy.

B. MISCELLANEOUS SITES

Patient numbers for the nongastrointestinal tumor sites are too small to arrive at definitive conclusions for an individual site on the basis of our data alone. In locally advanced sarcoma and gynecologic cases, 7 of 12 patients at risk are free of disease (5/9 sarcoma, 2/3 gynecologic) with 5/7 at least 12 months (sarcoma — 3, gynecologic — 2). When these data are combined with those from other institutions, tumors at these sites continue to appear appropriate for further study. While longer follow-up is needed in our group of pediatric patients, an IORT boost appears attractive, as it may allow the use of lower doses of external beam irradiation.

C. FUTURE NEEDS AND POSSIBILITIES

Many unanswered questions exist about using IORT in combination with external beam irradiation. Much information is needed regarding the necessary ratio of dose delivered with the external beam and IORT components, the dose needed for a suitable therapeutic ratio of tumor control to complications, the biologic equivalence of single fraction IORT boosts, and the role for radiation dose modifiers. Efforts are being made to gain some of these answers in both animal and human studies. Institutions involved in an NCI-IORT contract (MGH, Mayo Clinic, Howard University) are combining data to analyze patterns of failure and normal tissue tolerance as a function of treatment technique and dose levels. At present, we prefer to continue using external beam techniques to deliver 45 to 50 Gy in 1.8-Gy fractions to areas at some risk for local failure and plan to modify only the IORT dose and field size in boosting the dose to areas at maximum risk.

Some of the problems encountered in the Mayo Clinic and other pilot trials are due to the current limited availability of IORT facilities and could be overcome with a *dedicated*[19] or *semidedicated* facility.[3,4] This could be built as an operating room in the radiation therapy department or within or near the OR suite, the most ideal situation in our opinion. This would simplify the treatment of patients, necessitate fewer reoperations (refused by some patients and physicians), and would minimize transportation and sterility problems. It would also prevent the need to impede or delay routine outpatient treatments for a "potential" IORT case as occurs at present with nondedicated facilities.

The existence of a dedicated facility would also improve the ability to evaluate a larger number of disease sites and would allow one to consider treating selected subgroups in an adjuvant setting as opposed to our current criteria of residual, unresectable, or recurrent disease. It would be reasonable to combine IORT with "curative resection" with or without external beam irradiation in situations where the external beam dose needed for local control may approach or exceed normal tissue tolerance. Indications may include lesions with a high risk of tumor bed recurrence (selected colorectal, gastric, pancreatic, esophageal tumors, etc.) or tumors with a high risk of regional or aortic nodal failure (gynecologic,[20] genitourinary tumors, etc.). With early bladder tumors, it would be valuable to examine the Japanese experience of combining external and IORT — avoiding a cystectomy by boosting the dose to the gross lesion with IORT.[21]

The present results of IORT alone or in combination with external beam therapy and resection warrant continued careful scrutiny of the technique to determine its exact role in cancer care. While it appears that one may achieve an increased incidence of local tumor control at varied sites with improved safety based on current IORT pilot studies, this needs to be tested in appropriate randomized trials with many disease sites and various extents of disease. The best disease models for IORT would be those in which systemic failure is not an overwhelming problem (rectal, gynecologic, biliary tumors, low-grade sarcoma) or good systemic therapy exists (testicular cancer). With many other malignancies (stomach, pancreas, high-grade sarcomas, esophagus, lung, etc.), improvement in local control may result in an improvement in median survival and quality of life, but is not as likely to translate into improvement in long-term survival unless the systemic failure problem can be solved.

ACKNOWLEDGMENTS

The authors are indebted to Julie Boland and the Mayo Typing Service for assistance in preparation of the manuscript, and to the radiation oncology physicists and technicians, OR nurses, and many additional physicians who were involved in the treatment of the patients. This work supported in part by the National Cancer Institute, Contract CM-27528.

REFERENCES

1. **Gunderson, L. L., Tepper, J. E., Biggs, P. J., Goldson, A., Martin, J. K., McCullough, E. C., Rich, T. A., Shipley, W. U., Sindelar, W. F., and Wood, W. C.,** Intraoperative ± external beam irradiation, *Curr. Prob. Cancer,* 7, 1, 1983.
2. **Abe, M. and Takahashi, M.,** Intraoperative radiotherapy: the Japanese experience, *Int. J. Radiat. Oncol. Biol. Phys.,* 7, 863, 1981.
3. **Goldson, A.,** Preliminary clinical experience with intraoperative radiotherapy, *J. Natl. Med. Assoc.,* 70, 493, 1978.
4. **Goldson, A. L.,** Past, present and future prospects of intraoperative radiotherapy (IOR), *Semin. Oncol.,* 8, 59, 1981.
5. **Gunderson, L. L., Shipley, W. U., Suit, H. D., Epp, E. R., Nardi, G., Wood, W., Cohen, A., Nelson, J., Battit, G., Biggs, P. J., Russell, A., Rocket, A., and Clark, D.,** Intraoperative irradiation: a pilot study combining external beam photons with "boost" dose intraoperative electrons, *Cancer,* 49, 2259, 1981.
6. **Sindelar, S. T., Kinsella, T., Tepper, J., Travis, E. L., Rosenberg, S. A., and Glatstein, E.,** Experimental and clinical studies with intraoperative radiotherapy, *Surg. Gynecol. Obstet.,* 157, 205, 1983.
7. **Gunderson, L. L., Martin, J. K., Earle, J. B., Byer, D., Voss, M., Fieck, J., Kvols, L., Rorie, D., Martinez, A., Nagorney, D. M., O'Connell, M. J., and Weber, F.,** Intraoperative and external beam irradiation ± resection: Mayo pilot experience, *Mayo Clin. Proc.,* 59, 691, 1984.
8. **Wood, W., Shipley, W. U., Gunderson, L. L., Cohen, A. M., and Nardi, G. L.,** Intraoperative irradiation for unresectable pancreatic carcinoma, *Cancer,* 49, 1272, 1982.
9. **Gunderson, L. L., Cohen, A. M., Dosoretz, D. E., Shipley, W. U., Hedberg, S. E., Wood, W. C., Rodkey, G. V., and Suit, H. D.,** Residual, unresectable, or recurrent colorectal cancer: external beam irradiation and intraoperative electron beam boost ± resection, *Int. J. Radiat. Oncol. Biol. Phys.,* 1597, 1983.
10. **Shipley, W. U., Wood, W. C., Tepper, J. E., Warshaw, A. L., Orlow, E. L., Kaufman, D., Battit, G. E., and Nardi, G. L.,** Intraoperative electron beam irradiation for patients with unresectable pancreatic carcinoma, *Ann. Surg.,* 200, 289, 1984.

11. **Sarr, M. G., Gladen, H. F., Beart, R. W., Jr., and van Heerden, J. A.,** Role of gastroenterostomy in patients with unresectable pancreatic carcinoma, *Surg. Gynecol. Obstet.,* 152, 597, 1981.

12. **Kligerman, M. M., Urdaneta, N., Knowlton, A., Vidone, R., Hartman, P. V., and Vera, R.,** Preoperative irradiation of rectosigmoid carcinoma including its regional lymph nodes, *Am. J. Roentgenol.,* 114, 498, 1972.

13. **Dosoretz, D. E., Gunderson, L. L., Hoskins, B., Hedberg, S. E., Shipley, W. U., Blitzer, P. H., and Cohen, A. M.,** Preoperative irradiation for localized carcinoma of the rectum and rectosigmoid: patterns of failure, survival, and future treatment strategies, *Cancer,* 52, 814, 1983.

14. **Whittington, R., Dobelbower, R. R., Mohiuddin, M., Rosato, F. F., and Weiss, S. M.,** Radiotherapy of unresectable pancreatic carcinoma: a six-year experience with 104 patients, *Int. J. Radiat. Oncol. Biol. Phys.,* 7, 1639, 1981.

15. **Gunderson, L. L., Dosoretz, D. E., Hedberg, S. E., Blitzer, P. H., Rodkey, G., Hoskins, B., Shipley, W. U., and Cohen, A. M.,** Low-dose preoperative irradiation, surgery, and elective postoperative radiation therapy for resectable rectum and rectosigmoid carcinoma, *Cancer,* 446, 1983.

16. **Suit, H. D.,** Radiation biology: a basis for radiotherapy, in *Textbook of Radiotherapy,* 2nd ed., Fletcher, G. H., Ed., Lea & Febiger, Philadelphia, 1973, 75.

17. **McCullough, E. C., and Anderson, J. A.,** The dosimetric properties of an applicator system for intraoperative electron-beam therapy utilizing a Clinac 18 accelerator, *Med. Phys.,* 9, 261, 1982.

18. **Gunderson, L. L., Martin, J. K., Kvols, L. K., Nagorney, D. M., Fieck, J. M., Wieand, H. S., Martinez, A., O'Connell, M. J., Earle, J. D., McIlrath, D. C.,** Intraoperative and external beam irradiation ± 5FU for locally advanced pancreatic cancer. ASTRO Proceedings, *Int. J. Radiat. Oncol. Biol. Phys.,* 1985.

19. **Rich, T. A., Cady, B., McDermott, W. U., Kase, K. R., Chaffey, J. T., and Hellman, S.,** Orthovoltage intraoperative radiotherapy. A new look at an old idea, *Int. J. Radiat. Oncol. Biol. Phys.,* 10, 1957, 1984.

20. **Goldson, A., Delgado, G., and Hill, L.,** Intraoperative radiation of the paraaortic nodes in cancer of the uterine cervix, *Obstet. Gynecol.,* 52, 713, 1978.

21. **Matsumoto, L., Kakizoe, T., Mikuriyama, S., Tanaka, T., Kondo, I., and Umegaki, Y.,** Clinical evaluation of intraoperative radiotherapy for carcinoma of the urinary bladder, *Cancer,* 47, 509, 1981.

Chapter 27

THE RUSH-PRESBYTERIAN-ST. LUKE'S MEDICAL CENTER EXPERIENCE WITH INTRAOPERATIVE RADIATION THERAPY

Krystyna Kiel, Toby Kramer, and David L. Roseman

TABLE OF CONTENTS

I. INTRODUCTION

In December 1982, we began a program of intraoperative radiation therapy (IORT). There have been 85 patients treated through September 1986. Our facilities and treatment equipment necessitated development of unique techniques which may be applicable to other institutions. This chapter discusses our approach, techniques, and the preliminary results of our treatment.

Rather than build expensive new facilities, we elected to perform surgery in the operating room and radiation therapy in the radiation therapy department. We decided to limit the amount of time the patient spent outside the protected environment of the operating room. It has therefore become our practice to fix the radiation treatment field in the surgical suite rather than in the radiation therapy suite. The treatment machine, a THERAC-20 (AECL), delivers a scanning electron beam which provides dose homogeneity without "docking" an applicator to the gantry. Treatment is administered on the operating table, expediting the entire procedure.

In general, the sequence of events is as follows: (1) any required resections are performed, and surgical exposure of the IORT field is established; (2) retraction, shielding, and the placement of electron applicators is done in the operating room; (3) the patient is covered with a sterile sheet and transported on the operating table to the radiation therapy suite; (4) the patient on the operating table is positioned under the treatment machine and the position of the treatment applicator is confirmed; (5) treatment is delivered and the position of the applicator is again confirmed; (6) the patient is returned to the operating room; (7) anastamoses or other procedures are completed, and the surgical wound is closed in the usual fashion.

II. OPERATIVE CONSIDERATIONS

Resectable tumors are excised. After resection, organs and tissues are mobilized to establish maximal exposure of residual tumor, or of the tumor bed. Any necessary reconstruction is reserved until after the radiation treatment has been given. Retraction, shielding, and placement of applicators to direct the treatment beam are accomplished in the operating room. For unresectable lesions, unusual surgical manipulation may be necessary to expose the treatment area to spare radiosensitive uninvolved structures (i.e., division of the stomach to expose a pancreatic carcinoma). Self-retaining retractors are used not only to maintain exposure during surgery and irradiation, but also to fix the patient's position on the operating table during subsequent transport. Treatment applicators are likewise fixed to the operating table (Figure 1) to prevent accidental movement secondary to respiration or transport. Intraoperative ultrasonography has been useful in defining tumor position and thickness in three patients and appears to be helpful in some specific circumstances.

III. TRANSPORT CONSIDERATIONS

The operating table has been modified so the i.v. poles, EKG/pressure monitor, and oxygen cylinders are attached (Figure 1). The patient, with retractors, shields, and applicator in place, is covered with a sterile drape and transported. During transfer to the radiation therapy suite, the patient is supported with 100% oxygen using an "ambu" bag. On arrival in the treatment suite, the patient is attached to a standard anesthesia machine and automatic ventillation is reestablished. The patient is connected to external vital sign monitors, and video cameras are directed toward the respirator and patient.

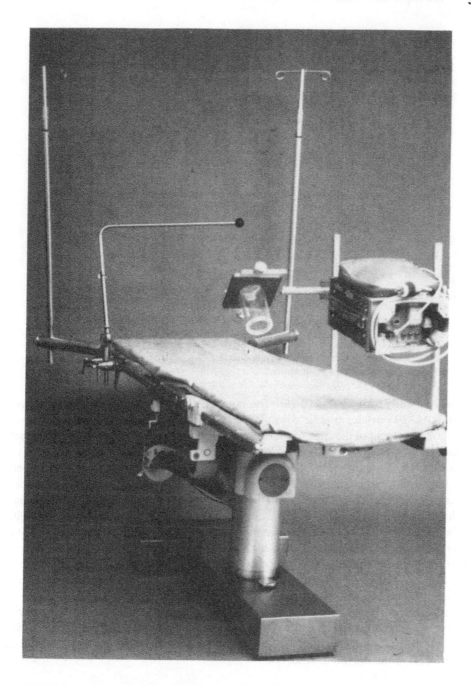

FIGURE 1. Operating room table with treatment applicator, i.v. poles, and portable monitor attached for transport and radiation treatment.

IV. TREATMENT CONSIDERATIONS

A series of treatment applicators was manufactured in our hospital. These included cylindrical applicators of various diameters (5, 5.5, 6, 6.5, 7, 7.5, 8, 8.5, and 9 cm), all sizes with flat and some with 20° beveled ends, and rectangular applicators, 6 × 9 and 9 × 12 cm. Rather than develop a device fixed to the gantry with the inherent disadvantages of "docking", shields were manufactured to be placed over the applicator (Figure 1). The field size is set slightly larger than the applicator diameter. Confirmation of leakage outside

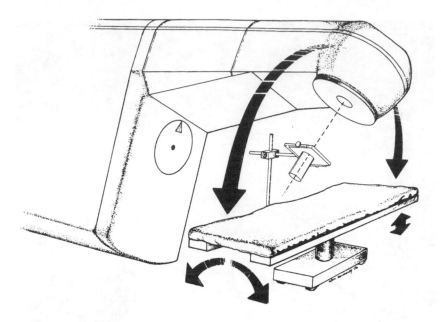

FIGURE 2.   The operating table is placed directly under the gantry. The table can be raised
to the appropriate source-target distance and rotated. The gantry is finally rotated to align
the beam with the treatment applicator.

the shield is made with the light field. The homogeneity of the scanning electron beam of
the THERAC-20 obviates precise coincidence of the field with the beam.

Precise alignment of the axes of the beam and applicator is necessary to avoid irradiation
of tissue outside the intended field. Alignment is done in three steps (Figure 2). (1) The
table is raised to the appropriate source-target distance. All applicators are manufactured 20
cm in length and the source-target distance is generally set at 100 cm to the top of the
applicator. (2) The table is laterally rotated; (3) the gantry is rotated. Precise alignment is
provided by a laser device developed by our physics team (Figure 3). A polished aluminum
plate is placed over the treatment applicator to allow reading of the source-target distance
and to reflect the two planar lasers. These lasers are set 90° apart. The incident beam projects
a line directly on the trimmer bars (which extend off the gantry to set field size). If the axes
of the applicator and electron beam are aligned, the reflected and incident beam will be
coincident in both axes of rotation.

The THERAC-20 delivers five electron energies, 6, 9, 13, 17, and 20 meV. Variable
thicknesses of shielding are available for each applicator for the various energies. Small
pieces of lead, cut in the operating room, are used to protect uninvolved sensitive structures
(e.g., ureters) in the treatment field.

V. RUSH EXPERIENCE

There have ben 85 patients treated with IORT at Rush-Presbyterian-St. Luke's Medical
Center (RPSLMC) from December 1982 through September 1986. All patients were felt to
be at high risk for local failure. External beam irradiation was planned unless the patient
had previously been treated with high-dose radiation therapy to the same area. However,
several patients refused external beam irradiation or the disease relapsed prior to the planned
start of treatment. The IORT dose was prescribed within general guidelines (10 to 15 Gy
for microscopic disease and 15 to 22.5 Gy for gross disease), but was decreased if mandated
by normal structures present in the IORT field (i.e., the full diameter of the duodenum,

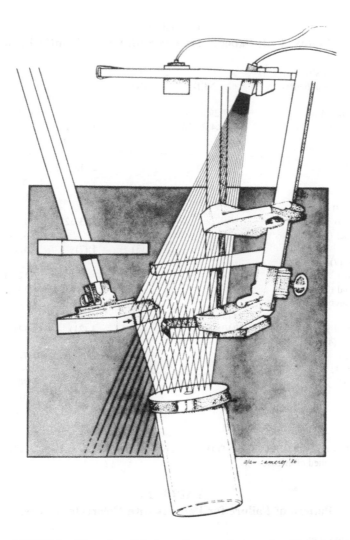

FIGURE 3. Illustration of the laser alignment device and treatment applicator. Two laser beams are focused in a planar fashion by cylindrical lenses mounted on a Lucite® tray that attaches to the gantry. This drawing shows a single beam projected onto the treatment applicator and trimmer bars and reflected from a polished aluminum plate which lies on the applicator. The incident beam projects a line (arrow) on the opposite trimmer bar. If the beam is not in direct alignment with the applicator, the reflected beam will project a line not coincident with the incident beam. Since the aluminum plate is perpendicular to the treatment applicator, coincidence of the lines in both axes verifies that the axis of the electron beam is identical with the axis of the treatment applicator.

both ureters) or by previous treatment. All IORT doses in this chapter are reported as maximum dose. Applicator sizes were chosen to provide a minimal margin around the target area. Electron energies were chosen to deliver a minimum tumor dose of 90% of the prescribed dose.

Table 1 lists our patients by cancer site and disease status. All patients had intraabdominal, pelvic, or retroperitoneal malignancies; 11 patients had known metastatic cancer at the time of the procedure, but were felt to be at high risk for disabling symptoms secondary to local progression of cancer.

TABLE 1
Disease Status of All Patients Treated with IORT (Months Follow-up)

Tumor site (number of patients)	NED	DID	AWD	DOD
Primary colorectal (6)	5 (27,29,30,33,36)	—	—	1 (10)
Recurrent colorectal (26)	5 (2,3,4,29,32)	—	4 (11,11, 11,28)	17 (1,3,6,6,6,6,8, 9,9,12,15,15,15, 16,17,22,25)
Pancreatic (21)	3 (8,10,11)	—	2 (13,23)	16 (3,4,5,5,6,6,7, 7,8,9,10,10,11, 13,14,23)
Biliary tract (9)				
Bile duct (5)	—	1 (19)	2 (3,32)	2 (3,9)
Gall bladder (4)	1 (22)	—	—	3 (6,13,25)
Gastric (7)	2 (2,40)	1 (3)	1 (7)	3 (4,5,15)
Gynecologic (7)				
Cervical (3)	1 (28)	—	—	2 (12,14)
Endometrial (2)	1 (15)	—	—	1 (13)
Leiomyosarcoma (1)	—	—	—	1 (5)
Ovarian (1)	1 (13)	—	—	—
Retroperitoneal sarcomas (4)	2 (10,41)	—	1 (21)	1 (14)
Genitourinary (4)				
Bladder (2)	1 (23)	—	—	1 (7)
Testicular (1)	—	1 (2)	—	—
Ureteric (1)	—	—	—	1 (20)
Melanoma (1)	—	—	—	1 (3)
Total (85)	22	3	10	50

Note: NED = no evidence of disease; DID = died of intercurrent disease; AWD = alive with disease; DOD = died of disease.

TABLE 2
Pattern of Failure for Patients with Colorectal Cancer

Residual disease (number of patients)	Local	Liver	Lung	Peritoneal	Other
Primary carcinomas (9)	—	1[a] (11%)	—	—	—
Microscopic (4)	—	—	—	—	—
Gross (3)	—	1[a] (11%)	—	—	—
Recurrent carcinomas (26)	10 (38%)	6 (23%)	5 (19%)	2 (8%)	4
Microscopic (11)	3 (27%)	2 (18%)	2[a] (18%)	—	—
Gross (15)	7 (47%)	4 (27%)	3 (20%)	2 (13%)	4[b]

[a] Includes one patient with metastases on presentation.
[b] Includes one patient surgically salvaged after abdominal wall failure.

VI. COLORECTAL CARCINOMA

Colorectal carcinoma was the most common disease in the IORT group. There were 23 patients treated for recurrent local disease, and 3 for recurrent disease in para-aortic nodes. Three patients had previously resected liver metastases and were clinically free of disease in that organ. Only one relapsed with spread to the liver at 6 months. One patient showed a solitary nodule on a lung CT scan consistent with a metastasis; another patient had known liver metastases. Six patients were treated for locally advanced colorectal carcinoma adherent to adjacent structures (three colon and three rectum).

TABLE 3
Incidence of Local Failure in Patients with Recurrent Colorectal Carcinoma

| | Residual disease | | |
External beam dose (Gy)	Microscopic	Gross	Total
<40	1/3	5/7	6/10
>40	2/8	2/8	4/16
Total	3/11	7/15	10/26

TABLE 4
Relationship Between Total Radiation Dose and Local Failure in Patients with Recurrent Colorectal Carcinoma

Total XRT dose[a] (Gy)	Proportion failed	
30—40	1/2	
41—50	2/4	
51—60	2/3	7/11
61—70	2/2	
71—80	0/5	
81—90	3/9	3/15
90+	0/1	

[a] Assumed RBE of IORT of 2. Total XRT dose = (IORT dose) multiplied by 2 + external beam dose.

The outcome of the patients with primary colorectal carcinoma was better than those with recurrent colorectal carcinoma (Table 1). Five of the six primary colorectal cancer patients are disease free more than 27 months after the procedure. The only patient who failed had liver metastases at the time of presentation, and the disease progressed in that organ.

Since local control is the primary goal of IORT, the pattern of failure was analyzed for the recurrent colorectal carcinoma patients (Table 2). The predominant site of failure was local. There appeared to be a relationship between the incidence of local failure and the ability to resect disease (Table 3). Of the patients with microscopic residual disease after resection, 27% failed locally vs. 47% of patients with gross residual disease. A relationship also appeared in the ability to deliver full-dose external beam therapy (>40 Gy): 25% vs. 60% (Table 3). The latter represents a group of patients with more advanced disease, many of whom had been treated previously. No patient's disease was locally controlled without resection or full-dose external beam irradiation in addition to IORT.

Table 4 suggests that the total dose (IORT plus external beam) is important in achieving local control. Assuming a relative biologic effect (RBE) of two for IORT, a total dose of 71 Gy or more was required to achieve local control.

Actuarial survival of the recurrent colorectal carcinoma patients is illustrated in Figure 4 for all patients, patients with resected disease, and patients with incompletely resected disease. There is no statistically significant difference between these groups, although there is a suggestion of improved survival for the patients with resected disease. These patients tended to have less bulky disease and to be treated with full-dose irradiation. Figure 5 illustrates the disease-free survival for these patients. Overall, this was 9% at 24 months.

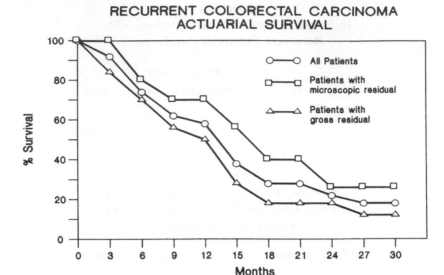

FIGURE 4.   Actuarial survival for patients with recurrent colorectal carcinoma.

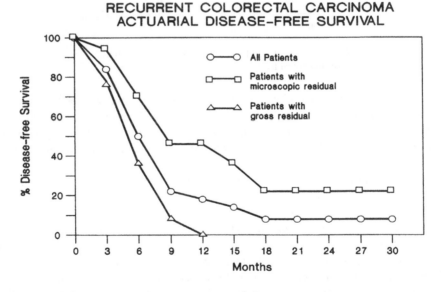

FIGURE 5.   Actuarial disease-free survival for patients with recurrent colorectal carcinoma.

VII. PANCREATIC CARCINOMA

There were 21 patients treated for pancreatic carcinoma; 5 patients had disease originating in or extending into the body or tail; 16 had disease limited to the head of the pancreas; 6 patients were treated immediately after resection; 15 patients underwent biopsy and only the appropriate bypass surgery. One patient had a single liver metastasis and a single peritoneal implant (both resected) at presentation and died at 3 months with progression of cancer at these sites. The remaining 20 patients had no evidence of distant metastasis.

Only three patients are disease-free at 8, 10, and 11 months (Table 1). Two of these patients had undergone resection. Several patients experienced an improved quality of life

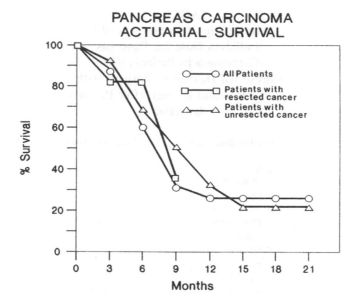

FIGURE 6.   Actuarial survival for patients with pancreas carcinoma.

TABLE 5
Pattern of Failure of Patients with Pancreas Carcinoma and Relationship to Type of Treatment

Treatment (number of patients)	Sites of failure				
	Local	Liver	Lung	Peritoneal	Unknown
Resection (6)	1 (17%)	2 (33%)	2 (33%)	2 (33%)	—
No resection (15)	9 (60%)	8 (53%)	2 (13%)	10 (68%)	1
Preoperative XRT[a] (7)	5 (71%)	2 (29%)	0	6 (86%)	—
No preoperative XRT (14)	5 (36%)	8 (57%)	4 (29%)	6 (43%)	1
Total (21)	10 (48%)	10 (48%)	4 (19%)	12 (57%)	1

[a]   6 patients received 5 Gy in 1 fraction; 1 patient received 46 Gy in 23 fractions.

and returned to work prior to relapse. The actuarial survival (Figure 6) for the entire group was 30% at 1 year and 14% at 2 years. The median survival was 9 months. There was no difference in survival between patients with resected disease and those with unresected disease.

Table 5 shows the pattern of failure for these patients. Most patients underwent follow-up CT scans. The predominant sites of failure were peritoneal, hepatic, and local. Only resection appeared to impact upon local failure. There were 7 who received preoperative irradiation (5 Gy in 1 fraction or 46 Gy in 23 fractions), but there appeared to be no impact on the pattern of failure. There is a suggestion that higher IORT and total dose improves local control for patients with gross disease (Table 6).

VIII. BILIARY TRACT CARCINOMA

Nine patients with carcinomas originating in the biliary system were treated with IORT, five with bile duct carcinomas and four with gall bladder carcinomas. Four of the five bile duct cancers were unresectable. The remaining patient's disease was resected and treatment

TABLE 6
Relationship of Local Control to
Radiation Dose for Pancreas
Carcinoma in Patients with
Unresected Disease or Patients with
Gross Residual Disease after Partial
Resection

Radiation dose (Gy)	Local failures
IORT dose	
10.0—12.5	2/3
12.5—15.0	2/2
15.1—17.5	2/3
17.6—20.0	3/6
>20.0	1/4
Total dose[a]	
<70	0/1
70—80	5/5
81—90	5/12

[a] Assuming RBE of 2 for IORT, total dose = IORT dose multiplied by 2 + external beam dose.

was directed to positive lymph nodes in the porta hepatis. All patients with gall bladder carcinoma had the disease resected; three received treatment to the port hepatis (including one patient with recurrent cancer) and one to both the porta hepatis and gall bladder fossa. Four patients received additional external beam irradiation. Most patients refused treatment after a prolonged hospital stay or when the cancer relapsed early. The only patient with no evidence of cancer at the time of this analysis received IORT and external beam radiation therapy.

Actuarial survival for the entire group with biliary tract carcinoma is 38% at 24 months. Median survival is 15 months. The only patient with recurrent squamous cell carcinoma of the gall bladder died at 6 months. Those patients with prolonged disease-free survival (three patients with disease-free survival longer than 12 months) returned to full activity. One patient died of biliary sepsis at 19 months without cancer.

Only one patient had a documented local failure, although two patients died of unknown causes (presumably of cancer). Two patients developed documented peritoneal seeding.

IX. GASTRIC CARCINOMA

Seven patients were treated with IORT to the celiac axis area following resection of gastric adenocarcinoma. Two patients had metastases at the time of exploration (one was resected). Only one patient had gross residual disease after resection. Three patients received further external beam irradiation.

Two patients are disease-free at 2 and 40 months. Neither patient was treated with external beam radiation therapy. One patient died at 3 months of intercurrent disease; autopsy demonstrated no recurrence of cancer. Only one local failure developed in this group, in a patient who did not receive external beam irradiation.

X. GYNECOLOGIC MALIGNANCIES

Seven gynecologic malignancies were treated with IORT. The primary sites of disease are listed in Table 1. Six patients were treated for local or nodal recurrences. The patient without recurrence was treated because of positive para-aortic lymphadenopathy. All the patients received external beam irradiation. One patient (with leiomyosarcoma) presented with a solitary lung metastasis.

Three patients remain disease free, including the patients with cancer of the uterine cervix. Two patients developed local failures, one with locally recurrent cervix cancer and one with locally recurrent leiomyosarcoma.

XI. RETROPERITONEAL SARCOMA

Two patients with initial presentation of retroperitoneal sarcoma and two patients with recurrent sarcoma were treated with IORT after apparently complete resection. The two patients with primary disease remain disease free. The two patients with recurrent disease failed within or at the margin of the IORT field.

XII. COMPLICATIONS

Many of the patients treated at RPSLMC had had several previous operative procedures and locally extensive carcinoma. Many of the complications encountered were secondary to the high surgical risk these patients presented and not directly related to the IORT itself.

There were 15 patients who developed acute complications that resulted in prolongation of hospitalization (Table 7). There was one postoperative death (at 3 months) from sepsis after gastric resection for carcinoma. No tumor was found at autopsy. Two patients developed pain in the pelvis shortly after surgery, probably related directly to the IORT.

There were 16 patients who developed complications more than 3 months following IORT (Table 8). Three patients developed biliary stasis related to tumor or biliary stents. One patient treated by IORT with an internal stent in place developed jaundice secondary to disintegration of the stent 2.5 years after the procedure. Needle biopsy documented local recurrence of cancer. One patient whose duodenum was partially treated by IORT for pancreas carcinoma and who had no gastrointestinal bypass procedure developed pain and partial gastric outlet obstruction secondary to duodenitis. Endoscopy revealed inflammation but no tumor. Two vascular complications occurred, an external iliac artery rupture and an iliofemoral thrombosis. A presacral abscess persisted in one patient for 37 months after IORT and resection of a locally extensive primary rectal carcinoma. One patient developed sacral osteonecrosis.

XIII. DISCUSSION

Our experience over the past 4 years has shown that IORT can be delivered safely, with a moderate risk of complications, to patients who are at high risk of local failure. Patients were selected who had already received previous radiation therapy and failed or who had a low likelihood of control with conventional doses of external beam irradiation with or without surgical extirpation.

With minimal surgical manipulation out of the operating room and radiation treatment on the operating table, there is minimal disruption of the radiation therapy schedule. This allows several patients to be scheduled for IORT on a given day. The procedure generally adds 1 h to the total anesthesia time. Patients can be scheduled at the time of initial exploration rather than requiring reoperation for IORT alone. Bypass procedures are done at the time

TABLE 7
Acute Complications (Within 3 Months) in 15 Patients

Complication	Primary site	Irradiated site
Fever	Uterine sarcoma	Pelvis
	Pancreas	Pancreas
	Bile Duct	Porta hepatis
Pneumonia	Colon	Pelvis
Sepsis — death	Stomach	Celiac axis
Small bowel obstruction	Sarcoma	Retroperitoneum
	Recurrent colon	Pelvis
Anastomotic leak	Stomach (2 patients)	Gastric bed
Wound dehiscence	Pancreas	Pancreas
	Biliary tract	Biliary tract
Prolonged ileus	Pancreas	Pancreas
Gastric outlet obstruction	Pancreas	Pancreas
	Biliary tract	Porta hepatis
Congestive heart failure	Stomach	Gastric bed
Pulmonary edema	Biliary tract	Porta Hepatis
Pulmonary embolus	Stomach	Gastric bed
Neurogenic bladder	Recurrent colon	Pelvis
Sciatic pain	Recurrent colon	Pelvis
	Primary colon	Pelvis

TABLE 8
Late Complications (More Than 3 Months Postop) in 16 Patients[a]

Complication	Primary site	Irradiated site	Dose (Gy)
Recurrent sepsis	Bile duct	Porta hepatis	22.0
	Gall bladder	Porta hepatis	16.5
Disintegrated biliary stent	Bile	Bile duct	22.0
Duodenitis	Pancreas	Pancreas	19.25
Celiac plexus pain	Stomach[a]	Gastric bed	22.0
	Pancreas[a]	Pancreas	19.8
	Pancreas	Pancreas	20.0
Vesicocolic fistula	Recurrent colon[a]	Pelvis	16.5
Vesicocutaneous fistula	Recurrent rectum[a]	Pelvis	26.5
Presacral abscess	Recurrent colon[a]	Pelvis	15.0
	Primary rectum	Pelvis	15.0
Sacral osteoradionecrosis	Recurrent colon[a]	Pelvis	16.3
External iliac artery rupture	Ureter[a]	Pelvis	15.0
Iliofemoral artery thrombosis	Recurrent rectum[a]	Pelvis	15.0
Leg weakness	Primary colon	Pelvis	20.0
Skin ulceration	Recurrent colon	Abdominal wall	26.0

[a]   Known local tumor recurrence or persistence.

of the initial operation, avoiding delay. Informed consent is obtained for all patients who are potential candidates for IORT. Only one fourth to one third of our potential patients undergo IORT.

Our preliminary results suggest an improvement in local control and survival in selected groups of patients. Three factors appear related to local failure: (1) primary vs. recurrent disease, (2) ability to perform resection, and (3) ability to deliver high-dose external beam radiation therapy. No disease was controlled in any patient who received IORT alone without resection.

Overall, 56% of our patients presented with primary disease. Of these patients, 27% developed local failure after IORT as compared to 38% of patients with recurrent cancer.

Patients with complete resection, suspected to have microscopic residual disease, failed locally in 17% of our cases vs. 27% of patients who underwent partial resection and 56% of patients who underwent no resection. These numbers are almost certainly low estimates since few autopsies were obtained. We feel, however, that these results are encouraging.

We conclude that IORT and external beam irradiation for patients with cancers below the diaphragm improves the probability of local control and disease-free survival. The risk of complications is moderate but acceptable. We feel that there exists a definite subset of patients, those with high risk of local tumor recurrence or progression, for which the potential benefits of this exciting technique outweigh the risk. Finally, we feel that our approach of using existing facilities for surgery and radiation therapy has proven to be reasonable and practical.

Chapter 28

INTRAOPERATIVE RADIATION THERAPY: THE MEDICAL COLLEGE OF OHIO EXPERIENCE

Ralph R. Dobelbower, Jr., Ahmed Eltaki, and Donald G. Bronn

TABLE OF CONTENTS

I. INTRODUCTION

The rationale for intraoperative radiation therapy (IORT) has been stated previously in Chapter 2 of this work. At the Medical College of Ohio (MCO) we have refrained from using IORT with radiosensitizers or chemotherapeutic agents so as to better assess the efficacy of IORT as a single treatment modality. In all cases we have employed intraoperative electron beam therapy (IOEBT). In general, we have employed IOEBT as a means of delivering a boost dose of radiation in addition to conventional external beam radiation therapy.

A team approach is essential to the application of IOEBT. The surgeon and the radiotherapist must agree regarding patient position on the operating table as well as the length and placement of the surgical incision preoperatively. This is necessary to give the best exposure of the tumor or the tumor bed.

In general, we have followed the philosophy of tumor resection before IOEBT when feasible. Normal tissues which cannot be retracted away from the field of treatment are protected by custom-fabricated sterilized lead shields of appropriate thickness (depending on electron energy).

A. TECHNIQUES

As a rule, the radiotherapist participates in the exploratory phases of surgery. He guides the surgeon toward adequate exposure of the tumor, the tumor bed, or regional nodes. The volume of interest is measured in three dimensions. An IOEBT applicator of appropriate size and shape is selected to provide a 0.5- to 1-cm margin around the tumor or the tumor bed. Applicators of various sizes and bevels are fit to the volume of interest to achieve the best possible application of the beam. The appropriate electron beam energy is selected according to thickness of the target volume (TV). Although the dose is prescribed to the

100% isodose line, an electron energy is selected so that the 80% isodose line falls at least 1 cm deep to the tumor or tumor bed. In each instance, in choosing a beam energy, the radiotherapist and physicist consult previously measured isodose distributions for the particular IOEBT applicator in use. The focus-surface treatment distance (FSD) ranges from 97 to 115 cm. Most often IOEBT is conducted at 100 cm FSD at the MCO. Extended FSD (>100 cm) is generally employed for pelvic applications, for deeply situated lesions, and in some situations where marked rotation of the linear accelerator gantry is required.

The MCO IOEBT protocols aim to utilize IOEBT to deliver a boost dose of radiation in conjunction with conventional fractionated external beam irradiation after maximal surgical resection. The external beam treatment usually includes potential lymph node drainage areas, and consists of 50 to 60 Gy in 1.8- to 2.0-Gy fractions delivered over 5 to 6 weeks using 6-million electron volt peak or 10 (meVp) or 10 meVp photon beams. Multiple fields, wedges, compensators and custom-shaped portals are employed as necessary to limit radiation dose to adjacent normal tissues.

Potential advantages of using a combined IOEBT-external beam approach include the possibility of improving local and regional tumor control. Also, using IOEBT as a sole treatment modality with higher single doses may increase the risk of local normal tissue damage.

B. PATIENT SELECTION

Patients selected for the MCO IOEBT protocols meet the following criteria:

1. No medical or other contraindication to exploratory surgery
2. Informed consent (written)
3. Unresectable tumor or high risk of local recurrence after resection, or local recurrence of tumor after surgery or irradiation.

Over the span of 4 years, we considered approximately 300 patients for IOEBT. Of these, we selected 150 patients for surgical exploration in the specially constructed IOEBT operating amphitheater in the Clement O. Miniger Radiation Oncology Center (COMROC) at the MCO; 109 (73%) of the 150 patients actually received IOEBT (Table 1).

The remainder of this chapter outlines the basis of and the early clinical experience with the MCO IOEBT protocols by disease site.

II. ADENOCARCINOMA OF THE PANCREAS

Cancer of the pancreas is the second most common neoplasm of the gastrointestinal tract and is the fifth leading cause of cancer death in the U.S. today.[1] It is estimated that over 27,000 new cases of cancer of the pancreas will be diagnosed this year in this country.[1]

Cure is an uncommon outcome of any form of treatment for adenocarcinoma of the pancreas. The disease extends beyond the capsule of the gland at the time of diagnosis in almost all cases, resulting in local or regional failure after surgery (indicating inadequate local treatment). In one recent cooperative group study, local recurrence was observed in 86% of patients after "curative" surgery.[2] Death from distant metastases is the exception rather than the rule.

The optimum approach to pancreatic cancer must take into consideration the clinical state of the patient and the stage of the disease. Less than 20% of patients with this diagnosis are candidates for a curative resection.[3] Operative mortality from the definitive surgical procedures for cancer of the pancreas ranges from 7 to 60%.[4,5]

Regionally extended surgical procedures have shown only slight increases in patient survival, but substantial increases in patient morbidity and mortality.[6] The overall 5-year survival rate for patients with resected disease is approximately 4%,[7] thus the risk of operative mortality exceeds the probability of cure in most centers.[4]

TABLE 1
Clinical Experience with Intraoperative
Radiotherapy at MCO

Primary tumor site	Number of patients	
	IOEBT	Explored
Pancreas	22	36
Rectum	23	25
Cervix	9	11
Sarcoma	7	7
Colon	6	17
Brain	6	6
Ovary	5	9
Stomach	5	8
Breast	5	6
Miscellaneous		
Kidney	3	3
Lung	2	4
Bile duct	2	3
Prostate	2	2
Head and neck	2	2
Anus	2	2
Endometrium	2	2
Urinary bladder	1	2
Melanoma	1	1
Sacral chordoma	1	1
Duodenum	1	1
Vagina	1	1
Malignant Schwannoma	1	1
Total	109	150

Nakase et al.[8] reviewed a series of 332 patients with adenocarcinoma of the pancreas explored surgically. Only 18% of patients proved to have resectable disease. The mortality rate was 25% and the 5-year survival rate was only 6%. Monge, at Mayo Clinic,[9] reported another study of 119 patients in which he observed a 10% resectability rate with a mortality rate of 25% and a 5-year survival rate of 8%.

The role of radiation therapy in the management of cancer of the pancreas has expanded considerably during the last decade. For locally advanced disease, this has resulted in improved median survival (about 1 year), but the 5-year survival rate for such patients remains less than 5%.[10]

Technological advances in radiation therapy treatment planning systems and treatment delivery systems permitted development of precision high-dose (PHD) external beam techniques.[11] Local control of disease was observed in only approximately one third of patients treated with PHD external beam therapy, but patient survival was found to be comparable to that of patients with resectable disease treated surgically via Whipple's procedure or total pancreatectomy, with a median survival of 10 to 12 months, but the 5-year survival rate was less than 10%.[12]

The radiation dose required to control pancreatic adenocarcinoma by external beam irradiation alone appears to be greater than the radiotolerance of the surrounding organs and tissues. This is also true for external beam irradiation by particle beams (neutrons, helium ions, etc.).[13]

Interstitial implantation of ^{125}I seeds, in addition to PHD external beam radiation therapy showed improvement in local control, but patient survival was not improved.[14] Administration of 5-Fluorouracil (5-FU) concurrently with external beam radiation therapy appears

TABLE 2
IOEBT — Adenocarcinoma of the Pancreas: Patient Data

36 Patients

Male	19
Female	17
Age	40—85 years (median: 63)
IOEBT	22
No IOEBT	14
Metastases	12
No tumor	2
(Pancreatitis, cyst)	

TABLE 3
IOEBT — Adenocarcinoma of the Pancreas: Symptoms

Symptom	Number of patients
Pain	18
Weight loss	13
Jaundice	12
Anorexia	9
Light-colored stool	8
Dark urine	6
Vomiting	3
Depression	2

to increase median survival over irradiation alone, but despite the positive result, few patients survive 2 years, and local control of the irradiated tumor remains an important clinical problem.[15] In an MCO study,[16] 12 patients with adenocarcinoma of the pancreas received combined therapy with ^{125}I implant, PHD photon external beam therapy, and systemic 5-FU. Median survival was 15 months, but morbidity was greater than that of PHD external beam therapy alone. Consequently, we commenced a study of IOEBT plus PHD external beam therapy for unresectable pancreatic adenocarcinoma.

A. PATIENT CHARACTERISTICS

Since 1983, the abdomens of 36 patients with a diagnosis of adenocarcinoma of the pancreas have been surgically explored at the MCO COMROC IOEBT operating amphitheater (Tables 1 and 2). Patient age ranged from 40 to 85 years (median: 63); 19 patients were male, 17 were female; 34 patients were white, 1 was black, and 1 was hispanic.

Presenting symptoms of the 34 patients with adenocarcinoma of the pancreas are shown in Table 3. The most common symptoms were pain, weight loss, and jaundice: 18 patients presented with pain, 13 patients with weight loss, and 12 with jaundice. Only one patient failed to manifest pain, weight loss or jaundice. There were 13 patients who lost an average of 20 lb in the immediate pretreatment period. Nine patients were anorexic, eight patients noted light-colored stool, and six, dark urine. Three patients presented with vomiting, and two with severe emotional depression.

Pretreatment studies included complete blood count, serum bilirubin and other standard liver function studies, chest radiography, upper gastrointestinal radiographs, computed tomography (CT) scans of the liver and pancreas, endoscopic retrograde cholangiopancreatography (ERCP), and radioisotope scans of the liver, spleen, and skeleton. Each patient underwent at least one abdominal laporatomy, at which time the diagnosis was established histologically before treatment, usually by direct biopsy of the pancreas. When possible, histologic confirmation of malignancy was obtained by biopsy of regional lymph nodes or extrahepatic extensions of the disease. Gastrointestinal and/or biliary decompressive bypass procedures were performed in all but two patients. Complete tumor resection was accomplished in three cases.

At the time of surgical exploration, 12 of the 36 patients were found to have distant metastasis or more than minimal hepatic metastasis; hence, no IOEBT was delivered. In one patient we were unable to histologically confirm a malignant process in spite of multiple biopsies of pancreas and common bile duct. Another patient was found to have a pancreatic cyst. In both of the latter two cases, the preexploration ERCP was highly suggestive of malignancy.

Three patients with Stage IV disease (hepatic metastasis) were treated with IOEBT as a palliative manuever because abdominal pain was a prominent presenting symptom.

B. STAGING

At the time of surgery for IOEBT, the stage of the disease was observed and recorded according to the following system.[16]

Stage I — Cancer confined to the pancreas. No extension of cancer beyond the capsule of the pancreas. No involved lymph nodes. No hepatic or distant metastasis.

Stage II — Cancer extending locally beyond the pancreas to involve contiguous structures. No involved lymph nodes. No hepatic or distant metastases.

Stage III — Metastatic cancer in regional lymph nodes. No hepatic or other distant metastasis.

Stage IV — Hepatic extension of cancer (either direct or hematogenous spread) or other distant metastasis.

In general, the pancreatic cancers were rather extensive. The size of the primary lesion ranged from $3 \times 4 \times 4$ to $7 \times 7 \times 8$ cm with an average of $6 \times 5.5 \times 5.2$ cm. The numbers of patients with different stages of cancer of the pancreas are shown in Table 4. One patient with Stage I cancer was treated with IOEBT as he was not a candidate for radical surgery because of advanced chronic obstructive bronchopulmonary disease and a previous history of multiple malignancies. There were 13 patients who had Stage II cancers, five had Stage III cancers, and 15 had Stage IV cancers. Only three patients with Stage IV disease were treated with IOEBT.

C. TREATMENT TECHNIQUES

The entire radiosurgical procedure was conducted in the MCO COMROC IOEBT operating amphitheater. After general anesthesia was administered, the abdomen was prepared and draped and exploratory laparotomy was conducted in the usual fashion. At the time of exploration, the abdominal viscera were carefully inspected and palpated in a search for abdominal metastatic disease. The primary lesion was surgically exposed, and extension to adjacent structures was noted and recorded. A biopsy was obtained from involved lymph nodes, local extensions of disease, or the primary tumor. The dimensions of the primary lesion and any local extensions of disease were measured and recorded. Intestinal and biliary bypass procedures were generally performed after IOEBT delivery.

1. IOEBT Delivery

Once the tumor was adequately exposed, hemostasis was obtained, and the tumor size measured, an assessment was made jointly by the radiotherapist and the surgeon regarding the appropriateness of IOEBT. The IOEBT dose was not delivered in the face of disease that could not be encompassed within a single treatment applicator, hepatic or peritoneal metastasis or massive local disease, unless pain was a prominent presenting symptom of the

TABLE 4
IOEBT — Adenocarcinoma
of the Pancreas: Stage

Stage	Number of patients
Stage I	1
Stage II	13
Stage III	5
Stage IV	15

TABLE 5
IOEBT — Adenocarcinoma of the Pancreas: Radiation
Dose, Electron Energy, and Applicator Size by Stage and
Size of Lesion

Stage	Number of patients	Lesion size (cm)	Dose (Gy)	Electron energy (meV)	Applicator
I	1	4 × 4 × 4	25	15	$1^3/_4$in. F[a]
II	13	3 × 4.5 × 5	20	12	2 in. 15°[a]
		3 × 5 × 5	20	15	4 in. 15°
		4 × 4.5 × 6	25	15	2.5 in. 15°
		4 × 4 × 5	25	18	2 in. 15°
		4.5 × 5 × 5	20	15	$2^2/_4$in. 30°[a]
		6.5 × 6.5	25	18	$2^3/_4$in. F
		7 × 7 × 8	25	18	$3^1/_2$ in. 30°
		3 × 4 × 3.5	25	15	$1^3/_4$ in. F
III	5	6 × 4 × 5	20	18	3 in. 30°
		3 × 4 × 4.5	15	15	4 in. 30°
		5 × 5 × 4.5	20	15	$2^3/_4$ in. F
IV	3	7 × 5 × 5	30	18	3 in. F
		5 × 4 × 5.5	25	15	$2^1/_2$ in. 30°
		3 × 5 × 5	20	15	2 in. 15°

[a]   F = flat end applicator; 15° = applicator with 15° beveled end; 30° = applicator with 30° beveled end.

disease. A Lucite® applicator of proper size was selected to encompass the tumor volume and a small margin of adjacent normal tissue. The energy of the electron beam, typically 15 or 18 meV, was selected according to the thickness of the tumor, except in patients with complete tumor resection where electron beam energies of 12 or 15 meV were used. The patient and the operating table were then moved underneath the treatment machine. The Lucite® applicator was telescoped out of the aluminum sleeve attached to the treatment head of the machine with the use of the right angle telescope. The table was then elevated to achieve a typical FSD of 100 cm. Once the radiotherapist, the surgeon, and the anesthesiologist were satisfied with the application and the patient's general condition, all personnel exited the treatment room for the period of dose delivery. An IOEBT dose of 15 to 30 Gy was delivered over a span of 5 to 12 min. Radiation dose, electron energy, and applicator size by stage and size of lesion are shown in Table 5. Early in the study, one patient received a dose of 30 Gy; thereafter, a dose of 25 Gy was usually employed for unresectable lesions. We have used a 20-Gy dose recently, as we participate in the Radiation Therapy Oncology Group (RTOG) prospective study of the use of IORT in pancreatic cancer. In most patients, an electron beam energy of 15 or 18 meV was employed. An electron beam energy of 12 meV was employed in one patient after complete tumor resection. In general, the depth of the TV is reduced by tumor resection. Two other patients with complete resection of pancreatic tumors were treated with 15-meV electron beams. In one patient with a lesion of the body of the gland that was completely resected via a distal pancreatectomy, the TV included clinically involved para-aortic lymph nodes not included in the surgical resection.

2. Surgical Procedures

After delivery of IOEBT, the patient was moved back to the operating area of the COMROC IOEBT operating amphitheater where biliary and gastrointestinal decompressive bypass procedures were performed as indicated. The preferred biliary bypass was chole-dochojejunostomy. Occasionally this procedure was not feasible. Additionally, in a few patients, alternative bypass procedures (cholecystojejunostomy) had been performed prior to referral to the MCO. A distal enteroenterostomy was performed in most patients. Gastrojejunostomy was usually performed. Recently, a feeding jejunostomy has sometimes been added.

3. External Beam Therapy

PHD external beam therapy[10] was initiated after recovery from surgery, generally within 4 to 6 weeks in all patients. The treatment technique consisted of four custom-shaped anterior, posterior, right and left lateral fields to irradiate the tumor volume, plus a 1- to 3-cm margin. The tumor was identified by radioopaque markers placed at the time of IOEBT and by CT scans. Alternatively, a three-field technique composed of a pair of wedged, custom-shaped lateral fields and a single, anterior custom-shaped field was used to irradiate the TV.

Great care was used in establishing the three-dimensional locations of the tumor and of surrounding normal tissues for PHD external beam therapy. Appropriate CT scans were routinely used to further delineate tumor margins and to localize the stomach, liver, and kidneys. Multiple body section images were taken at 5- to 10-m intervals. These scans were used to transfer the necessary anatomic information to the associated simulation films. Information from arteriograms, inferior venacavagrams, cholangiograms, and ERCP was also incorporated in the treatment plan when appropriate.

The cephalad and caudad margins of the TV were placed 2 cm beyond the excursion of the radioopaque markers with quiet respirations. The left TV margin was a generous 2 to 3 cm beyond the gross tumor margin along the pancreatic duct, as pancreatic cancers are known to spread along the pancreatic duct in occult fashion. Similarly, a 3-cm margin was used in the region of the hepatic hilus, since pancreatic cancers also spread along the common bile duct and to its surrounding lymph nodes. An anterior margin of 1 cm was used since the surgical approach was from the anterior, and it was this margin that was most reliably represented by radioopaque markers. Also, this margin was least sensitive to respiratory motion and patient rotation.

Placement of the posterior TV margin was dictated by the location of the anterior surface of the kidneys as visualized on the CT scan, or by lateral cross-table simulator radiographs during the nephrogram phase after intravenous injection of radiographic contrast material.

The tumor volume was generally encompassed by the 95% isodose curve for PHD external beam therapy. The external beam radiation treatment regimen used was a daily dose of 1.8 to 2.0 Gy, five fractions per week, for a minimum total external beam dose of 50 to 60 Gy over a 5.5- to 7-week period. A few patients received postoperative PHD external beam therapy at hometown facilities distant from the MCO. In most such cases, the simulation, treatment planning, and dose specifications were accomplished at the MCO treatment planning center.

Postoperative external beam therapy was terminated at a dose of 39.6 Gy in one patient when a CT scan showed a large pancreatic mass with multiple metastases in the liver and the spinal cord. Another patient's external beam therapy was terminated at a dose of 40 Gy

TABLE 6
**IOEBT — Adenocarcinoma of the Pancreas: Early
Complications**

Complication	Number of patients	
Anorexia, nausea, vomiting	3	
Splenic infarction, death, 9 days postoperatively	1 (?)	
Anastomotic leak	1	
Colonic fistula	1	Patients with complete
Postoperative fever	1	tumor resection

because surgical clips outlining the tumor were observed to be outside the field of irradiation. This was thought to be indicative of growth of the tumor during external beam radiation therapy. Three patients expired before PHD external beam therapy commenced.

D. RESULTS

No patient has been lost to follow-up. Follow-up ranges from 2 to 25 months.

1. Acute Morbidity

A total of 22 patients received IOEBT and 19 received PHD external beam therapy. In two patients, the PHD external beam therapy was terminated short of the planned dose of 50 to 60 Gy as described above. No intraoperative complications were observed in any patient treated. Early complications observed in patients who received IOEBT are shown in Table 6. One patient, within 1 week of IOEBT, developed splenic infarction complicated by splenic abscess and septicemia. She died 9 days postoperatively. This occurred early in the series, and we hypothesize that the infarction may have been due to compression of the splenic vasculature by the treatment applicator. The patient also had very extensive hepatic metastatic disease and IOEBT was delivered as a palliative maneuver.

Delayed gastric emptying after gastrojejunostomy constituted a significant problem in many patients. Nausea has been a frequent sequel to IOEBT, and, during PHD external beam therapy, anorexia and weight loss have been problems even though dietary supplements and pancreatic extracts were usually utilized.

Three patients with complete tumor resection developed early complications: one patient developed an anastomotic leak that healed with conservative treatment. That patient sustained an acute myocardial infarction and expired 2 months after IOEBT with no evidence of disease before postoperative external beam therapy commenced. One patient developed a colonic fistula, and a third patient was admitted to the MCO with postoperative fever.

Patients lost an average weight of 1.5 kg during the course of PHD external beam therapy. No patient lost more weight than 2.5 kg during this period. Patient nutrition was assessed by the radiation oncology nurse on a weekly basis, and patients were given dietary advice and encouragement as well as prescribed food supplements as needed.

2. Late Morbidity

Clinically significant hepatic, renal, or spinal cord damage was not observed. No patient developed diabetes as a result of treatment. Two patients with anorexia, nausea, and diarrhea lost an average of 5.5 kg (Table 7). Exocrine pancreatic insufficiency was suspected in these patients and treated empirically with pancreatic enzyme replacement, but no improvement was observed.

One patient was found to have an active ulcer in the gastric antrum, as well as an abdominal-cutaneous fistula. This patient had been previously treated for cancer of the pancreas with ^{125}I interstitial implant (140 Gy) and PHD external beam irradiation (60 Gy)

TABLE 7
IOEBT — Adenocarcinoma of the Pancreas: Late Morbidity of Combined IOEBT and External Beam Therapy

Complication	Number of patients
Anorexia, nausea, diarrhea, weight loss	2
Pancreatic exocrine insufficiency	2
Antral ulcer, fistula	1
Suspected aortoenteric fistula, pancreaticocuta-neous fistula	1

TABLE 8
IOEBT — Adenocarcinoma of the Pancreas: Patient Status

Patient	Status	Survival	Comment
R.R.	D	12 months	With disease
M.L.	D	9 days	Splenic infarction
C.V.	D	8 months	
A.G.	D	19 months	With disease
W.S.	D	10 months	With disease
M.W.	D	5 months	Extensive metastasis
L.P.	D	20 months	With disease
A.I.	D	2 months	
T.R.	A	24 months	With disease
J.B.	D	12 months	Liver metastasis
M.O.	D	5 months	
G.C.	D	1 month	
P.S.	D	7 months	
R.H.	A	12 months	
C.S.	D	4 months	
C.B.	D	5 months	
I.C.	A	9 months	
B.B.	A	4 months	
E.K.	A	3 months	Postoperative fever
A.C.	A	2 months	Colonic fistula, my-ocardial infarction
E.L.	A	1 month	

prior to developing local recurrence which was treated with IOEBT. One patient expired with massive upper gastrointestinal hemorrhage 5 months after IOEBT. Aortoenteric fistula was suspected, but an autopsy was not performed. She had received an IOEBT dose of 25 Gy using 15-meV electrons and PHD external beam radiation therapy to a dose of 50.4 Gy. This patient also developed a pancreaticocutaneous fistula postoperatively.

3. Palliation of Symptoms

Pain was relieved or improved in 17 of 18 patients presenting with same. Of 13 patients with weight loss, 6 showed a reversal of that trend and actually gained weight with treatment. Jaundice was relieved in all 12 patients presenting with biliary obstruction.

4. Survival

Patient status since IOEBT is shown in Table 8. Seven patients are alive as of November 1987. One of these patients has clinical evidence of hepatic metastasis and local recurrence of cancer. This patient received 40 Gy PHD external beam irradiation after 25 Gy IOEBT. His external radiation therapy was terminated after 40 Gy because the surgical clips outlining the tumor were outside the previous field and this was interpreted as an indication of tumor growth.

Of the 15 patients that died, 3 died from causes other than cancer: 1 of splenic infarction 9 days after IOEBT, and 2 others of unrelated causes 1 and 2 months after IOEBT, without clinical evidence of locally recurrent or metastatic cancer. The remaining 12 patients are presumed to have died of local progression of disease, although permission for post-mortem examination was not granted for any of those patients.

Except for hepatic metastases, distant metastases were observed in only three patients: one developed metastases in the spinal cord and liver — she had been treated for breast cancer by radical mastectomy 3 years before she developed an adenocarcinoma in the pancreas believed to be a second primary tumor. The development of spinal metastasis is unusual for pancreatic cancer, but common for breast cancer. Therefore, it is possible that the spinal (and perhaps also the hepatic) metastases were secondary to the breast cancer rather than the pancreatic cancer. It is not inconceivable that the entire disease picture was adenocarcinoma of the breast with extensive metastases including metastasis to the pancreas, although the breast and pancreatic lesions were histologically dissimilar. The second patient developed extensive metastatic disease in the pelvis, and the third patient developed pulmonary metastasis.

E. DISCUSSION

Cancer of the pancreas remains a major therapeutic challenge to the radiation therapist. PHD external beam therapy of upper abdominal tumors appears to be well-tolerated and produces not only satisfactory palliation, but also an occasional long-term survivor of unresectable cancer of the pancreas.

For patients with resectable disease, postoperative adjuvant radiation therapy may be of benefit.[2] Preoperative radiation therapy has been inadequately tested, and particle beam treatment seems associated with an increased complication rate.[13,17] Chemotherapy appears to be an effective adjunct to radiation therapy for patients with unresectable cancer of the pancreas.[12,18] Regardless of the surgical procedure employed and regardless of the use of adjuvant radiation therapy and chemotherapy, the overall survival rate for patients with cancer of the pancreas remains dismally low.[7,19] Furthermore, local recurrence continues to be a major problem.

IOEBT is a feasible method to deliver massive boost doses of radiation to unresectable pancreatic tumors (or to the beds of resected pancreatic tumors). When used in combination with appropriate biliary and gastrointestinal decompressive bypass surgery and PHD external beam therapy, palliation of pain and jaundice is the rule. The procedure, however, is not without significant risk, especially when used as an adjuvant to pancreaticoduodectomy. It remains to be seen whether patient survival can be improved with the delivery of massive boost doses by IOEBT. Only a few hundred patients with pancreatic cancer have been treated with IOEBT worldwide; hence, optimum dose, technique, and combination with other modalities are as yet unknown. A phase II RTOG protocol investigating IOEBT in combination with postoperative external beam radiation and adjuvant chemotherapy (5-FU) has been initiated.[20] Results of this study will hopefully shed more light on the value of IORT as regards palliation and patient survival in adenocarcinoma of the pancreas.

III. CANCER OF THE RECTUM

Surgical treatment for rectal cancer often fails because of occult residual disease. It is usually possible to obtain adequate surgical margins in the management of colon cancer,

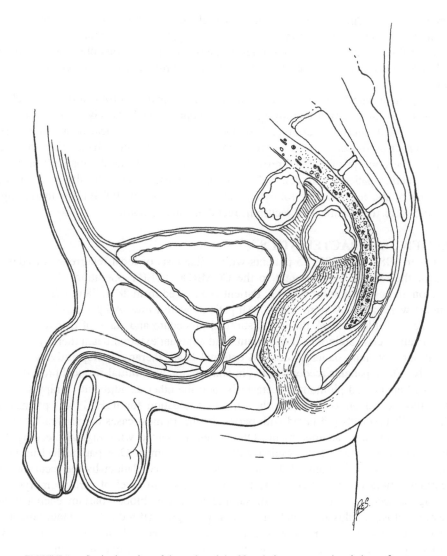

FIGURE 1.   Sagittal section of the male pelvis. Note intimate anatomic relations of rectum
to prostate, bladder, and presacral neurovascular plexus.

but in rectal cancer, because of the intimate anatomic relations of various pelvic structures
to the anterior and posterior rectal wall, it is often difficult to obtain satisfactory margins.
An adequate posterior margin is often difficult to achieve because of the proximity of the
bony sacrum and the presacral neurovascular plexus (Figure 1). Also, in the male, the urinary
bladder, seminal vesicles, and prostate gland lie just anterior to the rectum and often preclude
an adequate anterior margin without extensive debilitating surgery.

For the reasons noted above, local recurrence in the absence of distant metastasis continues to constitute a major area of treatment failure in rectal cancer. Approximately one
half of rectal cancer patients that are not cured of the disease fail in the pelvis without distant
dissemination of disease.[21] Approximately one half of rectal cancer patients that develop
distant metastases will also develop local pelvic recurrence of cancer.[22] Thus, local failure
is a component of disease recurrence in approximately three fourths of rectal cancer patients
that fail to achieve permanent tumor control. It follows that a significant improvement in
local control could translate into improved patient survival in this disease. Many authors
have suggested that this might be achieved for certain resectable rectal tumors by combining

surgery and irradiation.[23] For some groups of high-risk patients, external beam irradiation has been shown to be of benefit in an adjuvant setting,[24] but for patients with unresectable or recurrent disease the normal tissue tolerance emerges as a serious obstacle to cure since the radiation dose levels required to achieve local control generally exceed normal tissue tolerance.

In the patient with local gross recurrence of cancer, pain control can often be achieved with external beam radiation therapy in doses of approximately 50 Gy over 5 to 6 weeks, but this dose will rarely be curative. Patients with symptomatic local recurrence of rectal cancer after prior full-dose pelvic irradiation present even more challenging therapeutic problems. The concept of IOEBT provides a logistically and radiobiologically acceptable option in treating patients with residual, primarily nonresectable or locally recurrent adenocarcinoma of the rectum. The following illustrates the use of IOEBT for increasing the therapeutic ratio for treatment of recurrent rectal adenocarcinoma.

A. PATIENT CHARACTERISTICS

Between 1983 and 1987, 25 patients with a diagnosis of local recurrence of adenocarcinoma of the rectum were brought to the COMROC IOEBT operating amphitheater for exploration and evaluation for IOEBT. Patient age ranged from 28 to 78 (median: 64) years; 15 patients were male, 10 were female. All patients were white. All patients had undergone prior surgery. Table 9 shows the initial surgical procedure and stage of disease in patients with recurrent rectal carcinoma. Ten patients had adjuvant external beam therapy at the time of initial surgery: nine patients received external beam therapy postoperatively, one preoperatively. Three patients received 5-FU in conjunction with initial surgical procedure, two because of hepatic and pulmonary metastasis, and the other as adjuvant therapy.

The most common symptom at the time of evaluation for IOEBT was perineal pain (Table 10). Ten patients presented with perineal pain. In most cases the pain radiated to the leg. Nine patients were asymptomatic. One patient presented with vaginal bleeding due to involvement of the apex of the vagina with recurrent tumor. One patient had urinary incontinence due to involvement of the ureter and the urinary bladder by the recurrent mass. Pretreatment studies included complete blood count, serum level of carcinoembryonic antigen, digital rectal examination, stool sample for occult blood, barium enema with air contrast, proctosigmoidoscopy, and intravenous pyelogram (if indicated). Metastatic disease was searched for with chest Roentgenograms, CT scans, serum bilirubin and other standard liver function studies, as well as radioisotope scans of the liver and skeleton.

B. STAGING

The stage of the disease was retrospectively recorded according to the following system:[25]

A — lesion limited to the mucosa, lymph nodes negative
B_1 — lesion extending into but not through the muscular coat. Lymph nodes negative
B_2 — lesion extending through the muscular coat, without positive nodes
C_1 — lesion limited to the wall, with positive nodes
C_2 — lesion extending through all layers, with positive nodes

C. TREATMENT TECHNIQUES

Of the 25 patients, 23 underwent IOEBT. At the time of surgical exploration we were not able to confirm the clinical diagnosis of recurrent cancer in one patient, and in another we withheld IOEBT because of massive hemorrhage from the perineal incision. The latter patient was subsequently treated with external beam radiation therapy.

TABLE 9
IOEBT — Recurrent Rectal Cancer: Initial Surgical Procedure and Stage of Disease

Initial stage	Number of patients	Initial surgical procedure
A	1	Abdominoperineal resection
B_2	8	5 abdominoperineal resection; 3 low anterior resection
C_1	2	1 abdominoperineal resection; 1 Hartman's procedure
C_2	14	9 abdominoperineal resection; 1 Hartman's procedure; 4 low anterior resection

TABLE 10
IOEBT — Recurrent Rectal Cancer: Presenting Symptoms

Symptom	Number of patients
Perineal pain	10
Sciatica	3
Diarrhea	2
Urinary incontinence	1
Massive leg edema	1
Anemia and fatigue	1
Vaginal bleeding	1
Asymptomatic	9

1. Surgical Approach

There were 3 different approaches to the lesion utilized in the 23 patients who underwent IOEBT for recurrent rectal cancer (Table 11). The IOEBT was delivered to 13 lesions through a lower abdominal incision. Seven patients underwent abdominoperineal resection with IOEBT delivered through the abdominal incision and/or the perineal wound. For three patients, IOEBT was accomplished through a posterior intergluteal incision. In each of these three patients the disease was fixed to, or actually invading, the sacrum, necessitating a partial sacrectomy. Of 23 patients, 4 had distant metastases at the time of exploration and evaluation for IOEBT. Those patients were treated with IOEBT as a palliative maneuver, as perineal pain and back pain were prominent symptoms.

In general, the recurrences were rather extensive in terms of involvement of pelvic structures, although the actual sizes of the lesions were moderate. The size of the recurrent lesions ranged from $2 \times 2.5 \times 2$ to $5 \times 5 \times 5.7$ cm (average, $4.5 \times 4.5 \times 5.5$ cm). After exposure of the recurrent mass (and prior to any resection), areas of gross recurrent tumor were confirmed by biopsy. Table 12 shows the extent of resection performed at time of IOEBT, doses delivered and beam energy.

2. IOEBT Delivery

After complete or partial resection of the mass, if resectable, or exposure of the unresectable mass, the proposed IOEBT field was defined by the radiosurgical team. Areas free of macroscopic tumor, but at high risk for microscopic residual disease, were determined by correlation with preoperative assessment, adherence of tumor to contiguous structures at the time of surgery, and frozen-section analysis of the surgical specimen.

TABLE 11
IOEBT — Recurrent Rectal Cancer:
Radiosurgical Approach to Lesion

Approach	Number of patients
Lower abdominal	13
Abdominoperineal	7
Posterior (intergluteal)	3

TABLE 12
IOEBT — Recurrent Rectal Adenocarcinoma:
Radiation Doses and Electron Energies

Complete resection (8 patients)		Partial resection (8 patients)		Unresectable tumor (7 patients)	
15 Gy	6 meV	20 Gy	15 meV	20 Gy	18 meV
15 Gy	9 meV	25 Gy	15 meV	25 Gy	18 meV
15 Gy	9 meV	25 Gy	15 meV	25 Gy	18 meV
15 Gy	9 meV	15 Gy	18 meV	25 Gy	18 meV
20 Gy	12 meV	25 Gy	18 meV	25 Gy	18 meV
20 Gy	12 meV	25 Gy	18 meV	25 Gy	18 meV
20 Gy	12 meV	25 Gy	18 meV	25 Gy	18 meV
20 Gy	15 meV	25 Gy	18 meV		

TABLE 13
IOEBT — Recurrent Rectal Cancer: Areas Irradiated

Areas irradiated	Number of patients
Sacral hollow, in 3 patients tumor extended distally involving the coccyx	12
Rectal wall	4
Lateral pelvic wall	6
Vagina	2
Prostate and bladder	2
Multiple sites (sacral hollow, vagina)	1

The electron energy was selected on the basis of estimated (or measured) thickness of the tumor or tumor bed. The range was 6 to 18 meV. When treating a tumor bed after complete resection, the energy usually employed was 9 or 12 meV. In one instance, a 6-meV beam was used to irradiate a superficial area at risk, and in five patients with partial tumor resection, the 18-meV beam was used to irradiate to greater depth, despite the resection of approximately 85 to 90% of the tumor. Sacrectomy was done in those four patients, and the feeling that the sacral stump might still harbor residual tumor cells necessitated irradiation thereof with an 18-meV beam (Table 12).

For lesions in the mid and upper rectum, as well as other proximal bowel locations, insertion of the applicator was via abdominal incision in most cases. Treating the presacral area was done in some cases by angulating the applicator cephalad. For lesions in the lower rectal region, it was necessary to insert the applicator via the perineal incision. For lesions involving the sacrum, we usually performed a partial sacrectomy through a posterior inter-gluteal incision. The applicator was inserted through the incision after sacrectomy with the gantry in the near-horizontal position. The areas treated with IOEBT boost are listed in Table 13.

TABLE 14
IOEBT — Recurrent Rectal Adenocarcinoma:
Applicators Employed

Applicator	Number of applications	Flat	Bevel 15°	Bevel 30°
1.00 in., cylindrical	2	1	1	
1.25 in., cylindrical	1		1	
1.50 in., cylindrical	7	1	6	
1.75 in., cylindrical	2	1	1	
2.00 in., cylindrical	5	1	2	2
2.25 in., cylindrical	1			1
2.75 in., cylindrical	3	1	1	1
3.00 in., cylindrical	1			1
4.00 in., cylindrical	1	1		
8 × 10 cm, rectangular	1	1	1	1

Note: Some patients required two applications (e.g., via perineal wound and abdominal wound).

An IOEBT applicator of appropriate size and bevel which defined the treatment field was selected (Table 14). The applicators most frequently used ranged from $1^1/_2$ to $2^3/_4$ in. in internal diameter. The applicators with 15° beveled ends were particularly useful in these anatomic sites.

3. External Beam Therapy

Of 23 patients, 6 had not received external beam therapy at the time of the initial surgery. They received 45 Gy in a 4- to 5-week period after the IOEBT. The pelvis was generally treated with a four-field technique using 10-meVp photons.

D. FOLLOW-UP

No patient has been lost to follow-up.

E. RESULTS
1. Acute Morbidity

There were 23 patients with locally recurrent rectal cancer who completed the planned therapy, either resection and IOEBT, IOEBT alone, or IOEBT and external beam radiation therapy with or without resection.

There were few operative complications observed. The acute and chronic IOEBT complications are summarized in Table 15. One patient developed an enterocutaneous fistula in the suprapubic region within 4 weeks of IOEBT. Biopsy of the cutaneous edges of the fistula showed local recurrence of tumor. Another patient developed a perineal sinus, which healed completely with conservative treatment. Immediately after treatment, one patient who received 25 Gy to the presacral and coccygeal area with an 18-meV electron beam through a 2-in. 15° beveled-end applicator developed pelvic phlebitis and urinary retention. Later, the same patient developed urinary incontinence.

One patient developed diarrhea within 2 weeks of IOEBT. This patient later developed vulvitis and vaginitis during the course of external beam therapy.

One patient with recurrent cancer invading the sacrum developed urinary incontinence immediately following IOEBT of the proximal sacral stump after high sacrectomy. One additional patient developed a pelvic abscess which resolved completely with antibiotics.

Of 14 patients, 4 developed permanent leg and back pain after receiving an IOEBT

TABLE 15
IOEBT — Recurrent Rectal Adenocarcinoma:
Complications

Complication	Number of patients
Urinary incontinence	2
Nausea and vomiting	2
Pelvic phlebitis and urinary retention	1
Diarrhea	1
Enterocutaneous fistula	1
Perineal sinus	1
Pelvic abscess	1
Vulvitis and vaginitis (during external beam therapy)	1
Permanent leg and back pain	4

TABLE 16
IOEBT — Recurrent Rectal Adenocarcinoma: Local Failure

Disease category	Number of patients	Local failure number of patients (%)	Time from IOEBT (months)
Complete resection	8	2 (25)	13, 14
Partial resection	8	3 (37)	6, 9, 9
No resection	7	4 (57)	2, 2, 3, 3

boost dose to the presacral area and/or to the pelvic sidewall. These patients received radiation boost doses of 20 or 25 Gy with electron beam energies of 6 to 18 meV. This suggests that delivering high single doses to the presacral area or pelvic sidewall may lead to the development of such pain.

2. Late Morbidity
A vesicovaginal fistula developed in one patient. This was associated with local failure 11 months after IOEBT. Another patient developed severe leg edema under similar circumstances. No patient died of radiation complications. Clinically significant renal or spinal cord damage was not observed.

3. Palliation of Symptoms
Pain was relieved completely in all of the ten patients presenting with perineal pain. It was partially improved in one patient presenting with back pain radiating to her lower leg. A single patient with massive leg swelling showed partial relief therefrom.

4. Local Control
In this group of patients with locally advanced recurrent disease, it was observed that when surgical debulking could not be accomplished, the rate of local recurrence was higher and occurred earlier than in those patients with complete or partial resection of the recurrent disease (Table 16). Four of seven patients (57%) with no resection developed local recurrence 2 to 4 months after IOEBT. In the group of patients with partial resection of the recurrent disease, three of eight patients (37%) developed local failure 6 to 9 months from the date of treatment. In patients with complete tumor debulking, two of eight patients (25%) developed local failure 13 to 14 months from the date of IOEBT.

TABLE 17
IOEBT — Recurrent Rectal Cancer: Patient Status

Status	Number of patients	Survival (months)
Alive 6/23 (26%)		
Disease free	5	4, 8, 11, 13, 36
With disease	1	18 (local failure)
Dead 17/23 (74%)		
Disease free	3	12, 16, 30
Local disease	9	2, 4, 4, 5, 5, 7, 9, 11, 15
Distant metastasis	5	8, 14, 16, 20

5. Survival

Patient status since IOEBT is shown in Table 17. Six patients are alive as of November 1987. Five patients have no clinical evidence of local recurrence or distant metastasis of cancer. One of these patients has survived 37 months since IOEBT and has no evidence of disease. This particular patient had complete resection of the disease with prostatectomy and cystectomy, and he received 25 Gy to the tumor bed. One patient survives with clinical evidence of local recurrence 19 months after the IOEBT. Of the 17 patients that died, 9 died with clinical evidence of local failure of the disease, although permission for post-mortem examination was not granted for any of the patients that died. Five patients were observed to have distant metastases, mainly in the lung.

F. DISCUSSION

Local recurrence with or without distant metastasis is the major cause of treatment failure in patients with cancer of the rectum, especially in the late stages of this disease (B_2 and C).[26] Surgical resection of the recurrent disease in the pelvis is usually difficult due to extension of the disease into the surrounding pelvic structures (i.e., pelvic sidewall, prostate, ureter, urinary bladder, etc.). External beam radiation therapy in the range of 45 to 50 Gy may be effective in controlling microscopic residual adenocarcinoma of the rectum, but in order to maximally control gross residual tumor, doses greater than 60 Gy should be employed. In this situation, small bowel tolerance is an obstacle to delivery of such doses.[27]

In a joint study, 52 patients with initially unresectable rectal cancer were treated at Massachusetts General Hospital or Mayo Clinic.[28] These patients received 50.4 Gy preoperatively at 1.8 Gy/fraction. An intraoperative dose of 10 to 20 Gy was delivered through a perineal incision. For those patients in whom complete resection of gross disease was possible, the local failure rate was reduced to nearly zero, and the 3-year survival rate was nearly doubled in comparison to historic controls.

IOEBT is a feasible and safe method to deliver a massive boost dose to unresectable rectal tumors (or to the bed of resected rectal tumors when used in combination with appropriate surgical debulking of recurrent tumors). Salvage of patients with recurrent rectal cancer is difficult even with resection and IOEBT. Our data suggest that IOEBT is effective in palliating pain due to recurrent rectal cancer and that the rate of local recurrence as well as the timing of same is a function of the extent of surgical resection. To avoid the development of distant metastases, more effective systemic therapy is needed.

IV. CANCER OF THE COLON

Cancer of the colon represents the second most common malignant tumor affecting men and women in the U.S.[1] The overall 5-year survival after treatment for this tumor has remained essentially unchanged for the past 40 years.[29]

Despite the fact that radical surgical resection remains the primary therapeutic modality for curative management of adenocarcinoma of the colon, data from clinical[21,30] and autopsy series indicate that local recurrence is often a significant problem after surgical resection.[31] When all stages of disease are considered together, from 35 to 45% of patients undergoing a potentially curative resection for colorectal carcinoma will have a relapse of disease;[32] therefore, the limited ability of surgical excision to provide long-term cure of colorectal cancer, especially in patients with unresectable or recurrent disease, is a very important reason to seek effective adjuvant therapy to enhance survival. For patients with unresectable or recurrent disease, combinations of conventional external beam irradiation and surgery do not always control the disease locally nor improve the survival.

To increase the chances of local control and improve survival rates, high radiation doses must be delivered. Normal tissue tolerance emerges as a serious obstacle to cure, since the radiation dose levels required to achieve local control generally exceed normal tissue tolerance. The concept of IOEBT provides a logistically and radiobiologically acceptable option in treating patients with residual primarily nonresectable or locally recurrent adenocarcinoma of the colon, but expectations of improvement in overall survival must be tempered by knowledge of the biologic propensity of this cancer to produce hepatic metastases. The following describes our experience at the MCO using IOEBT in the treatment of adenocarcinoma of the colon. Our clinical material consists largely of patients with known or suspected intra-abdominal recurrence of colon cancer.

A. PATIENT CHARACTERISTICS

Between 1983 and 1987, 17 patients with a diagnosis of primary unresectable (2 patients) or local recurrence (15 patients) of adenocarcinoma of the colon were brought to the COM-ROC IOEBT operating amphitheater for exploration and evaluation for IOEBT. Patient age ranged from 27 to 84 (median: 59) years. Ten patients were male, seven were female. All patients were white. Only 6 of the 17 patients underwent IOEBT because of the frequent discovery of extensive disease at surgery. We found our ability to accurately assess the extent of the disease preoperatively rather limited despite CT scans, colonoscopy, barium enema with air contrast, etc. At the time of exploration, four patients had widespread intra-abdominal disease, another four patients had distant metastases (liver and retroperitoneal extensions of disease). Three patients had localized resectable disease with no need for IOEBT. Three of the six patients that received IOEBT had undergone prior hemicolectomy. Two had adjuvant external beam therapy at the time of initial surgery. One of the six had been treated initially with external beam therapy as adjuvant treatment to a dose of 50.4 Gy. One of the six presented primarily with extensive primary disease.

The most common symptoms at the time of evaluation for IOEBT were back pain and change in bowel habit. In addition to the studies noted above, pretreatment evaluations included complete blood count, serum level of carcinoembryonic antigen, stool occult blood, chest Roentgenograms, serum bilirubin, and other standard liver function studies, as well as radioisotope scans of liver and bone.

B. TREATMENT TECHNIQUES
1. Surgical Procedure

At the time of IOEBT, the diagnosis was confirmed histologically. The IOEBT was delivered to the five patients through anterior abdominal incisions.

After complete resection (two patients) or exposure of the unresectable mass (four patients), the proposed IOEBT field was defined by the radiosurgical team. Areas free of macroscopic tumor, but at high risk for microscopic residual disease, were determined by correlation with preoperative assessment and frozen-section analysis of the surgical specimen.

2. IOEBT Delivery

The electron energy was selected on the basis of estimated (or measured) thickness of the tumor or tumor bed. The electron beam energy ranged from 9 to 18 meV. In two patients with complete resection, the energy employed was 9 or 15 meV. An electron beam energy of 18 meV was employed in all four patients with unresectable tumor. The IOEBT doses were 20 or 25 Gy. An IOEBT applicator of appropriate size and bevel, which defined the treatment field, was used. One of the six patients (with a second recurrence of cancer after two surgical resections) received interstitial intraoperative hyperthermia at 43°C for 60 min (RF 500 kHz), followed immediately by IOEBT. Three patients received 45 Gy adjuvant external beam therapy after IOEBT.

C. RESULTS

1. Acute Morbidity

Six patients with locally recurrent (five patients) or primary extensive colon cancer (one patient) completed the planned therapy of either resection and IOEBT, IOEBT alone, or IOEBT and external beam radiation therapy and hyperthermia. There were no operative complications. One patient who received 25 Gy IOEBT with 18-meV electrons developed acute vomiting and diarrhea which completely improved with medical treatment.

2. Late Morbidity

None of the patients developed late radiation complication. One patient died 10 months after the IOEBT due to intestinal obstruction. Although no autopsy was done, local recurrence of cancer was thought to be the cause.

3. Survival and Local Control

Three of the six patients are still alive as of October 1987. Two of those patients are clinically disease free for a period of more than 6 months since IOEBT. The third patient has clinical evidence of local tumor recurrence 1 year after IOEBT. Two patients died with local failure 10 months after IOEBT.

D. DISCUSSION

The prognosis for patients with colon cancer that is treated only with surgery is clearly related to the extent of tumor spread at the time of diagnosis. Regional lymph node involvement reduces the operative cure rate to the range of 25%.[31] Although preoperative irradiation has allowed surgeons to resect more advanced tumors, gross residual disease cannot be controlled with the usual external beam dose of 45 to 50 Gy. Residual disease must be boosted to doses of at least 60 to 70 Gy for local control. Unfortunately, this high dose is associated with a higher small bowel complication rate when therapy is delivered with external radiation beams.

The results with systemic chemotherapy in colorectal cancer have also been poor. The Gastrointestinal Tumor Study Group (GITSG) found no benefit when patients were treated with adjuvant chemotherapy with 5-FU and Semustine, nonspecific immunotherapy with the methanol extraction residue of bacillus Calmette-Guerine, or a combination of these treatments.[33] Because of the morbidity associated with uncontrolled local disease and the high recurrence rate associated with incomplete resection, a new modality of treatment is needed.

Our experience suggests that even with modern diagnostic techniques including colonoscopy, CT scan, and air contrast radiographic studies, our ability to accurately assess the extent of recurrent colon cancer preoperatively is quite limited. Only one third of the cases that we selected for abdominal exploration were ultimately judged suitable for IOEBT. Perhaps laporoscopy would be helpful in screening patients with recurrent colon cancer being considered for IOEBT.

V. CANCER OF THE STOMACH

Most available information regarding the use of IOEBT for the treatment of gastric cancers come from the Japanese studies, specifically the work of Abe and Takahashi.[34] Abe has pointed out that for IOEBT of inoperable gastric cancer, a large volume dose is required, making it impossible to sterilize the tumor in one exposure within the tolerance limits of normal structures supporting or surrounding the tumor. This is why he has repeatedly emphasized that in order to cure gastric cancer, the primary tumor must be removed surgically prior to delivery of IOEBT. He performed a prospective randomized study of the value of IOEBT as an adjuvant to surgical resection for gastric cancer. His work is reported in detail in Chapter 16 of this book. Our modest experience with gastric cancer is reported here.

A. PATIENT CHARACTERISTICS

Eight patients with a diagnosis of adenocarcinoma of the stomach were brought to the COMROC IOEBT operating amphitheater for exploration and evaluation for IOEBT. Patient age ranged from 22 to 80 (median: 52) years. All patients were white. Five were male and three were female.

B. TREATMENT

At the time of surgical exploration, three of the eight patients were found to have extensive disease; hence, no IOEBT was delivered. In the remaining five patients, the tumor was removed surgically. A dose of 12.5 to 15 Gy was delivered intraoperatively with a 6-meV electron beam followed by 45 Gy external beam therapy to the tumor bed and periaortic lymph nodes with 10-meVp X-rays at 2 Gy/fraction.

C. RESULTS

One patient developed an enterococcus abscess within 10 days of IOEBT and was treated with antibiotics. Complete resolution was observed. No patient demonstrated late radiation complication.

Three patients are alive as of August 1987, with no evidence of local or distant recurrence of the disease. One of the three patients has survived more than 2 years from the time of IOEBT. The other two patients died within 10 months after the IOEBT with local recurrence of the disease.

VI. EXTRAHEPATIC BILIARY DUCT CARCINOMA

Despite the tendency of this cancer to grow slowly and manifest its presence early by obstructive jaundice, the overall survival is dismally low. Local failure is the rule especially for proximally situated lesions. Transcatheter intraluminal brachytherapy techniques[35] have been shown to be effective when combined with external beam therapy, but the technique has seen limited application due to major complications, including infection and ulceration. The multicentric nature of biliary cancers and their propensity toward intraductal spread also contribute to the high local recurrence rate.

Abe and Takahashi[34] reported their experience in treating 59 patients with locally advanced lesions by delivering a single IOEBT dose of 25 to 40 Gy. At the time of the report, 16 of the 59 patients were alive, with the longest survival time being 18 months. The mean survival in this study was 10 months. Gunderson[36] has treated a small group of biliary cancer patients with IOEBT as a boost treatment in addition to external beam therapy and observed a trend toward increased local control and improved survival in comparison to historical experience. The MCO experience with IOEBT for biliary cancer is also limited.

A. MCO EXPERIENCE

Three patients with biopsy-proven adenocarcinoma of the extrahepatic biliary tract have been brought to the IOEBT operating amphitheater in the COMROC for exploration and consideration of IOEBT. Pretreatment studies included complete blood count, serum chemistries, CT scanning, ultrasonogram, transhepatic cholangiography, and ERCP.

One 70-year-old patient was treated with 20 Gy IOEBT with a 12-meV electron beam following an extended Whipple procedure. External beam therapy (50 Gy, 10-meVp X-rays, 1.8 Gy/fx) was delivered postoperatively. He developed severe nausea and vomiting 1 week after IOEBT. This totally resolved with medical treatment. The patient is still alive without evidence of cancer 12 months after IOEBT.

One 81-year-old patient received a dose of 22 Gy intraoperatively with a 9-meV electron beam after partial resection of the tumor. No external beam therapy was delivered due to rapid deterioration of the patient's condition. She developed local recurrence and liver metastases 4 months after treatment. She survived 7 months from the day of IOEBT.

The third patient, a 72-year-old, received 50 Gy external beam therapy before exploration for IOEBT. At the time of reexploration, distant metastases were found and no IOEBT was delivered. The patient survived 5 months from the beginning of the external beam therapy.

VII. ANAL CANCER

At the MCO, two patients, ages 67 and 88, with extensive local recurrence of epidermoid carcinoma of the anal canal, after being treated primarily with abdominoperineal resection, were treated with an IOEBT dose of 25 Gy with an 18-meV electron beam to the perineum after incomplete resection, followed by 40 Gy fractionated external beam therapy to the whole pelvis. One patient received adjuvant chemotherapy. No intraoperative complications were observed, the patient who received adjuvant chemotherapy developed severe cystitis during the chemotherapy. The other patient who presented with vaginal bleeding before the IOEBT experienced complete resolution after the treatment. Neither patient has developed local or distant recurrence of the disease (5 and 42 months) since the IOEBT.

VIII. CANCER OF THE DUODENUM

One patient, age 47 years, with advanced primary adenocarcinoma of the duodenum was treated with 15 Gy IOEBT with a 9-meV electron beam following extended Whipple procedure and 45 Gy postoperative external beam therapy. No intraoperative complications were observed. The patient developed severe nausea and vomiting during the course of postoperative external beam therapy. This required hospitalization and parenteral alimentation. The patient died 13 months after IOEBT, with local recurrence of disease.

IX. CANCER OF THE UTERINE CERVIX

The incidence of invasive cancer of the uterine cervix has been steadily decreasing in North America since the turn of the century, putatively because of screening procedures.[37]

Irradiation is the mainstay of therapy in patients with FIGO[38] Stages IIB, III, and IV. For those with Stage I and IIA disease, comparable results are obtained with either irradiation or radical hysterectomy. However, there are patients for whom external beam radiation therapy alone has limitations: those with bulky pelvic lymph node metastases, lymph node metastases outside the usual pelvic radiation portals (para-aortic nodes), and/or bulky parametrial lesions with involvement of the pelvic sidewall and lesions that are nonresponsive to conventional radiation therapy. Several studies have shown that patients with para-aortic node metastases treated with extended field external beam radiation therapy up to the diaphragm have experienced an increased incidence of major complications, particularly in the gastrointestinal tract.[39] Also, external beam radiation therapy after retroperitoneal exploration of the periaortic lymph nodes has not been convincingly shown to improve survival.[40]

The problem of para-aortic lymph node metastasis in the management of cancer of the uterine cervix continues to be significant. It has been repeatedly demonstrated that where the primary disease is more advanced than FIGO Stage I, the incidence of para-aortic node metastasis exceeds 10%.[41] The para-aortic lymph nodes are the most common loci of disease in patients who die of extrapelvic extension of disease with local control of cancer in the pelvis. The para-aortic lymph nodes are, in fact, the most frequent site of extrapelvic metastasis in patients with carcinoma of the cervix.[41] The problems of identification and treatment of para-aortic lymph node metastases are, however, considerable. Lymphangiography is relatively nonspecific for accurate detection of metastases.[42] Pretreatment laparotomy is much more reliable, but can predispose the patient to severe morbidity in terms of radiation complications and, in some cases, mortality.

It is important that the effectiveness of any new treatment modality be assessed not only with respect to its ability to control the tumor, but also with respect to toxicity. The use of IOEBT permits delivery of massive doses of radiation to pelvic and/or para-aortic deposits of disease without affecting other important tissues and organs such as the bowel, bladder, or rectum.

For cancer of the uterine cervix, as for most gynecologic tumors, central pelvic persistent disease is not the major cause of treatment failure, since a very high, well-defined dose can be safely delivered to the tumor via intracavitary applicators or interstitial implants of radioisotopes in conjunction with external beam therapy. Some patients with locally advanced cervical cancer may have disease fixed to the pelvic sidewall, where it can be difficult to deliver an adequate radiation dose by conventional radiation therapy techniques. A few tumors fail to respond to conventional radiation therapy.

As mentioned above, the major potential advantage of IOEBT in gynecologic tumors may be in the treatment of para-aortic nodal metastases. Chism and others,[43] have shown an increasing incidence of para-aortic metastases with increasing stage of the primary disease (Stage I, 3/63 or 5%; Stage II, 10/61 or 16%; Stage III, 22/58 or 38%).

Several investigators have treated patients with para-aortic nodal metastases with curative intent. The results suggest evidence of the ability to cure a subset of 15 to 20% of patients if a dose of 55 to 60 Gy is employed, but the high complication rates seen in several series[38,44] suggest that different radiotherapeutic techniques must be employed if aggressive treatment to this area is to be done on a large scale. For these reasons, we have employed IOEBT in the management of patients with recurrent cancer of the uterine cervix and, following the logic of Delgado and associates,[45] also those with locally advanced primary lesions (FIGO Stages IIIB and IVA). The IOEBT has been used in conjunction with standard abdominal exploration and para-aortic lymphadenotomy after conventional external beam and intracavitary radiation therapy.

A. PATIENT CHARACTERISTICS

Between 1983 and 1986, 11 patients with a diagnosis of squamous cell carcinoma of the uterine cervix were brought to the COMROC IOEBT operating amphitheater for exploration and evaluation for IOEBT. Patient age ranged from 29 to 58 (median: 41) years. Ten patients were white, one was black. Of the 11 patients, 9 had primary lesions and two had recurrent cancer (Table 18).

All patients underwent preoperative clinical staging procedures that included physical examination, chest X-ray, intravenous pyelogram, cystoscopy, barium enema, proctoscopy, bipedal lymphangiogram, and a CT scan. When the lymphangiogram suggested cancer in the lymph nodes, percutaneous needle biopsies were performed. Metastases in para-aortic

TABLE 18
IOEBT — Cervical Carcinoma: Disease Stage
and Para-aortic Node Status

Stage	Number of patients	Para-aortic nodes	
		Negative	Positive
IIB	2	0	2
IIIB	7	2	5
IVB	1	0	1
Recurrent	1	0	1

lymph nodes and at the pelvic wall were confirmed histologically at laparotomy in all cases. The most common presenting symptoms were vaginal bleeding and discharge. Five of the ten patients presented with pelvic and leg pain associated with leg swelling.

At the time of surgical exploration, 2 of the 11 patients were found to have very extensive local disease precluding IOEBT. Later, one of the two developed liver metastasis and the other developed extensive peritoneal metastasis.

Of the remaining patients, all received IOEBT after conventional external beam therapy and intracavitary irradiation, except one patient who received IOEBT prior to external beam irradiation because her pretreatment abdominal CT scan suggested an epigastric mass (that proved to be normal bowel at surgery).

B. STAGING

Each patient's cancer was staged according to the following system.[46]

Stage 0: Carcinoma *in situ*, intraepithelial carcinoma.
Stage I: Carcinoma strictly confined to the cervix. Extension to the corpus disregarded.
  Ia: Microinvasive carcinoma.
  Ib: All other cases of Stage I.
Stage II: Carcinoma extending beyond the cerivx, but not onto the pelvic wall. Carcinoma involving the vagina, but not the lower third.
Stage III: Carcinoma extending onto the pelvic wall. On rectal examination, there is no finger free space between the tumor and the pelvic wall. Tumor involving the lower third of the vagina. All cases with hydronephrosis or nonfunctioning kidney.
  IIIa: No extension onto the pelvic wall.
  IIIb: Extension onto the pelvic wall and/or hydronephrosis and/or nonfunctioning kidney.
Stage IV: Carcinoma extending beyond the true pelvis or involving the mucosa of the bladder or rectum.
  IVa: Spread to mucosa of bladder or rectum (biopsy proven).
  IVb: Spread to distant organs.

One patient presented with pelvic and leg pain due to recurrence of cervical carcinoma at the pelvic sidewall and in para-aortic lymph nodes. This was confirmed histologically at surgery. This patient had been treated elsewhere for Stage IIB cervical carcinoma with external beam radiation therapy and intracavitary Radium 2 years before. IOEBT was administered to the sites of recurrence for palliation. Another patient presented with leg swelling in addition to pelvic and leg pain. This patient with Stage IVb cervical carcinoma had been treated with external beam irradiation, intracavitary radioisotope application, and systemic chemotherapy. She received IOEBT to the para-aortic area as a palliative treatment.

C. TREATMENT TECHNIQUES
1. External Beam Therapy

Initially, and in an attempt to shrink the bulk of the central tumor, external beam radiation therapy was often delivered at a dose of 40 to 50 Gy to the pelvis in daily dose increments of 1.8 to 2.0 Gy. Four or five fractions were given per week for 4 to 5.5 weeks. A four-field arrangement was almost always used in all patients. This commonly shrank the tumor and reduced infection and tumor volume, and often the pelvic anatomy returned toward normal; this facilitated the introduction of intracavitary radioisotope to deliver high doses of radiation to the cervix and vagina. Each of two applications was left in place for sufficient time to deliver 25 Gy to Point A, our commonly used dose specification point (where the ureter crosses the uterine artery.)

Point A lies 2 cm above and 2 cm lateral to the cervical os. Usually Point A received a total dose of 85 to 90 Gy with standard treatment, and the pelvic sidewalls were treated to doses as high as 65 Gy in conventional fashion.

2. Surgical Procedures

After completion of the external beam irradiation and intracavitary treatment, each patient was brought to the COMROC IOEBT operating amphitheater for exploration and evaluation for IOEBT. A long paramedian incision was made from the symphysis pubis to the xiphoid process. After opening the peritoneal cavity, peritoneal washings for cytology were done followed by complete intraperitoneal exploration. The peritoneum overlying the root of the mesentery was incised so that the vena cava and aorta were exposed, the fatty tissue containing the lymph nodes anterior and lateral to the vena cava was carefully dissected and removed. After this, lymph nodes anterior and lateral to the aorta were dissected. When the lymph nodes were large and fixed to the vena cava, only biopsies were performed. The nodes or biopsies were sent for frozen section examination. Before administering IOEBT, the uninvolved visceral structures were retracted out of the field.

3. IOEBT Delivery

The lowest possible effective electron beam energy was selected to give an homogenous dose distribution throughout the TV while minimizing the dose to the spinal cord (Table 19). For unresectable para-aortic lymph node metastases (biopsy only), a dose of 20 or 25 Gy was delivered with a 12-meV electron beam. If the para-aortic lymph nodes showed no metastatic tumor on frozen section examination, an IOEBT dose of 10 or 15 Gy was administered with a 6- or 9-meV electron beam, the energy depending on the thickness of the retroperitoneal TV. Similarly, when histologically positive nodes were completely re-sected from the para-aortic region, a dose of 15 or 10 Gy was administered with a 12- or 9-meV electron beam, the energy again dependent upon the thickness of the retroperitoneal TV. An 8 × 10-cm rectangular applicator was usually employed for para-aortic node irradiation. In two patients, a $3^1/_2$-in. circular applicator with a 15° beveled end fit the local anatomy better than the rectangular applicator.

After the para-aortic nodes were irradiated, the pelvis was carefully explored. If residual disease was encountered, the rectosigmoid and the bladder were retracted medially so as not to be included in the IOEBT field. A treatment applicator was applied to the area to be treated after ascertaining that the pervious para-aortic IOEBT field was not overlapped, and a single dose of 20 or 25 Gy was delivered. High doses of 20 or 25 Gy were employed for the treatment of pelvic wall disease and pelvic lymph nodes with electron beam energies of 9 to 18 meV. The electron energy was selected according to the thickness of the TV.

Eight of nine patients presenting with primary disease received IOEBT to the para-aortic area. Six of these patients had histologically positive para-aortic nodes; two did not (Table 20). Four of the former and one of the latter also received IOEBT to the pelvic nodes,

TABLE 19

**IOEBT — Advanced Cervical Cancer: Doses, Electron Beam
Energies, and Size of Applicators**

Site	Dose (Gy)	Energy (meV)	Applicator	Number of patients
Para-aortic area				
Negative nodes	10	6	8 × 10 R	1
	15	9	8 × 10 R	1
Positive nodes				
Complete surgical removal	10	12	8 × 10 R	1
	15	9	$3^1/_2$ in. 15°[a]	1
	15	12	8 × 10 R	1
Biopsy only	20	12	$3^1/_2$in. 15°	1
	20	12	8 × 10 R	1
	25	12	8 × 10 R	1
	25	12	$2^1/_4$in. 30°[a]	1
Pelvic area				
Lymph nodes	20[b]	9	8 × 10 R	1
	20[c]	12	4in. 30°	1
	20[c]	18	2in. F[a]	1
Pelvic wall	25[c]	15	3 in. 30°	1
	25[c]	18	$3^1/_2$in. 15°	1

[a] $3^1/_2$ in. 15° = $3^1/_2$-in. circular applicator with 15° beveled end; $2^1/_4$-in. 30° = $2^1/_2$-in. circular applicator with 30° beveled end; 2in. F = 2 in. circular applicator with flat end.

[b] Surgically removed.

[c] Biopsy only.

TABLE 20

IOEBT — Advanced Cervical Cancer: Patient Status

	Primary cancer			
	Positive para-aortic nodes	Negative para-aortic nodes	Recurrent cancer	Total
Number alive	3	2	1	6[a]
Number dead	3			3
Total	6	2	1	9

[a] Alive 4 to 30 months after treatment.

obturator nodes, iliac nodes, parametria, and/or pelvic sidewalls. The one patient with recurrent pelvic sidewall disease after radiation therapy of her primary cervical cancer received IOEBT to the para-aortic and pelvic areas.

D. RESULTS

1. Acute Morbidity

No intraoperative complications were observed in any patient. Three patients that received IOEBT to the para-aortic area developed mild nausea and vomiting within 1 month of treatment. Two patients who received IOEBT to the pelvic area developed mild diarrhea. None of the patients developed prolonged ileus. Table 21 shows complications affecting the patients after IOEBT for cancer of the uterine cervix. One patient had hemorrhagic cystitis of more than 10 days duration. Another patient had proctitis with rectal bleeding. Both

TABLE 21

IOEBT — Advanced Cervical Cancer:

Morbidity

Complication	Number of patients
Hemorrhage cystitis	1
Proctitis and rectal bleeding	1
Acute vaginitis	1
Leg pain	1

problems resolved completely with medical treatment. One patient, who had received IOEBT prior to external and intracavitary radiation treatment, had acute vaginitis which subsided completely with medical treatment.

2. Late Morbidity

No patient died of late radiation complications. Clinically significant renal, intestinal, or spinal cord radiation damage was not observed. No patient developed leg edema. One of three patients that received an IOEBT boost dose to the presacral area or pelvic sidewall developed permanent leg and back pain.

3. Survival

Table 20 shows the survival of the patients in this study. Six of the nine patients have survived 4 to 30 months after IOEBT. Three of the nine patients died of local recurrence of the disease 9 to 26 months after IOEBT. Of the six patients with primary cancer with positive para-aortic nodes, three died from local recurrence as mentioned before. Two of the three surviving have no clinical evidence of disease, and one is alive with recurrent cancer.

Both patients with primary cancer and negative para-aortic lymph nodes are still alive with no clinical evidence of the disease. One patient with recurrent disease, treated both to the recurrence site and the para-aortic nodes, is alive with clinical evidence of local pelvic recurrence.

E. DISCUSSION

Recurrence of carcinoma of the uterine cervix, except for a few central ones in patients with early stage disease, is almost always fatal.[47] Therefore, it is imperative to deliver doses of radiation that will provide maximum tumor control with an acceptable number of complications. The survival rate for patients with advanced disease is low, especially when the pelvic and para-aortic nodes are involved.[40] Although external beam irradiation can successfully control microscopic disease, its value in the treatment of bulky deposits of disease is limited, since the relatively low radiotolerance of surrounding organs (bowel, kidney, spinal cord, etc.) precludes delivery of high doses to the para-aortic and pelvic regions.

Thus, conventional radiation therapy for the late stages of cervical cancer has limitations. It does not necessarily enhance survival and it may produce gastrointestinal complications. The use of IOEBT permits high-dose irradiation of diseased areas without irradiation of adjacent radiosensitive normal structures. This way, areas of frequent failure such as the para-aortic and pelvic lymph nodes, as well as the parametria, may receive additional radiation doses without affecting the rectosigmoid or bladder. In our group of patients, we observed no operative mortality, but our patients did encounter some acute and delayed morbidity as noted above. Two of the nine patients had conventional external beam radiation therapy (45 to 50 Gy) followed by an 8-Gy boost to the affected pelvic sidewall in addition to two intracavitary applications plus 25 Gy IOEBT to the affected pelvic sidewall. One of these two patients developed mild proctitis with rectal bleeding. This resolved completely with medical treatment. Relief of symptoms in the group of patients with uterine cervical cancer was satisfactory. Five patients with leg and ankle edema experienced partial relief postoperatively; also, they experienced partial alleviation of back and leg pain.

X. CANCER OF THE OVARY

Ovarian cancer is a complex disease. Despite the fact that ovarian cancer is less common than cervical or endometrial cancer, it produces more deaths than both combined.[1]

All current treatment methods for ovarian cancer are potentially toxic. To achieve for each patient the maximum gain from treatment, it is essential that each of the various therapeutic modalities is used optimally. To reach this objective requires careful evaluation of outcome for various management strategies. In general, the response to chemotherapy may be affected by the presence of minimal residual disease (2 cm) at initial surgery, tumor grade, and prior chemotherapy exposure.[48] Surgery is essential, both diagnostically, to determine sites of involvement, and therapeutically, to resect gross deposits of disease, so that postsurgically only minimal residual disease is left to be treated with chemotherapy or radiation.

There have been numerous reports of ovarian cancer response to chemotherapy, together with arguments for the curative potential of that modality.[49] With the introduction of combination chemotherapy, particularly combinations incorporating cisplatinum, such reports have increased.[50] Presently, there are insufficient published data to convince all clinicians that chemotherapy achieves the same long-term survival advantages as radiation therapy given with an appropriate technique.[51]

A number of investigators have examined the value of abdominopelvic irradiation for such patients. Although abdominopelvic irradiation has been shown to improve survival for approximately one third of patients with cancer of the ovary,[52] still the greatest challenge from this disease comes from the large proportion of patients who present with extensive bulky disease, who are at high risk of having recurrent disease even after the various adjuvant modalities have been optimally employed, and especially from those with recurrent disease. A dose of 50 to 55 Gy to the lower abdomen and pelvis can control more than 90% of microscopic deposits of disease.[53] On the other hand, dose limitations of surrounding normal tissues (i.e., liver, bowel, kidneys) compromise control of macroscopic residual or recurrent disease, especially in the upper abdomen. The following illustrates the use of IOEBT for increasing the therapeutic ratio for treatment of both bulky primary and recurrent ovarian carcinoma.

A. PATIENT CHARACTERISTICS

Between November 1983 and July 1985, eight patients with a diagnosis of local recurrence of epithelial carcinoma of the ovary, and one patient with extensive primary epithelial carcinoma of the ovary, were brought to the COMROC IOEBT operating amphitheater for exploration and evaluation for IOEBT. Patient age ranged from 13 to 80 (median: 51) years. All the patients were white.

Initial evaluation included a careful history and physical examination, chest X-ray, intravenous pyelogram, barium enema, complete blood count, proctoscopy, and pelvic CT scan. Also, needle biopsy was often done to confirm the diagnosis before surgery.

The most common presenting symptoms were a sensation of pressure in the pelvis and increased abdominal girth. One patient presented with a localized mass in the chestwall 1 year after total abdominal hysterectomy and bilateral salpingo-oophrectomy (TAH & BSO) and systemic chemotherapy.

TABLE 22
IOEBT — Ovary: Treatment Factors

Patient number	Dose (Gy)	Energy (meV)	Applicator size	Site	Extent of resection	External beam X-ray and chemotherapy
1[a]	25	18	5in. flat	Presacral	Incomplete	36 Gy and chemotherapy
2	25	15	2in. flat	Rt. hemipelvis		
	20	6	2in. flat	Sigmoid colon	Incomplete	41.4 Gy
	15	9	2$^1/_2$in. 15°	Perioartic		
3	20	12	2$^1/_2$in. 15°	Pelvic sidewall	Incomplete	32 Gy
4[a]	20	9	1$^1/_2$in. 15°	Pelvic sidewall	Complete	Chemotherapy only
5	15	15	3in. 30°	Chest wall	Incomplete	

*   These patients developed permanent leg and/or back pain.

B. TREATMENT TECHNIQUES
1. Surgical Procedure

Initially, all patients had surgical treatment consisting of TAH & BSO. All of the patients had omentectomy or omental biopsy, assessment of pelvic and periaortic nodes, and cytological examination of peritoneal fluid.

2. IOEBT Delivery

At the time of surgical exploration in the COMROC IOEBT operative suite, four of the nine patients were found to have extensive disease, and it was evident that there was more disease than could be controlled with IOEBT and external beam radiation therapy; hence, no IOEBT was delivered. Survival of those patients ranged from 2 to 6 months postoperatively.

The other five patients were treated with IOEBT. The IOEBT dose to pelvic lesions was 20 or 25 Gy administered with electron beams with energies from 9 to 18 meV, the energy of the beam a function of the thickness of the TV. One patient with extensive local pelvic recurrence also received 15 Gy to the para-aortic area as a prophylactic procedure, even though a para-aortic lymph node biopsy was negative (Table 22).

3. External Beam Therapy

Total abdominal irradiation (which included the entire peritoneal surface and diaphragm) was initiated after recovery from surgery, generally within 4 to 6 weeks, and carried to a total dose of 30 Gy at 1.5 Gy/fraction. In one patient, external beam treatment was terminated at a dose of 7.2 Gy because of severe diarrhea. In three patients, an additional course of external beam radiation therapy was administered to the whole pelvis using total doses of 32 to 41.4 Gy.

C. RESULTS
1. Acute Morbidity

No intraoperative complications were observed in any of the patients in this series. One patient suffered a pulmonary embolus within 24 h postoperatively. This responded well to anticoagulant therapy. One patient developed acute peritonitis that was successfully treated with intravenous chloramphenicol. Another patient developed severe diarrhea during whole abdomen irradiation, necessitating termination of external beam treatment at a dose of 7.2 Gy.

2. Late Morbidity

No patient died of radiation complication, nor developed any late complication. Two of five patients treated with an IOEBT boost of 20 to 25 Gy delivered to the presacral region or pelvic wall developed permanent back and leg pain starting within 3 weeks after the radiation treatment. Both these patients also received chemotherapy, suggesting an enhancement of the effect of irradiation on neural tissue (Table 22).

3. Survival

Patient survival ranged from 9 to 25 months, with an average of 18.6 months. Two patients who did not receive whole-abdomen irradiation developed peritoneal metastases. One patient died with clinical evidence of local recurrence on the pelvic wall. One of the five patients developed metastatic adenocarcinoma in multiple areas in the chestwall. She received external beam radiation therapy to those areas. Another patient developed metastatic disease in the supraclavicular and mediastinal areas. She also received external beam radiation therapy to both areas.

D. DISCUSSION

The greatest challenge from ovarian cancer comes from the large proportion of patients who present with extensive bulky disease or develop locally recurrent disease. To achieve maximum gain from any treatment modality, it is necessary to use each modality optimally. Conventional radiation therapy is limited most of the time by the radiation tolerance of the small bowel.

Previous studies provide only limited information about the results and complications of using large, single-fraction irradiation to palliate symptomatic pelvic and gynecologic cancers. In a study by Adelson et al.,[54] 42 patients received external beam radiation in single or multiple fractions of 10 Gy (3 maximum) to the pelvis. Most patients had advanced disease. Of 42 patients, 40 had received preirradiation chemotherapy. Ten patients required gastrointestinal surgical procedures, and in six, radiation injury was believed to be the main contribution to complications. Also, hemorrhagic cystitis or proctitis occured 6 to 18 months after irradiation in four patients. Obviously, the risk of tissue injury from radiation increases as the irradiation dose exceeds the tolerance of the surrounding normal tissue (i.e., small bowel, urinary bladder, rectum).

In our small series of patients we observed none of these complications, as the rectum and bladder were excluded from the IOEBT boost dose volume. However, two of five patients developed permanent leg and back pain when the radiation dose was delivered to the pelvic wall or the presacral area. This observation correlates with the National Cancer Institute work of Kinsella et al.[55] in which five patients from a group of 40 that received IOEBT to pelvic or retroperitoneal tumor developed clinical signs of lumbosacral or sciatic neuropathy within 9 months of receiving 20 to 25 Gy. In an attempt to investigate this clinical observation, the same group investigated the effect of IOEBT of 20 to 75 Gy on the lumbosacral plexus and sciatic nerve of 21 dogs. They found an approximately linear relationship between radiation dose and time to onset of hind limb paresis, they also suggested that peripheral nerve may be a dose-limiting normal tissue in clinical studies of IOEBT. Clinical results from our small group of patients raises the possibility of chemotherapy enhancing the neurotoxic effect of IOEBT.

XI. CANCER OF THE BREAST

Breast cancer is the most common malignancy in females in the U.S. today.[1] Over the past decade there has been a growing trend to manage this disease with local excision of the lesion followed by radiation therapy rather than surgical amputation of the breast. This

```
                                                                 Boost Dose
Conventional ——→ Excisional → Axillary →External ————→ ¹⁹²Ir or
Regimen:          Biopsy      Sampling  Beam Treatment  Electron Beam
                                                        or Tangents


MCO Regimen: →Excisional → Axillary →External
              Biopsy      Sampling  Beam Treatment
                          plus
                          IOEBT
                          Boost
```

--Shorter Overall Treatment Course

--Minimize Possibility of Geographic Miss

--Better Sparing of Skin and Lung

--Radiobiological Higher Boost Dose

--Less Expensive (¹⁹²Ir, Hospital Stay)

--No Radioisotope Exposure

--Homogeneous dose distribution

FIGURE 2.   Comparison of conventional definitive radiation therapy for breast cancer and the concept of IOEBT boost dose to tumor bed. The advantages using IOEBT are listed.

is only applicable in early stages of the disease. The usual course of events is as follows: after the breast lump is removed, an axillary node dissection is performed. The breast and adjacent node-bearing regions are then treated with external beam radiation therapy. Then the dose to the tumor bed is boosted by surgical implantation of radioisotope or by external beam techniques, including electron beam therapy.

At the MCO, we have begun to employ IOEBT as the modality for delivering a boost dose to the tumor bed. This is done at the time of axillary node dissection or lumpectomy.

A. PATIENT CHARACTERISTICS AND TREATMENT TECHNIQUES

Between 1984 and 1987, six white females, age 37 to 60 years, with a diagnosis of infiltrative ductal carcinoma of the breast, were brought to the COMROC IOEBT operating amphitheater for lumpectomy and lymph node dissection. The IOEBT boost dose was delivered to the tumor bed immediately after lumpectomy or after reopening the lumpectomy scar. The IOEBT dose was 10 or 15 Gy, and the electron beam energy was either 6 or 9 meV, depending on the thickness of the TV. All the patients received 45 or 50 Gy additional external beam radiation therapy to the breast and regional lymph nodes.

B. RESULTS

All the patients are alive as of November 1987, with no evidence of local or distant recurrence. Excellent cosmesis is the rule.

C. DISCUSSION

In comparison to standard treatment, the procedure described above has several advantages (Figure 2): the patient is spared one hospitalization and one anesthetic for the boost dose. The overall treatment time is shortened, as the radiation boost dose is delivered at the time of axillary node dissection. The overall cost is less because of savings in physician fees, hospitalization, and in purchase of the radioisotope. Radiation exposure to hospital personnel occasioned by radioisotope implant is eliminated. The dose to the skin is minimized because radiation is delivered through the surgical incision. The lung is protected by choosing an appropriate electron beam energy. As well, one can probably deliver a radiobiologically higher dose to the tumor bed with this procedure, and, perhaps most importantly, the chances of a geographic miss are minimized because of direct surgical exposure of the tumor bed at the time of IOEBT.

Clearly, this approach to the definitive radiotherapeutic management of mammary carcinoma deserves further investigation. Obviously, it will require many years to assess the long-term effects of such breast conservation treatment.

XII. ENDOMETRIAL CARCINOMA

Two patients, age 66 and 70, with recurrent adenocarcinoma of the uterus have been treated with IOEBT at the COMROC. Both patients developed recurrent disease in the pelvis after being treated with intracavitary radium therapy followed by TAH & BSO. The first patient received IOEBT to a dose of 25 Gy with an 18-meV electron beam followed by 45 Gy external beam therapy. The patient developed distant metastases 6 months after IOEBT and local recurrence 7 months after IOEBT. The second patient was treated with IOEBT after partial resection of the lesion. Here we employed a dose of 25 Gy with a 12-meV electron beam followed by 45 Gy external beam therapy. She developed neck node metastasis 2 months after IOEBT. She subsequently developed bone and brain metastasis and died 8 months after IOEBT, but with no clinical evidence of local tumor recurrence.

XIII. VAGINAL CANCER

One patient, age 60 years, with locally extensive vaginal carcinoma was treated with 50 Gy external beam therapy combined with interstitial ^{192}Ir hairpins implanted into the right lateral vaginal wall and the right parametrium to deliver an additional 30 Gy to point A. When the disease recurred it was treated with an IOEBT dose of 17.5 Gy with an 18-meV electron beam delivered to the right pelvic sidewall. The periaortic region also received 17.5 Gy with a 12-meV electron beam after periaortic lymphadenectomy. No intraoperative complication was observed. The patient developed local recurrence in the right parametrium 7 months after the IOEBT.

XIV. SARCOMAS

Soft tissue sarcomas are uncommon tumors which may occur in any anatomic site. The locally infilterative behavior of soft tissue sarcomas accounts for the high incidence of local failure (42 to 93%)[56] after surgical resection. Also the proximity of the tumor to vital structures often limits complete resection (e.g., retroperitoneal sarcoma). External beam radiation therapy, pre- or postoperative, employed in conjuction with wide tumor resection for soft tissue sarcomas of the extremities can be highly effective. Local control rates above 85% have been reported with doses in the range of 60 to 75 Gy.[57,58]

In a prospective randomized controlled IOEBT study, the first of its kind, Kinsella et al.[59] treated 35 patients with sarcomas; 15 patients received resection, moderate dose external beam therapy (35 to 40 Gy), and IOEBT along with misonidazole, a radiation sensitizer (3.5 g/M^2); 20 patients received standard therapy (resection and external beam therapy, 50 to 55 Gy). The investigators observed no difference in disease-free survival (20 months) or local recurrence between the two groups of patients, but did observe three patients who developed neuropathy as a result of nerves being included in the IOEBT fields. Of 20 patients that received standard treatment, 7 developed disabling radiation enteritis as compared to 1 of 15 receiving IOEBT.

TABLE 23
IOEBT — Soft Tissue Sarcoma: Tumor Location and
Histopathology

Tumor location	Number of patients	Pathology
Chestwall	3	2 fibrous histiocytoma; 1 chondrosarcoma
Pelvis	2	1 liposarcoma; 1 fibrous histiocystoma
Retroperitoneum	1	1 liposarcoma
Paravertebral	1	1 liposarcoma

The Japanese experience includes the treatment of 29 patients at 7 institutions.[60] Treatment was generally a combination of surgical resection and IOEBT to doses of 30 to 45 Gy. Of these patients, 21 were alive at the time of analysis, and 5 had survived for more than 5 years. The local control rate was 73%. By comparison, our experience at the MCO is modest.

A. PATIENT CHARACTERISTICS

Seven patients with extensive primary soft tissue sarcomas (two patients) or local recurrence of same (five patients) in different sites (Table 23) were brought to the IOEBT operating amphitheater in the COMROC. Patient age ranged from 29 to 71 (median: 62) years. All patients were white. Four were male and three were female.

B. TREATMENT TECHNIQUES

After partial or complete resection (five patients) or exposure of the unresectable mass (two patients), the proposed IOEBT field was defined by the radiosurgical team. A dose of 15 to 25 Gy was administered with electron beams ranging from 6 to 18 meV in energy, depending on the thickness of the residual tumor. Four of the seven patients received external beam therapy (45 to 55 Gy) after the IOEBT.

C. RESULTS

No patient was lost to follow-up. Follow-up ranged from 7 to 35 months. No intraoperative complications were observed in any patient treated. One patient with extensive recurrent malignant fibrous histiocytoma in the pelvis received 25 Gy to three different areas: left and right pelvic sidewalls and presacral area. The patient developed persistant severe diarrhea and radiation cystitis which resolved completely with conservative management. Another patient with primary liposarcoma in the pelvis developed permanent leg numbness and tingling sensations after receiving 25 Gy IOEBT with an 180-meV electron beam. Three patients are alive as of November 1987 (7, 15, 35 months) after IOEBT. They are disease free with no local recurrence. The other four patients developed local recurrence 4 to 10 months from the time of IOEBT and expired.

Patients with complete tumor resection (two patients) and partial tumor resection (one patient) have local control of disease, while the four patients without tumor resection developed local recurrence and died, again emphasizing the importance of surgical resection in the management of this disease.

XV. BRAIN TUMORS

Standard external beam radiation therapy is known to have a significant biological effect on malignant cells and a salutary clinical effect on patients with cerebral malignancies.

Limitation of dosage that results in failure of eradication of brain tumors is related to the radiobiological tolerance of the tissues (scalp, bone, brain) that surround the target malignancy. if these tissues can be spared by direct application of high tumor doses, it may have a beneficial effect. IOEBT can accomplish this goal by application of a large single dose of radiation directly to tumor tissue exposed by surgery in the radiation therapy suite.

Brain tumors are most likely to have the smallest number of viable cells shortly after surgical decompression and external irradiation by standard techniques. Radiobiologically, this is the "ideal" time to apply IOEBT to the remaining viable tumor cells, as discussed in detail by Greenblatt and Rayport in Chapter 13 of this book.

In addition to malignant gliomas, other proven malignancies of the cerebrum or cerebellum may be appropriate for IOEBT, including single brain metastasis. Very deep tumors are not appropriately treated by IOEBT, because the overlying brain could be damaged by the electron beam. However, this does not exclude application of IOEBT to tumors that do not reach the surface, as long as the overlying cortex is nonfunctional and potentially expendable. The tumor size must be within the range of the maximum depth of the electron beam.

A. PATIENT CHARACTERISTICS

At the MCO, we have treated six patients with IOEBT for brain tumors. All were white, all were female. Two patients had solitary metastasis in the brain; one from unknown primary, the other from malignant melanoma; two had astrocytoma; two had glioblastoma multiforme. Greenblatt and Rayport discuss the early patients in detail in Chapter 13 of this book.

1. Treatment Techniques

All patients underwent primary tumor debulking followed by external beam radiation therapy to a total dose of 40 to 56 Gy. A craniotomy was executed in the COMROC IOEBT operating amphitheater. Computerized tomography and magnetic resonance imaging scans were used to select the proper position of the head for surgery, plan the procedure, and to choose the appropriate electron beam energy. After good exposure of the tumor and wide resection, if possible, IOEBT was applied using an appropriate applicator. A dose of 15 or 20 Gy was administered in most cases, as gross residual tumor remained. The electron beam energy ranged from 6 to 18 meV, depending on the thickness of the TV. One of the six patients received external beam therapy after IOEBT. The treatment was terminated before completion due to the development of severe brain edema which was attributed to the combination of IOEBT and external beam irradiation.

2. Results

No intraoperative complications were observed in any of the patients, but one patient died 2 days after IOEBT. Autopsy showed acute tonsillar herniation with posterior cerebral hemorrhage with diffuse cerebral edema. Another patient who developed local recurrence 1 year after IOEBT using a dose of 15 Gy with an electron beam energy of 15 meV, received another IOEBT boost dose of 20 Gy with a 9-meV electron beam. She developed aphasia with severe headaches and generalized fatigue and expired within 1 month.

No patient died of late radiation complications. One patient with glioblastoma multiforme and one patient with metastatic disease survived more than 1 year after IOEBT (13 months). The other two patients survived for 3 months after IOEBT.

3. Discussion

In a pilot study from Tokyo, Matsutani[61] treated 15 patients with glioblastoma multiforme with an aggressive combined modality protocol as follows: (1) surgical excision of tumor; (2) conventional external beam therapy, 35 to 60 Gy; (3) wide resection and IOEBT of 10 to 20 Gy with 8 to 20 meV; and (4) additional external beam therapy, as necessary, to bring the total external beam radiation dose to 60 Gy. He reported a median survival time of 80 weeks from first operation to tumor progression, as well as 1- and 2-year survival rates of 100 and 62%, respectively. Matsutani's work is presented in detail in Chapter 14 of this book.

Goldson et al.[62] treated 12 patients (10 with astrocytoma, 2 recurrent meningioma) with 15 Gy IOEBT using 9- to 12-meV electron beams in conjunction with 30 to 50 Gy conventional external beam irradiation. The patients with meningioma did well. Three patients with astrocytoma died within 3 months of IOEBT of causes that may have been related to the IOEBT.

Abe and Takahashi[60] reported 36 patients with brain tumors (19 were primary, 15 were recurrent, and 2 were metastatic). Histological distribution was as follows: ten glioblastoma, three astrocytoma, two metastatic adenocarcinoma, and one fibrosarcoma. The patients were treated with IOEBT doses of 10 to 25 Gy in addition to 30 to 40 Gy external beam therapy. Of the 36 patients, 9 were alive at the time of this report. Survival was generally poor, and complications of therapy were not well-addressed.

XVI. MISCELLANEOUS TUMORS

IORT can be applied to practically any unresectable malignant neoplasm or to the bed of nearly any resected tumor where there is a high likelihood of local recurrence. The indications for treatment and technical considerations for IOEBT vary considerably among different anatomic tumor locations as well as among various tumor types. At the MCO, we have treated a potpouri of tumors of the urinary tract, lung, head and neck, and other sites with IOEBT.

A. RENAL CELL CARCINOMA

Three patients with biopsy-proven advanced primary or locally recurrent renal cell tumor were brought to the IOEBT operating amphitheater in the COMROC. One patient with an unresectable right renal mass was treated with IOEBT using a dose of 20 Gy to the lower half and 25 Gy to the upper half of the mass with 18-meV electron beams after intraoperative interstitial hyperthermia (43°C) for 60 min. The patient developed local recurrence 5 months after the IOEBT.

Two patients presented with renal cell carcinoma with possible direct invasion of the paravertebral area. One who presented with leg edema and lower back pain radiating down the lower extremity was treated with an IOEBT dose of 25 Gy with a 15-meV electron beam directed to the tumor in the left renal fossa followed by 40 Gy external beam therapy. The patient survived for 3 months after the treatment and died with disease. He experienced partial relief of the back pain. The other patient presented with cord compression and had a decompression laminectomy and 45 Gy external beam therapy to the spine. He then developed local recurrence in the paraspinal area with lower back pain. He then was treated with an IOEBT dose of 20 Gy with a 12-meV electron beam and intraoperative interstitial hyperthermia (43°C for 60 min). He experienced complete pain relief with local control for 9 months after the treatment. He subsequently expired with widespread metastatic disease at about the same time that local recurrence of cancer caused paraplegia.

B. CANCER OF THE PROSTATE

Cancer of the prostate is the second most common malignancy and the third most common cause of cancer death in men.[1]

At the time of diagnosis, only 10% of patients are candidates for radical prostatectomy.[63] Approximately 40 to 50% of patients have localized tumors at the primary site without extracapsular extension.[64] Total surgical removal is followed by local recurrence in 21 to 29% of patients.[65]

External beam radiation therapy has been successfully used to definitively treat prostate cancer localized to the gland and even when spread to regional lymph nodes, but local recurrence of disease is a substantial problem with this treatment modality also.[66] In 1972, IOEBT was first performed by Takahashi for inoperable carcinoma of the prostate.[67] His experience is reported in Chapter 21 of this work.

Two patients with biopsy-proven adenocarcinoma of the prostate have been brought to the IOEBT operating amphitheater in the COMROC. Pretreatment studies included complete blood counts, serum chemistries, chest X-rays, intravenous pyelography, retrograde urography, bone scintigraphy, and CT scanning.

One 70-year-old patient with Stage C disease was treated with transurethral prostatectomy followed by IOEBT. At 4 weeks after initial surgery, he received a dose of 25 Gy intraoperatively with a 15-meV electron beam followed by 45 Gy external beam therapy with 10-meVp X-rays at 1.8 Gy/d.

The other patient, age 73, with locally recurrent disease, received a dose of 20 Gy with 15-meV electrons in conjunction with 50 Gy external beam therapy.

For IOEBT, each patient was placed in the exaggerated lithotomy position. The prostatic tumor was exposed with a perineal incision, and the prostate was secured within the circular acrylic treatment applicator with a urethral probe. No serious complications were observed in bladder, urethra, or rectum. Both patients have been followed at regular intervals by radiotherapists and urologists. Evaluation of the response of the prostatic tumors was based on digital rectal examination and CT scan. As of November 1987, both patients have complete local control with no evidence of tumor regrowth or recurrence 28 and 12 months, respectively, from the time of IOEBT.

Clearly, additional work needs to be done to establish the minimal necessary dose of IOEBT and the optimal combination of IOEBT with full-pelvic radiation therapy for prostate cancer.

C. CANCER OF THE URINARY BLADDER

Transurethral resection is the most popular modality of treatment of superficial bladder cancer at the present time. The recurrence rate within 5 years after the initial resection is reported as high as 80%,[68] and 40 to 50% of recurrences occur within the first year. Prophylactic intravesicle installation of chemotherapeutic agents (principally Thiotepa[69] or Doxorubicin[70]) has not been completely satisfactory.

Matsumoto et al.[71] reported clinical results from 116 patients with superficial bladder cancer treated to doses of 25 to 30 Gy intraoperatively with 4- to 6-meV electrons followed by 30 to 40 Gy whole-bladder external beam irradiation in 15 to 20 d. Their results are reported in Chapter 19 of this work as is Shipley's analysis of same in Chapter 20.

Two patients, age 65 and 76, with local recurrence of transitional cell carcinoma have been brought to the COMROC IOEBT operating amphitheater for exploration and consideration for IOEBT. In one patient the lesion was resected, hence no IOEBT was delivered. The other patient had a second recurrence of tumor following radical cystectomy and prostectomy combined with external beam therapy at a dose of 65 Gy. He was treated with 20 Gy IOEBT with a 12-meV electron beam to the pelvic sidewall and another 10 Gy with 6-meV electrons delivered to the abdominal wall. No intraoperative complications were observed. The patient has survived 9 months after IOEBT with no local recurrence of disease, but he developed bone metastases 6 months after IOEBT.

D. CANCER OF THE LUNG

Initial clinical intraoperative experience indicates that the radiotolerance of mediastinal structures must always be respected when treating tumors of the chestwall, lung, and mediastinum.[72] Four patients with a diagnosis of advanced primary or extensive local recurrence of adenocarcinoma of the lung were brought to the IOEBT operating amphitheater in the COMROC for treatment. At the time of exploration for IOEBT, one of the four patients was discovered to have extensive primary disease beyond the scope of radiation treatment, and another was found to have a benign lesion; hence, no IOEBT was delivered in either case. The other two patients were treated with IOEBT.

A 43-year-old white man with adenocarcinoma of the left upper lobe developed a highly symptomatic paravertebral mass, eroding the bodies of the 11th and 12th thoracic vertebrae. He has been treated previously with 45 and 40 Gy external beam therapy to the chest and spine, respectively. The recurrent paravertebral mass was treated with IOEBT to a dose of 25 Gy with a 15-meV electron beam combined with intraoperative interstitial hyperthermia (43°C for 60 min). The recurrent chestwall mass was treated with an IOEBT dose of 20 Gy with 12-meV electrons. The upper lobe received 20 Gy with a 15-meV electron beam combined with intraoperative interstitial hyperthermia (43°C for 60 min). The patient experienced complete pain resolution after he received treatment to the paravertebral mass. Radiological evidence of new bone formation was observed at the site of the bony erosion. He survived for 21 months after IOEBT, disease free at both sites. Later, he developed distant metastases elsewhere and expired.

The other patient was a 61-year-old white man with primary locally advanced pulmonary adenocarcinoma. He underwent IOEBT to a dose of 15 gy with a 12-meV electron beam directed to the anterior superior mediastinum and a dose of 15 Gy with a 12-meV electron beam to the right hilum. The patient expired within 2 months of the IOEBT due to medical problems other than the cancer. We were unable to adequately assess tumor response in this case.

E. CANCER OF HEAD AND NECK SITES

Garrett et al.[73] treated more patients with head and neck primary tumor sites with IOEBT than all other investigators combined. They employed doses ranging from 10 to 100 Gy. Their results are reported in Chapter 15 of this work.

Two patients with extensive, locally recurrent, poorly differentiated epidermoid carcinoma in the neck and mandibular areas were brought to the COMROC IOEBT operating amphitheater for treatment. One patient with extensive, locally recurrent, poorly differentiated epidermoid carcinoma of the mandibular gingiva with cortical bone erosion was treated with an IOEBT dose of 10 Gy with a 6-meV electron beam to the tumor bed after complete resection of the tumor, followed by 55 Gy conventional external beam therapy.

The other patient with extensive, locally recurrent, poorly differentiated epidermoid carcinoma from an unknown primary site was treated with an IOEBT dose of 25 Gy with 15-meV electron beam to the residual tumor. No external beam therapy was delivered after the IOEBT because the patient had received 60 Gy external beam therapy after the initial surgery.

The first patient is still alive 2 months after the IOEBT with no evidence of disease. The other one expired 18 months after the IOEBT with metastatic disease, but with no evidence of local recurrence.

F. MALIGNANT MELANOMA

Although the fact that melanoma cells *in vitro* demonstrate a large shoulder on the radiation dose response curve is disputed by some researchers,[74] it is the rationale for using large radiation fractions in the treatment of this disease. There does exist some biologic rationale for the use of IOEBT in the management of this malignancy in selected cases in certain clinical situations. One patient, age 42 years, with recurrent malignant melanoma in left external iliac lymph nodes, was treated with partial tumor resection and 20 Gy IOEBT with an 18-meV electron beam followed by 30 Gy external beam therapy at 6 Gy/fraction, once weekly for 5 weeks. No intraoperative complications were observed, and the patient is alive 11 months after the IOEBT, with no evidence of the disease.

G. CHORDOMA

One patient, age 59 years, with primary advanced presacral chordoma was treated with almost complete resection and 15 Gy IOEBT with an 18-meV electron beam. This was delivered to the sacrum, and a dose of 10 Gy with a 9-meV electron beam was delivered to the margin of the resected area and the sciatic nerve. No intraoperative complications were observed. The patient is alive 9 months after IOEBT with no evidence of disease and no neuropathy.

H. MALIGNANT SCHWANNOMA

One patient, age 34 years, was treated elsewhere with external beam therapy for Hodgkin's disease to a dose of 40 Gy with mantle fields and 40 Gy with an inverted Y-field for a period of 3 months; 2 years later he received whole-brain radiation therapy, 50 Gy over a period of 4 weeks, for recurrent Hodgkin's tumor in the posterior fossa; 10 years later he developed a paravertebral mass within the prior radiation fields that proved to be a malignant Schwannoma. This was treated by laminectomy of $T_{3,4,5}$ and T_6 and 20 Gy external beam therapy. That was followed by 20 Gy IOEBT with a 12-meV electron beam in conjunction with intraoperative interstitial hyperthermia (43°C for 60 min). During the delivery of the IOEBT, the spinal cord in the treated area was protected with custom-designed shields (three layers of lead sheets) about 0.48 cm thick. The patient died 3 months after the IOEBT with local and distant disease, but the cord compression was partially relieved by the procedure, and the patient did regain some movement of the lower extremities.

XVI. CONCLUSIONS

The Medical College of Ohio experience in IORT reflects the international experience of medical centers where a dedicated facility permits patient accrual based on the expertise and interests of the surgeons, medical oncologists, and radiation oncologists which comprise the multimodality team essential for the proper therapeutic implementation and evaluation of IORT.

The concept of IORT is intellectually pleasing and intuitively acceptable as normal tissues are physically spared and cancerous tissues are directly exposed to high-dose electron beam irradiation. However, it is clearly evident that IORT is not a panacea, and its true therapeutic capability and role are yet to be established. It is possible at this point to conclude that IORT should not be viewed as an isolated mode of treatment. The initial disappointments in early IORT trials have been based on an unrealistic expectation of the role of IORT as a sole modality to the exclusion of comprehensive surgery and external beam radiation therapy.

The MCO experience reflects an appreciation of the role of IORT as an adjunctive tool, the future success of which will depend on innovative applications as part of a comprehensive multimodality approach which includes the more traditional methods of radiation therapy, surgery, and chemotherapy. Future broad areas of investigation that need to be studied will include the effect of preresection IORT delivered to gross disease followed by complete resection and a second IORT dose to the tumor bed for microscopic residual disease. The role of IORT in the routine treatment of adjacent high-risk lymphatic sites is another broad area of investigation that needs to be pursued for a variety of different primary cancers. Finally, the enhancement of local control via regional or systemic chemotherapy in addition to IORT and external beam radiation therapy needs to be extensively evaluated for a number of primary sites.

The true definition of the role of IORT in the management of malignant disease will be highly dependent on the results of future trials that are generated at dedicated IORT facilities which have equally dedicated interdisciplinary staffs. IORT studies which are pursued in a less rigorous manner will fail to properly evaluate this modality. The MCO experience has resulted from a dedicated interdisciplinary effort and has provided us with clear directions for future IORT studies which are necessary for a full understanding of this potentially powerful modality.

ACKNOWLEDGMENTS

The authors acknowledge Mrs. D. Ann Hollon, R.N.R.T.(T.) for assistance in collating data and Miss Sandra K. Price for clerical preparation of this manuscript.

REFERENCES

1. **Silverberge, E. and Lubera, J. A.,** Cancer statistics 1988, *Cancer J. Clin.*, 38, 5, 1988.
2. **Kalser, M. H. and Ellenberg, S. S. for the Gastrointestinal Tumor Study Group,** Pancreatic cancer adjuvant combined radiation and chemotherapy following curative resection, *Arch. Surg.*, 120, 899, 1985.
3. **Tepper, J., Nardi, G., and Suit, H.,** Carcinoma of the pancreas: review of MGH experience from 1963. Analysis of surgical failure and implications for radiation therapy, *Cancer*, 37, 1519, 1976.
4. **Borgelt, B. B., Dobelbower, R. R., Jr., and Strubler, K. A.,** Betatron therapy for unresectable pancreatic cancer, *Am. J. Surg.*, 135, 76, 1978.
5. **Ellison, E. C., VanAman, M. E., and Carey, L. C.,** Preoperative transhepatic biliary decompression in pancreatic and periampullary cancer, *World J. Surg.*, 8, 862, 1984.
6. **Fortner, J. G.,** Surgical principles for pancreatic cancer: regional total and subtotal pancreatectomy, *Cancer*, 47,(Suppl. 6), 1712, 1981.
7. **Hirayama, T., Waterhouse, T. A. H., and Fraumeni, J. F., Jr., Eds.,** Cancer risks by site *(Union Int. Contre Cancer) UICC Tech. Rep. Ser.*, 41, 78, 1980.
8. **Nakase, A., Matsumoto, Y., Uchida, K., and Honjo, I.,** Surgical treatment of cancer of the pancreas and the periampullary region — cumulative results in 57 institutions in Japan, *Ann. Surg.*, 185, 52, 1977.
9. **Monge, J. J., Judd, E. S., and Gage, R. P.,** Radical pancreatoduodenectomy: a 22-year experience with the complications, mortality rate, and survival rate, *Ann. Surg.*, 160, 711, 1964.
10. **Dobelbower, R. R., Jr., Borgelt, B. B., Strubler, K. A., Kutcher, G. J., and Suntharalingam, N.,** Precision radiotherapy for cancer of the pancreas: technique and results, *Int. J. Radiat. Oncol. Biol. Phys.*, 6, 1127, 1980.
11. **Dobelbower, R. R., Jr. and Milligan, A. J.,** Treatment of pancreatic cancer by radiation therapy, *World J. Surg.*, 8, 919, 1984.
12. **Dobelbower, R. R., Jr.,** The radiotherapy of pancreatic cancer, *Semin. Oncol.*, 6, 378, 1979.
13. **Dobelbower, R. R., Jr.,** Therapy by irradiation, in *The Exocrine Pancreas: Biology, Pathology, and Diseases,* Go, V. L. W. et al., Eds., Raven Press, New York, 1986, 699.
14. **Whittington, R., Dobelbower, R. R., Jr., Mohiuddin, M., Rosato, F. E., and Weiss, S. M.,** Radiotherapy of unresectable pancreatic carcinoma: a six year experience with 104 patients, *Int. J. Radiat. Oncol. Biol. Phys.*, 7 (12), 1639, 1981.
15. **Gastrointestinal Tumor Study Group,** Comparative therapeutic trial of radiation with or without chemotherapy in pancreatic carcinoma, *Int. J. Radiat. Oncol. Biol. Phys.*, 5, 1643, 1979.
16. **Dobelbower, R. R., Jr., Merrick, H. W., III, Ahuja, R. K., and Skeel, R. T.,** ^{125}I interstitial implant, precision high-dose external beam therapy, and 5-FU for unresectable adenocarcinoma of pancreas and extrahepatic biliary tree, *Cancer*, 58, 2185, 1986.
17. **Pilepich, M. V. and Miller, H. H.,** Preoperative irradiation in carcinoma of the pancreas, *Cancer*, 46, 1945, 1980.
18. **Komaki, R., Wilson, J. F., Cox, J. D., and Kline, R. W.,** Carcinoma of the pancreas: results of irradiation for unresectable lesions, *Int. J. Radiat. Oncol. Biol. Phys.*, 6, 209, 1980.
19. **Whittington, R., Solin, L., Mohiuddin, M., Cantor, R. I., Rosato, F. E., Biermann, W. A., Weiss, S. M., and Pajak, T. F.,** Multimodality therapy of localized unresectable pancreatic adenocarcinoma, *Cancer*, 54, 1991, 1984.

20. **Dobelbower, R. R.,** Intraoperative radiation therapy, *Rev. Brasil. Cancerol.,* 1988, in press.
21. **Gunderson, L. L. and Sosin, H.,** Areas of failure found at reoperation (second of symptomatic look) following "curative surgery" for adenocarcinoma of the rectum, *Cancer,* 34, 1278, 1974.
22. **Rao, A. R., Kagan, A. R., Chan, P. M., Gilbert, H. A., Nussbaum, H., and Hintz, B. L.,** Patterns of recurrence following curative resection alone for adenocarcinoma of the rectum and sigmoid colon, *Cancer,* 48, 1492, 1981.
23. **Sischy, B.,** The place of radiotherapy in the management of rectal adenocarcinoma, *Cancer,* 50, 2631, 1982.
24. **Mohuidden, M., Kramer, S., Marks, G., and Dobelbower, R. R., Jr.,** Combined pre and postoperative radiation for carcinoma of the rectum, *Int. J. Radiat. Oncol. Biol. Phys.,* 8, 133, 1982.
25. **Astler, V. B. and Coller, F. A.,** The prognostic significance of direct extension of carcinoma of the colon and rectum, *Ann. Surg.,* 139, 846, 1954.
26. **Rich, T., Gunderson, L. L., Galdabini, J., Lew, R., Cohen, A. M., and Donaldson, G.,** Clinical and pathologic factors influencing local failure after curative resection of carcinoma of the rectum and rectosigmoid, *Cancer,* 52, 1317, 1983.
27. **Cohen, A. M., Gunderson, L. L., and Wood, W. C.,** Intraoperative electron beam radiation therapy boost in the treatment of recurrent rectal cancer, *Dis. Colon Rectum,* 23, 453, 1980.
28. **Gunderson, L.,** Colorectal cancer, paper presented at the First Int. Symp. on Intraoperative Radiation Therapy, Dana Center, Medical College of Ohio, Toledo, May 15 and 16, 1986.
29. **Sugarbaker, P. H., MacDonald, J. S., and Gunderson, L. L.,** Colorectal cancer, in *Cancer: Principles and Practice of Oncology,* DeVita, V. T., Jr., Hellman, S., and Rosenberg, S. A., Eds., Lippincott, Philadelphia, 1982, 643.
30. **Russell, A. H., Tong, D., Dawson, L. E., and Wisbeck, W.,** Adenocarcinoma of the proximal colon. Sites of initial dissemination and patterns of recurrence following surgery alone, *Cancer,* 53, 360, 1984.
31. **Welch, J. and Donaldson, G. A.,** The clinical correlation of an autopsy study of recurrent colorectal cancer, *Ann. Surg.,* 89, 496, 1979.
32. **Willett, C., Tepper, J. E., Cohen, A., Orlow, E., Welch, C., and Donaldson, G.,** Local failure following curative resection of colonic adenocarcinoma, *Int. J. Radiat. Oncol. Biol. Phys.,* 10, 645, 1984.
33. **Gastrointestinal Tumor Study Group,** Adjuvant therapy of colon cancer — results of a prospective randomized trial, *N. Engl. J. Med.,* 36, 737, 1984.
34. **Abe, M.,** Intraoperative radiation therapy for gastrointestinal malignancy, in *Clinical Management of Gastrointestinal Cancer,* DeCosse, J. J. and Sherlock, P., Eds., Martinus Nijhoff, Boston, 1984, 327.
35. **Herskovic, A. M., Engler, M. J., and Noell, K. T.,** Radical radiotherapy for bile duct carcinoma, *Endocuriether. Hypertherm. Oncol.,* I, 119, 1985.
36. **Gunderson, L.,** Personal communication, October 1986.
37. **Guznick, D. S.,** Efficacy of screening for cervical cancer: a review, *Am. J. Public Health,* 68, 125, 1978.
38. **Perez, C. A., Breaux, S., Bedwinek, J. M., Madoc-Jones, H., Camel, H. M., Purdy, J. A., and Walz, B. J.,** Radiation therapy alone in the treatment of carcinoma of the uterine cervix. II. Analysis of complications, *Cancer,* 54, 235, 1984.
39. **Haie, C., Pejovic, M. H., Gerbaulet, A., Horiot, J. C., Pourquier, H., Delouche, J., Heinz, J. F., Brune, D., Fenton, J., Pizzi, G., Bey, P., Brossel, R., Pillement, P., Volterrani, F., and Chassagne, D.,** Is prophylatic para-aortic irradiation worthwhile in the treatment of advanced cervical carcinoma? Results of a controlled clinical trial of the EORTC radiotherapy group, *Radiother. Oncol.,* 11, 101, 1988.
40. **Delgado, G., Caglar, H., and Walter, P.,** Survival and complications in cervical cancer treated by pelvic and extended field radiation after para-aortic lymphadenectomy, *Am. J. Roentgenol.,* 130, 141, 1978.
41. **Berman, M., Keys, H., Creasman, W., Disia, P., Bundy, B., Blessing, J.,** Survival and patterns of recurrence in cervical cancer metastatic to periaortic lymph nodes, *Gynecol. Oncol.,* 19, 8, 1984.
42. **Diver, M. S., Wallace, S., and Castro, J. R.,** The accuracy of lymphangiography in carcinoma of the uterine cervix, *Am. J. Roentgenol.,* 111, 278, 1971.
43. **Chism, S. E., Park, R. C., and Keys, H. M.,** Prospects for para-aortic irradiation in treatment of cancer of the cervix, *Cancer,* 35, 1505, 1975.
44. **Fletcher, G. H. and Rutledge, F. N.,** Extended field technique in the management of the cancers of the uterine cervix, *Am. J. Roentgenol.,* 114, 116, 1972.
45. **Delgado, G., Goldson, A. L., Ashayeri, E., Hill, L. T., Petrilli, E. S., and Hatch, K. D.,** Intraoperative radiation in the treatment of advanced cervical cancer, *Obstet. Gynecol.,* 63, 246, 1984.
46. **Kottmeier, H. D., Ed.,** Annual report, in *The Results of Treatment in Carcinoma of the Uterus, Vagina and Ovary,* Vol. 15, International Federation of Gynecology and Obstetrics, Stockholm, 1973.
47. **Prasasvinichi, S., Glassburn, J. R., and Brady, L. W.,** Treatment of recurrent carcinoma of the cervix, *Int. J. Radiat. Oncol. Biol. Phys.,* 4, 957, 1978.
48. **Ozols, R. F. and Young, R. C.,** Chemotherapy of ovarian cancer, *Semin. Oncol.,* 2, 251, 1984.
49. **Horowitz, C. and Brady, L. W.,** Carcinoma of the ovary, in *Principles and Practice of Radiation Oncology,* Perez, C. A. and Brady, L. W., Eds., Lippincott, Philadelphia, 1987, 988.

50. **Bell, D. R., Woods, R. L., Levi, J. A., Fox, R. M., and Tattersall, M. H.**, Advanced ovarian cancer: a randomized trial of chlorambucil versus combined cyclophosphamide and cis-diamminedichloroplatinum, *Aust. N.Z. J. Med.*, 12, 245, 1982.

51. **Bush, R. S.**, Ovarian cancer: contribution of radiation therapy to patient management. Erskine Memorial Lecture, 1983, *Radiology*, 153, 17, 1984.

52. **Dembo, A. J., Bush, R. S., Beale, F. A., Bean, H. A., Pringle, J. F., and Sturgeon, J. F. G.**, The Princess Margaret Hospital Study of ovarian cancer: stages I, II, and asymptomatic III presentations, *Cancer Treat. Rep.*, 63, 249, 1979.

53. **Schray, M. F., Cox, R., and Martinez, A.**, Lower abdominal radiotherapy for stages I, II, and selected III epithelial ovarian carcinoma: 20 years experience, *Gynecol. Oncol.*, 15, 78, 1983.

54. **Adelson, M. D., Wharton, J. T., Delclos, L., Copeland, L., and Gershenson, D.**, Palliative radiotherapy for ovarian cancer, *Int. J. Radiat. Oncol. Biol. Phys.*, 13, 17, 1987.

55. **Kinsella, T. J., Sindelar, W. F., DeLuca, A. M., Pezeshkpour, G., Smith, R., Maher, M., Terrill, R., Miller, R. Mixon, A., Harwell, J. F., Rosenberg, S. A., and Glatstein, E.**, Tolerance of peripheral nerve to intraoperative radiotherapy (IORT): clinical and experimental studies, *Int. J. Radiat. Oncol. Biol. Phys.*, 11, 1579, 1985.

56. **Shieber, W. and Graham, P.**, An experience with sarcoma of the soft tissues in adults, *Surgery*, 52, 295, 1962.

57. **Lindberg, R. D., Martin, R. G., Romsdahl, M. M., and Barkley, H. T.**, Conservative surgery and postoperative radiotherapy in 300 adults with soft-tissue sarcomas, *Cancer*, 47, 2391, 1981.

58. **Wood, W. C., Suit, H. D., Mankin, H. J., Cohen, A. M., and Proppe, K.**, Radiation and conservative surgery in the treatment of soft tissue sarcoma, *Am. J. Surg.*, 147, 537, 1984.

59. **Kinsella, T., Sindelar, W., Glatstein, E., and Rosenberg, S.**, Preliminary results of a prospective randomized trial of intraoperative (IORT) and low dose external beam radiotherapy *vs.* high dose external beam radiotherapy as adjunctive therapy in resectable soft tissue sarcomas of the retroperitoneum, *Int. J. Radiat. Oncol. Biol. Phys.*, 12, 1983, 1986.

60. **Abe, M. and Takahashi, M.**, Intraoperative radiotherapy: the Japanese experience, *Int. J. Radiat. Oncol. Biol. Phys.*, 7, 863, 1981.

61. **Matsutani, M.**, Brain tumors, paper presented at the First Int. Symp. on Intraoperative Radiation Therapy, Dana Center, Medical College of Ohio, Toledo, May 15 and 16, 1986.

62. **Goldson, A. L., Streeter, O. D., Jr., Ashayeri, E., Collier-Manning, J., Barber, J. B., and Fan, K. J.**, Intraoperative radiotherapy for intracranial malignancies. A pilot study, *Cancer*, 54, 2807, 1984.

63. **Jewett, H. J.**, Radical perineal prostatectomy for palpable, clinically localized, non-obstructive cancer: Experience at the Johns Hopkins Hospital 1909—1963, *J. Urol.*, 124, 492, 1980.

64. **Scott, W. W. and Schrimer, H. K. A.**, Carcinoma of the prostate, in *Urology*, Vol. 2, 3rd ed., Campbell, and Harrison, Eds., W. B. Saunders, Philadelphia, 1970, 1177.

65. **Whitmore, W. F.**, The rationale and results of ablative surgery for prostatic cancer, *Cancer*, 16, 1119, 1963.

66. **Bagshaw, M. A.**, Current conflicts in the management of prostatic cancer, *Int. J. Radiat. Oncol. Biol. Phys.*, 12, 1721, 1986.

67. **Takahashi, M., Okada, K., Shibamoto, Y., Abe, M., and Yoshida, O.**, Intraoperative radiotherapy in the definitive treatment of localized carcinoma of the prostate, *Int. J. Radiat. Oncol. Biol. Phys.*, 11, 147, 1985.

68. **Althasen, A. F., Prout, G. R., Jr., and Daly, J. J.**, Non-invasive papillary carcinoma of the bladder associated with carcinoma *in situ*, *J. Urol.*, 116, 575, 1976.

69. **Veenema, R. J., Dean, A. L., Jr., Uson, A. C., Roberts, M., and Longo, F.**, Thiotepa bladder instillations: therapy and prophylaxis for superficial bladder tumors, *J. Urol.*, 101, 711, 1969.

70. **Pavone-Macaluso, M.**, Intravesical treatment of superficial (T1) urinary bladder tumors. A review of a 15-year experience, in *Diagnosis and Treatment of Superficial Urinary Bladder Tumors*, Montedison Lakemedel, Stockholm, 1978, 21.

71. **Matsumoto, K., Kakizoe, T., Mikuriya, S., Tanaka, T., Kondo, I., and Umegaki, Y.**, Clinical evaluation of intraoperative radiotherapy for carcinoma of the urinary bladder, *Cancer*, 47, 509, 1981.

72. **Goldson, A. L.**, Past, present, and future prospects of intraoperative radiotherapy (IORT), *Semin. Oncol.*, 8, 59, 1981.

73. **Garrett, P., Pugh, N., Ross, D., Hamaker, R., and Singer, M.**, Intraoperative radiation therapy for advanced or recurrent head and neck malignancies, *Int. J. Radiat. Oncol. Biol. Phys.*, 13, 785, 1987.

74. **Overgaard, J.**, The role of radiotherapy in recurrent and metastatic malignant melanoma: a clinical radiobiologic study, *Int. J. Radiat. Oncol. Biol. Phys.*, 12, 867, 1986.

Chapter 29

PARTICIPATION OF COMMUNITY FACILITIES IN INTRAOPERATIVE RADIATION THERAPY

Gerald E. Hanks and Harvey B. Wolkov

TABLE OF CONTENTS

I. HISTORICAL DEVELOPMENT

Intraoperative radiation therapy (IORT) was first begun in nonuniversity or private hospitals in the U.S. in 1983. Radiation oncology trainees from the established programs were the first to bring this technology to the community, and they not only continued treating the common disease sites, such as colon and pancreas, but also introduced the procedure as an adjuvant in head and neck cancer and elsewhere. The next community facilities to be involved were those where there is a strong clinical research background, which seems to be very important for introducing such a complex new modality.

A survey conducted in the spring of 1985 attempted to identify all the IORT users in the U.S. A summary of the response (as of March 1985) is shown in Table 1; 29 facilities were using IORT and an additional 28 planned to introduce the procedure during 1985. They were equally divided between federal/university hospitals and community hospitals. This astonishing increase in the utilization of IORT has prompted the organization, in October 1985, of an IORT Users Group in the U.S.

II. WHY THE COMMUNITY?

It is critical for community hospitals to be involved in IORT for the reasons shown in Table 2. The Patterns of Care Study has demonstrated that more than 80% of radiation therapy is administered in nonuniversity or community centers, and involvement of the community is the only way the procedure will be available to more than the small subset of patients seen in the few U.S. universities or federal centers with IORT experience.

During the 1980s we have seen an explosion in medical technology and procedures in the U.S. This has been accomplished by the training of large numbers of specialists and subspecialists. The university is no longer the sole locus for complex procedures, many have been transferred to community hospitals along with the personnel necessary to perform them. This will also be true for IORT as patients continue to demand that even the most complex procedure be readily available for them in their own community.

Many community radiation oncology practices have achieved the technical sophistication that is necessary for conducting IORT and have also gained experience in clinical research through participation in community oncology programs or with the various national clinical trial groups. This background of clinical research is important to develop IORT in a scientific and nonentrepreneurial basis.

Lastly, the question of efficacy of IORT as compared to the current best treatments has not been answered. Large numbers of patients will be required when Phase III trials begin, and all of these patients cannot be expected to come from the university sector.

III. PREREQUISITES FOR AN IORT PROGRAM

The prerequisites necessary for an IORT program are similar for a community or a university facility. The starting point is skilled and interested physicians in surgery, radiation oncology, and anesthesia. Their intent must be in developing and maintaining an ongoing program directed at assisting patients while continuously evaluating the efficacy of IORT. Programs should not exist without a dedication to clinical research.

Support facilities must be available with a cooperative nursing and operating room staff, surgical oncology unit, and a hospital administration willing to support the procedure. The radiation oncology facility must have high-energy electrons and the full-time physics support necessary to perform the complex evaluations of dose distributions needed to treat patients safely.

The facility must have a large number of cancer patients to provide a pool from which

TABLE 1
Intraoperative Radiation Therapy U.S. Facility Survey March 1985

	Active program	Planned by January 1986	Totals
Federal or university hospitals	15	13	28
Community hospitals	14	15	29
Total	29	28	57

TABLE 2
IORT: Why the Community Must be Involved

- 80% of patients are treated there
- Patients demand dissemination of high-technology procedures
- The community is experienced in clinical research through community oncology programs
- Determining the efficacy of IORT will require that many patients enter clinical trials

TABLE 3
IORT: Steps to Introducing the Procedure

- Identify key personnel
- Literature review
- View existing program
- Hospital administration approval
- Approval of Hospital committees
- Equipment purchase
- Physics — dosimetry preparation
- Quality control and data analysis

can be selected the small fraction of patients who may be helped by IORT. The institutions and physicians involved must have experience in clinical trials and access to data registry and retrieval and patient outcome analysis.

IV. PROCEDURE FOR INTRODUCING IORT

We have found the procedure outlined in Table 3 to be valuable in introducing IORT in a community hospital. When the key personnel have been identified, one must carefully review the literature and visit and observe the procedure as performed in existing programs. The hospital administration must agree to proceed with the program, at least in a pilot experience. The DRGs may reduce the potential hospital income, welfare programs will not pay for the special aspects of IORT, and Medicare will pay only a fraction of IORT costs. These are very real economic concerns for any hospital in the U.S. in 1985, and the administration will perhaps wish to proceed with a pilot program that allows them to evaluate the economic impact of IORT. Obviously, this program can greatly contribute to the hospital's public image, helping to keep its beds full and to attract other complex care procedures.

The medical staff needs reassurance that the procedure can be performed safely and that it has some efficacy. One may need to inform and educate a host of groups, including medical oncology, general surgery, gynecologic surgery, infection control, radiology, anesthesiology, nursing administration, and others. It is better to spend the time repetitiously discussing IORT with an excessive number of committees than to hurry the procedure through the approval process. If established procedures are bypassed and a complication occurs, the progress of the program can be seriously impeded.

The position of the hospital institutional review board (IRB) is unclear. The procedure may be introduced as a "new procedure", not a research procedure as outlined by federal and state guidelines. In that circumstance, the IRB does not have the right of review and approval. When a formal research protocol study is begun, IRB approval is necessary, so it seems best to keep the IRB informed from the start as their approval will be required when formal clinical trials begin.

A substantial amount of special equipment is needed to introduce an IORT program, such as Surgi-Lifts®, special portable monitors, changes in the radiation therapy treatment room to provide for the exhaust of nitrous oxide, special applicators for directing the electron beam treatment, and others. The cost of these is modest in terms of modern medical costs and does not normally exceed $25,000.00. The physicians and personnel must then become familiar with their use, and the physicists must have a substantial period of time to perform the complex dosimetry necessary to safely use a broad spectrum of electron treatment applicators.

V. QUALITY CONTROL AND DATA ANALYSIS

Quality control and continuing data analysis can be assisted by establishing pre-IORT planning conferences, identifying the parties responsible for data recording, conducting joint follow-up clinics, and periodically reviewing the outcome of IORT and reporting the results of that outcome. The pretreatment conference is very important and must be interdisciplinary, consultative, and provide a focus whereby all the clinically relevant material can be brought together with the surgeon, the radiation oncologist, the diagnostic radiologist, and the pathologist to make the necessary preprocedure decisions. It is best to follow patients in joint clinics with both the surgeons and radiation oncologists in attendance so that there can be an ongoing monitoring of complications and benefits from the procedure.

VI. EXAMPLE OF RESULTS FROM A COMMUNITY IORT PROGRAM

IORT with electrons was first used in the western U.S. in December of 1983 at the Radiation Oncology Center of Sutter Community Hospitals of Sacramento, California. Since that time 50 patients have been treated (Table 4).

A continuing problem for facilities without dedicated units is the number of patients explored but not treated with IORT. This was 40% in our series. The usual problem is an inability to accurately define the true extent of the disease before surgery, as shown in Table 5. A maximal effort should always be made to lower this number by very careful preoperative evaluation.

Outcome for the 50 patients treated prior to September 8, 1985, is shown in Table 6. Several observations can be made from these preliminary data. The failure rate within the IORT field has been satisfactory with only 9 local failures in 50 patients (18%), suggesting that the procedure contributed to local control. The first sites of progression were most commonly in the liver (6/21) and/or lung (3/21), this emphasizes the need to carefully evaluate these organs prior to treatment. Table 6 also shows that operative complications were observed in only 2 of the 50 patients (4%), a figure consistent with those surgical procedures observed without IORT in our hospital.

TABLE 4
IORT: Sutter Radiation Oncology
Center Treatment Sites
12/8/83—9/8/85

Gynecologic	10
Colorectal	12
Pancreatic	12
Gastric	6
Biliary	3
Genitourinary	3
Sarcomas	2
Others	2
Total	50

TABLE 5
IORT: Patients Explored for IORT but not Treated

Sutter Radiation Oncology Center 12/8/83—9/8/85

Disease site	Number	Reason[a]
Gynecologic	8/18	Ext. L.D. — 4
		Hemostasis — 1
		No proven tumor — 3
Colorectal	8/20	P.S. — 4
		L.D. — 3
		No proven tumor — 1
Pancreatic	8/20	L.M. — 4
		P.S. — 1
		Benign cyst — 2
		Ovarian CA — 1
Gastric	1/7	L.M. — 1
Biliary tree	1/4	Ext. L.D. — 1
Genitourinary	1/4	Ext. L.D. — 1
Retroperitoneal sarcoma	3/4	P.S. — 2
		Ext. L.D. — 1
Lung	1/1	Ext. L.D. — 1
Total	31/78 (40%)	

[a] L.D. = local disease; P.S. = peritoneal seeding; L.M. = liver metastases; Ext. L.D. = extensive local disease.

VII. CLINICAL TRIALS IN THE COMMUNITY

It is very important that the major effort of community and university programs be ultimately directed toward the performance of ongoing prospective clinical trials. Under this circumstance, informed consent will be assured and patients will be treated by a national consensus-based treatment program. Locally derived, single-institutional protocols will never answer the necessary questions and can only serve as Phase I-II pilot studies. They frequently do not provide adequate informed consent and protection for the patient. In addition, national clinical trials require external quality control, review of the physical and medical aspects of the treatment, and require a structured follow-up. These points all help to develop a stronger, more scientifically based program with improved patient protection. Efficacy must be proven if IORT is to have a broad-based usage. We must know whether IORT is of palliative or

TABLE 6
IORT: Survival and Sites of Failure

Sutter Radiation Oncology Center 12/8/83—9/8/85

	Total	Died	Disease progression site[a]	IORT field failure	Complications
Gynecologic	10	3	3 (PS) (LM + Lg) (LM)	5	0
Colorectal	12	2	6 (LM — 5) (wound)	0	2[b]
	12	10	7 (LM — 5) (LM + Lg)	3	0
Gastric	6	3	2 (LM) (ana)	1	0
Biliary	3	3	2 (LM — 2)	1	0
Kidney	2	2	2 (PS) (LM)	0	0
Bladder	1	0	0	0	0
Retroperitoneal sarcoma	2	0	0	0	0
Other	2	0	0	0	0
Totals	50	23	22	10	2

[a]   PS = peritoneal seeding; LM = liver metastases; Lg = lung; ana = anastomosis.
[b]   1 — wound infection; 1 — delayed wound healing.

TABLE 7
IORT Protocols Radiation Therapy
Oncology Group

Pancreatic carcinoma
Gastric carcinoma
Retroperitoneal sarcoma
Recurrent or inoperable rectal carcinoma
Recurrent cervical carcinoma
Extrahepatic biliary duct carcinoma

curative benefit and how it compares to the best current combinations of surgery and radiation therapy for these same diseases.

The Radiation Therapy Oncology Group (RTOG) introduced six protocols in 1985 as shown in Table 7. These protocols will assess patients as Phase II nonrandomized trials for at least 12 to 18 months. During and at the conclusion of that time period, prospective randomized trials will be designed in each of the sites for which there are prospects for answering a specific question. By early 1987, a sufficient number of facilities must be participating to provide the large number of patients necessary to answer the clinical questions; this cannot be done without involving community patients. The requirements for participation will be strict, but the rewards of that participation great.

VIII. THE EFFECT OF CHANGES IN REIMBURSEMENT

Table 8 illustrates the main points where changes in the economics of medicine in the U.S. may influence reimbursement from IORT. There is concern that DRGs will stifle the development of inpatient clinical research, including IORT, unless some changes are made. The Medicaid program in California does not pay for the additional costs of IORT, although the hospital receives its usual low rate of reimbursement for the majority of the charges. The Medicare program will support about two thirds of the cost of IORT and the prospects are that that will become less rather than more.

TABLE 8
IORT Economic Considerations

- Effect of DRGs is unknown
- Medicare reimbursement 65% cost
- Medicaid reimbursement 0—50% cost
- HMOs view IORT as "experimental"

Health maintenance organizations (HMOs) are reluctant to approve payment for IORT for two reasons: first, it is a procedure generally performed out of their own hospital which represents out-of-pocket expense, and second, if it is classified as clinical research, their policy restrictions generally prohibit payment. As we have seen with HMOs and complex procedures, such as organ and bone marrow transplantation, they will respond to appropriate public and governmental pressure.

VIV. CONCLUSION

IORT is a promising innovation in combined modality therapy for selected cancers. The originators of the procedure in the U.S. and abroad have demonstrated preliminary evidence of efficacy and the important hazards, toxicity, and complications that may result from the procedure. The time has come for university and community oncologists to begin to prove the efficacy of IORT in RTOG Phase III clinical trials.

Chapter 30

INTRAOPERATIVE RADIATION THERAPY IN AUSTRIA

K. Glaser, E. Bodner, M. Url, and H. Frommhold

TABLE OF CONTENTS

I. INTRODUCTION

The role of intraoperative radiation therapy (IORT) in the treatment of malignancies of the abdomen, thorax, brain, and extremities is increasing. An impressive summary of the different areas in which IORT is used was given at the First International Symposium in Toledo, OH, which surely served as an essential impulse for the preparation of this chapter.

Compared to the patient numbers of U.S. or Japanese centers, the Austrian experience with IORT is limited. Nevertheless, there are differences in our way of preoperative patient selection and method management which allow us to simplify both the planning and practice of IORT.

A. HISTORICAL SUPPLEMENT

A detailed report on the history of IORT has already been given. We would also like to mention Czerny (Heidelberg), who in 1911 radiated an inoperable stomach cancer using γ-rays. Radium, as the source of radiation, was enclosed in a block of lead which was brought in as close a contact to the tumor as possible (Figure 1). IORT serves as an example that modern therapeutic strategies sometimes are based on long-recognized principles.

B. THE PROBLEM OF PANCREATIC CANCER

In 1984, approximately 700 Austrians developed cancer of the pancreas (about 10 out of 100,000 inhabitants).[1] As in the rest of the world, the results of our therapeutic endeavours are poor. Remarkable developments in diagnostic procedures and the reduction of operative risks have not improved the outlook. Resectability rates remain low at 10 to 30%.[2] About half of the cases with "radical" resection develop local resection.[3] Median survival following radical resection is 14 months; less than 5% of all the patients who underwent resection of their tumors survived 5 years.[4,5] Jaundice and disturbances of the gastroduodenal passage can be palliated satisfactorily, whereas tumor-related pain, especially with body and tail tumors, is not influenced by surgical measures. In our search for promising methods of tumor palliation, we came across publications by U.S. authors who had achieved pain and growth reduction in pancreatic tumors using IORT.[6-8]

After studying the indication, method, and equipment of IORT while on a sabbatical at Massachusetts General Hospital,* we were able to begin in Innsbruck in May 1984.

II. OUR INDICATIONS FOR IORT

According to recent experience, we consider IORT suitable for the following situations in general surgery:

1. Locally nonresectable pancreatic carcinoma without distant metastases (regional lymph node metastases are no hinderance as long as they can be included in the radiation field).[6,9-11]
2. Irradiation of tumors adjacent or with a very close relation to the upper abdominal vasculature directly before resection.
3. Irradiation of the tumor bed immediately after radical resection with the intention of eliminating microscopic residual disease.[12]
4. As an exception in cases with minor local tumor spread unknown before laparotomy; if the operation was started in the radiation therapy room, we take advantage of the preparatory work in order to at least reduce pain (known metastases prior to operation exclude patients from IORT).

---

* We would like to thank Drs. Warshaw, Tepper, Cohen, and Shipley for their inestimable support.

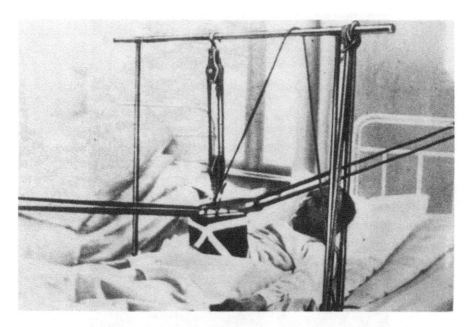

FIGURE 1.   Irradiation of an advanced stomach cancer (Czerny, Heidelberg, 1911).

5.   Irradiation of resectable pancreatic tumors if, due to contraindications such as age or severe underlying diseases, Whipple's procedure is not performed.
6.   Unresectable rectal cancer after preoperative external beam radiation therapy.[13]

III. METHODS

A. LOCAL CIRCUMSTANCES

Although the operating theater and the radiation therapy room in our hospital are in the same building, they are two stories apart. As in many other institutions, this necessitates cautious transportation of anesthetized patients with temporarily closed wounds.

B. PATIENT SELECTION

The linear accelerator is usually fully occupied for treatment of ambulatory or hospitalized patients. If, according to the surgical-radiation team, IORT is indicated, the radiation therapy room has to be blocked from regular use. Therefore, it is particularly important to be informed as to the exact extent of the malignancy preoperatively in order to avoid intraoperative cancellations because of tumors not within our indication groups 1 to 3.

In our approach to patient selection we put strong emphasis on the following two diagnostic procedures.

1. Abdominal Ultrasound

At our institution, preoperative ultrasound is routinely performed by the surgeon. We were able to predict local resectability or inoperability of a pancreatic tumor in over 90% of the cases.[14] Location of the tumor in relation to the upper abdominal vasculature is a special point of interest. Deformation, invagination, or lack of a visual border between the tumor and venous axis are signs of a nonresectable cancer of the pancreas (Figure 2). The presence of ascites indicates spread to the peritoneum.

2. Laparoscopy

Both ultrasound and CT scan may fail to detect small liver metastases. For this reason, preoperative laparoscopy is essential in our opinion (Figure 3).

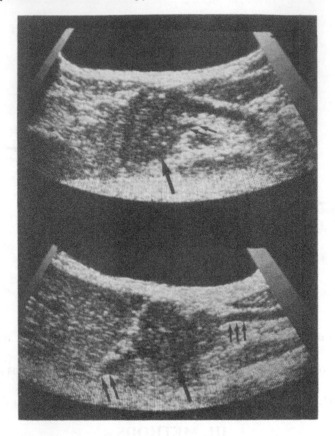

FIGURE 2.   (Top) The tumor (↑) infiltrates and deforms the superior
mesenteric vein (↑ ↑). (Bottom) Tumor spread around the mesenteric-
portal junction. Tumor (↑), portal vein (↑ ↑), superior mesenteric
vein (↑ ↑ ↑).

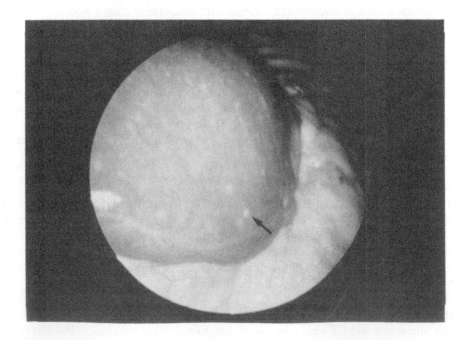

FIGURE 3.   Small subcapsular liver metastases (↑) detectable with neither ultrasound nor CT.

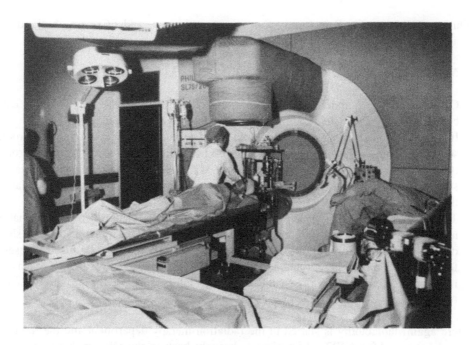

FIGURE 4. The linac room serves as an operating room.

Preoperative CT scan is to aid the radiation physicists and to help outline a radiation plan. It also serves as a basis for further documentation of the course of disease. Most of the time, patients undergo preoperative ERCP, sometimes gastroscopy or an upper GI series. Since it is possible to detect anatomical abnormalities of the hepatic artery using ultrasound, angiography is applied only in very selected cases.

C. SURGICAL INTERVENTION

Laparotomy serves primarily to confirm diagnosis and to establish the exact tumor stage and local resectability. Liver, peritoneal cavity, and lymphatic nodes are examined for extrapancreatic tumor spread. In case of doubt, diagnostic biopsies for frozen section are taken. Prior to IORT, pathologic confirmation of the diagnosis is obtained by intraoperative fine-needle biopsy; the results being available in 10 to 15 min. The waiting period can be used for preparation of the radiation field. We try to avoid preoperative percutaneous fine-needle biopsy because of the potential implantability assumed with pancreatic carcinoma.[16,17]

D. RADIOTHERAPEUTIC INTERVENTION

The high-velocity electrons from a linear accelerator (Philips® SL 75-20) are used in a single dose of 20 to 25 Gy. Eight electron energy stages can be selected between 5 and 20 meV in order to adapt the maximum dose to the particular topographic situation.

In correlation to the diameter and depth of the tumor, assessed by preoperative CT scan, ultrasound, and operative findings, the electron energy is chosen in a way that the tumor is positioned within the 80% isodose curve. Beveled or regular radiation applicators are available in diameters from 5 to 9 cm.

Special measures are taken to prepare the radiation therapy room to function as an operating room (floor disinfection, sterile cloths for the accelerator head, portable light, suction, surgical supplies, etc.) (Figure 4).

It must be strictly observed that surrounding tissue (hollow viscera and abdominal organs) be pushed aside by the applicator in placing it over the tumor. This assures that these structures lie outside the radiation field, thus preventing damage.

During IORT, usually 3 to 6 min, the patient, respirator, and ECG are observed via television monitors.

E. SIMPLIFICATION OF THE METHOD

1. Consequent use of abdominal ultrasound and laparoscopy enabled us to avoid cancellations of IORT at the time of laparotomy in 80% of the patients.
2. In case of a nonresectable tumor, laparotomy takes place in the radiation therapy room so that the anesthetized patient must only be transported once to the operating room (OR) in order to perform bypass operations. If there is no need for further palliative surgical measures (body and tail tumors), the operation is terminated in the radiation therapy room.
3. The ultrasound image of some tumors shows a very close relation between the malignancy and the superior mesenteric vein or mesenteric-portal junction over a short distance without deforming the blood vessel. We classify them as "borderline cases" for a Whipple procedure: resection of the tumor may be possible, but the risk of leaving microscopic residual disease on the vessel is high because of the proximity of the tumor.

Here again, laparotomy is started in the radiation therapy department and the tumor is irradiated *in situ*. After IORT, the patient is brought back to the OR for thorough tumor exploration. If radical operation is feasible, the tumor is resected; if not, bypass anastomoses are performed. As far as we know, this tactical approach has not as yet been reported in the literature.

In both instances, IORT was administered to regional lymphatic nodes and the tumor or tumor bed. Only once was patient transportation necessary, thus considerably reducing the expenditure of time and manpower. In addition, occupation of the radiotherapy room is limited to a minimum, and treatment of ambulatory patients can be continued after the linac room has been cleaned.

The above-mentioned strategy may also be applied in cases where the tumor is classified as clearly resectable, intending to limit nidation of malignant cells which may be spread during surgical manipulations.

F. EXTERNAL BEAM IRRADIATION

Radiosensitivity of pancreatic carcinoma has been clearly demonstrated *in vitro*.[18] The effect of a single high radiation dose on the tumor tissue has also been examined several times.[19] According to the findings, IORT leads to a massive necrosis of tumor cells followed by replacement with connective tissue, with nests of vital tumor cells remaining between collagen fibers.[10] Therefore, it seems reasonable to carry out external beam irradiation in addition to IORT.[20,21] Preoperative irradiation is often impossible because of increasing jaundice. Furthermore, patients often reject postoperative irradiation, and in some cases, irradiation must be stopped because of poor tolerance or severe side effects. In spite of this, we make an effort to perform postoperative external beam irradiation in daily fractions of 2 Gy to the tumor area with a total maximum dose of 40 to 46 Gy.

IV. PATIENT MATERIAL

From May 1984 to July 1986, 60 patients with pancreatic carcinoma were admitted to our hospital. IORT was administered in 17 cases (Table 1). The patients (seven male, ten female) ranged in age from 49 to 80 years, with a median age of 72 years. All of them suffered from ductal adenocarcinoma of the pancreas. In all the cases, microscopic tumor

TABLE 1

Patient	Age	Sex	Tumor location and size (cm)	TNM/Stage[a]	IORT dose (Gy)	Operation
1	58	F	Head, 4	$_cT_4N_xM_o$/ —	20	Gastroenterostomy
2	69	M	Isthmus-body 4 × 5	$_pT_4N_xM_1$/III	20	Exploratory laparotomy
3	49	M	Head, 5	$_cT_4N_xM_0$/ —	20	Cholecystectomy, cholodoco- and gastrojejunostomy
4	72	F	Head, 4 × 5	$_cT_4N_xM_0$/ —	20	Cholecystectomy, cholodoco- and gastrojejunostomy
5	73	M	Head, 4 × 5	$_pT_2N_0M_0$/I	20	Whipple procedure
6	66	F	Head-isthmus, 4 × 3	$_cT_4N_xM_0$/ —	20	Cholectystoduodenostomy
7	75	F	Head, 3.5	$_cT_4N_xM_0$/—	20	Cholodoco- and gastrojejunostomy
8	73	F	Body-tail 4 × 5	$_pT_4N_1M_1$/III	20	Exploratory laparotomy
9	72	F	Head, 3 × 4	$_cT_4N_xM_0$/ —	25	Biopsy of pancreatic tail, cholodocojejunostomy
10	66	F	Head, 3	$_cT_4N_xM_0$/ —	25	Cholodoco- and gastrojejunostomy
11	77	M	Head, 3.5 × 3	$_pT_4N_0M_0$/I	20	Whipple procedure
12	67	M	Head, 2 × 2	$_pT_4N_0M_0$/I	20	Whipple procedure
13	72	F	Body 4	$_pT_4N_1M_0$/II	25	Exploratory laporatomy
14	73	F	Body 4 × 5	$_pT_4N_2M_2$/III	15	Partial excision of gastric wall
15	56	M	Head, 3	$_pT_2N_0M_0$/I	20	Whipple procedure
16	80	M	Body, 5	$_pT_4N_2M_2$/III	20	Partial resection of stomach and transverse mesocolon, cholecystectomy
17	77	F	Head, 5 × 6	$_cT_4N_xM_0$/ —	20	Cholodoco- and gastrojejunostomy

[a] TNM — classification and staging according to Fortner.[22] Stage I: T_1—T_4, N_0M_0; Stage II: T_1—T_4, N_{1-2}, M_0; Stage III: T_1—T_4, N_{0-3}, M_{1-4}; c: clinical staging; p: pathological staging.

diagnosis was obtained with intraoperative fine-needle biopsy (in eight cases by additional histologic specimen).

In 11 cases, the tumor was located in the head, twice in the isthmus, and 4 times in the body or tail of the organ. Nine patients can be classified in the above-mentioned indication group 1, two patients were treated in spite of distant metastases (group 4), and two patients showed direct extension of the tumor to contiguous structures (stomach and transverse mesocolon). In four cases, irradiation was carried out along with a radical resection, among which the tumor was radiated *in situ* prior to resection in three of the patients.

V. RESULTS

There were no intraoperative mishaps or anesthesia problems during IORT.

A. EARLY COMPLICATIONS

As shown in Table 2, one patient had to undergo relaparotomy because of hemorrhage from the mesocolon transversum. Leakage of the pancreatojejunostomy was observed in one patient who had received IORT prior to resection. He developed a pancreaticocutaneous fistula which healed under conservative treatment. We saw no disorders of wound healing

TABLE 2
Early and Late Complications of 17 Patients
Following IORT

Early complications	No. of patients
Rebleeding (relaparotomy)	1
Cutaneous fistula after leakage of pancreatojejunostomy	1
Hemorrhagic gastritis	1
Apathy	6
Nausea, vomiting	2
Elevation of liver function tests (temporary)	2
Venous thrombosis	1
Late complications	2
Duodenal obstruction	1
Duodenal ulcerations	1
Epiploiditis of the mesentery	1

which could be ascribed to the IORT. Six patients showed noticeable somnolence and apathy starting between the second and fourth postoperative day and lasting at the most until the third postoperative week. There were no perioperative deaths.

The number of early complications did not differ from that of comparable operations without IORT.

B. LATE COMPLICATIONS

As shown in Table 2 all the patients had follow-up investigations at 3-month intervals, with routine ultrasound, blood samples, in most cases CT, and (rarely) gastroscopy. Two patients had specific late complications which may be related to IORT. In Case 7, a female patient developed massive duodenal obstruction 14 months after operation with recurrent episodes of intestinal bleeding. Due to extensive mucosal edema, the pylous could hardly be passed with the gastroscope. Gastric emptying occurred via the gastrojejunostomy performed during the prior operation (Figure 5). Bleeding ceased under H_2-blocker therapy. In Case 6, duodenal ulcerations developed in a female patient 3 months after IORT. These resolved with conservative measures. At 9 months following IORT, this patient was reoperated due to an unrelated cause. During operation, marked swelling of the mesentery was found. A histologic specimen showed the presence of nonspecific inflammatory reaction of the peritoneum typed as "granulomatous epiploiditis" (Figure 6).

Both patients received additional external beam irradiation (20 and 46 Gy).

C. PAIN REDUCTION

Of the 13 patients who received palliative treatment, 10 suffered from characteristic abdominal and back pain. In nine cases, pain was favorably influenced; five patients were free of pain after IORT, and in four, pain was alleviated.

This subjective improvement lasted up to 6 months in those patients who died in the meantime. Of the living four patients out of this group, three are almost free of pain; in one case, pain was simply reduced after IORT.

D. SURVIVAL TIME

Three of the four patients with radical resection are alive without evidence of disease after 21.5, 15.5, and 6 months. One patient died from local recurrence and liver metastases 12 months after operation. Nine patients who received palliative treatment died 9, 9, 8.5, 7, 6, 4, 3, 3, and 1.5 months after IORT (median: 6 months), including two cases treated

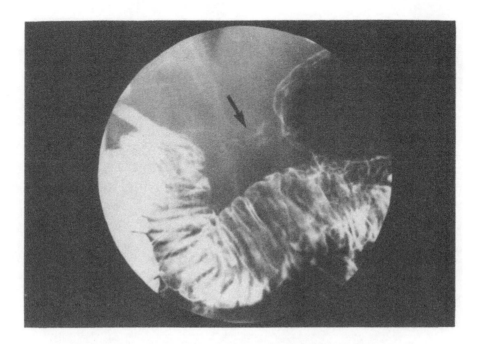

FIGURE 5.   Duodenal stenosis (↑); gastric emptying via gastrojejunostomy.

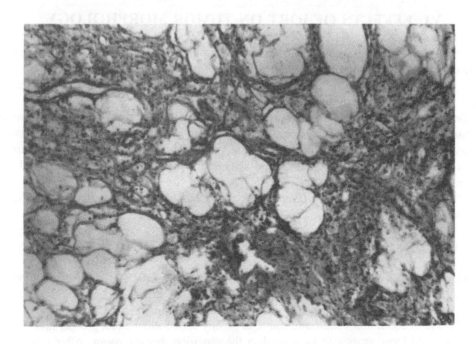

FIGURE 6.   Lymphocytic infiltration of mesenteric connective tissue.

in spite of distant metastases and one patient with contiguous extension of the disease to the stomach wall and transverse mesocolon.

Two patients of this group are alive without evidence of disease 19 and 16 months after IORT, respectively. One patient is doing well 6 weeks following IORT. In one case, because of a poor clinical condition, tumor progression is assumed 2 months after IORT.

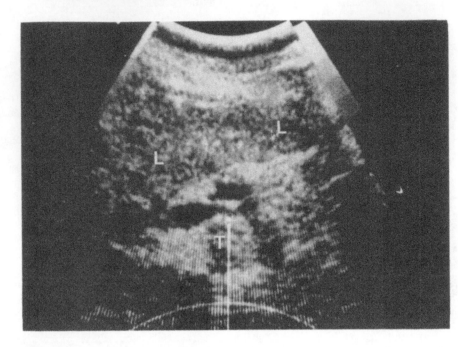

FIGURE 7.   Narrowing of the mesenteric-portal junction. L: liver; T: tumor in the uncinate process.

VI. EFFECTS OF IORT ON TUMOR MORPHOLOGY

Due to the absence of controlled trials, we do not know if patients receiving IORT have a longer life expectancy than comparable patients not treated with IORT. What we do know is the fact that IORT does influence tumor growth as can be demonstrated by changes of tumor morphology in CT and ultrasound images.

One patient with nonresectable pancreatic carcinoma showed a noticeable narrowing of the confluence and superior mesenteric vein caused mainly by tumor in the uncinate process (Figure 7). An ultrasonic follow-up examination 1 year later showed shrinkage of the tumor, now with a more reflective echo pattern (possibly due to increased fibrosis) and no evidence of venous obstruction (Figure 8).

CT images of another tumor taken 1 year apart showed no local tumor growth (Figure 9, Figure 10).

VII. PRELIMINARY COMMENT CONCERNING METHOD

Planning and performance of IORT require close cooperation of surgeons, radiotherapists, and anesthesiologists. Organizational and personnel efforts transporting the anesthetized patient from the OR to the linac room and back are remarkable.

The use of abdominal ultrasound and laparoscopy allows more exact preoperative patient selection, and laparotomy can be started in the radiation therapy room. After IORT, the tumor will either be resected or bypassed. There is only need for one patient transportation from the linac room to the OR. In cases of body or tail pancreatic carcinoma, where bypassing is not usually necessary, the operation can be terminated in the linac room.

Evidence of local tumor control and the reduction of tumor growth can be observed, this possibly explaining the satisfactory pain palliation following IORT. However, the central problem of long-term survival is the metastatic spread to distant lymph nodes or the liver. This spread does not seem to be markedly influenced by the local tumor control obtained with IORT.

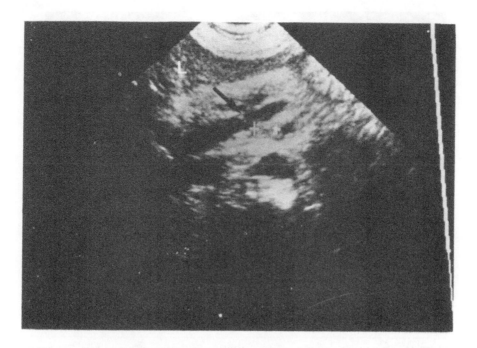

FIGURE 8.   Normal venous lumen (↑) and shrinkage of the tumor (+ +) 1 year after IORT. L: liver; ↑ : mesenteric-portal junction.

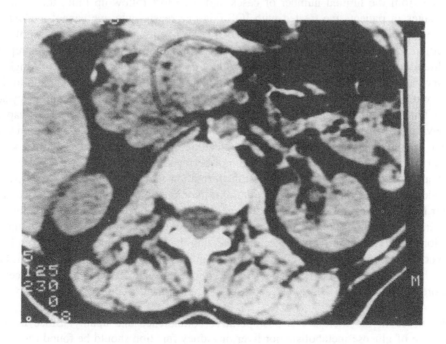

FIGURE 9.   Pancreatic carcinoma prior to IORT.

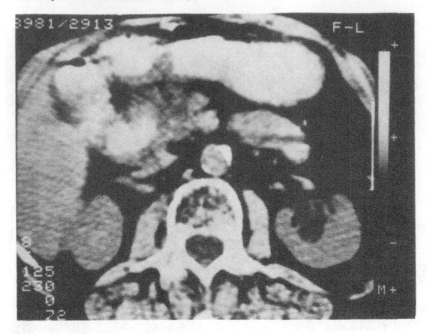

FIGURE 10.   Good local control: 1 year after IORT, no tumor growth can be seen. The tumor seems smaller and differs in morphology.

Aside from the limited number of cases and the short follow-up time, the variety of tumor stages in patients we treated with IORT is one reason why we cannot evaluate the influence of IORT on survival (median survival of 6 months in the palliative group).

Median survival time for patients after IORT and palliative surgical measures reported in the literature is 16.5 months, the longest follow-up being 41 months. A clearly higher 1-year survival rate exists in patients with radical operation and IORT in comparison to those who were only resected. However, the rates of the two groups coincide again after 1 year.[12]

It is not difficult to judge the general and focal tissue effects of IORT nor its capacity for relieving pain. Apparently wound healing is not disturbed. The only complication which required operative revision was secondary bleeding in an area of detached mesocolon. However, this is a surgical problem and cannot be regarded as a result of irradiation. One case of anastomosis insufficiency and fistula formation was observed out of four patients who underwent tumor or tumor bed irradiation in conjunction with Whipple's procedure.

Our low complication rates and the absence of perioperative deaths are compatible with reports in the literature. On the other hand, the cases of obstructive duodenitis and duodenal ulcerations demonstrate the importance of protecting the stomach and intestines from IORT. However, this is not always possible with tumors in close proximity to the duodenum. Other authors have also observed isolated cases of duodenal stenosis and bleeding ulcers.[8,20] Therefore, we consider it absolutely necessary to perform gastroenterostomy as part of the primary operation.

Not noted in the literature is postoperative somnolence and apathy. Since neither a disturbance of glucose metabolism nor liver or kidney function should be found responsible for these occurrences, we consider them a result of the radiation therapy.

With regard to influencing the severe back pain often associated with advanced forms of pancreatic cancer, we see IORT as an enhancement of our treatment possibilities. We can count on freedom from pain or distinct improvement in same in 70 to 80% of the cases.

Regarding tumor stage, modes of treatment, and our experiences with IORT of pancreatic cancers, we consider our results comparable to those of other centers using this method and are encouraged by the low mortality rate resulting from this therapy.

VIII. FUTURE PLANS

In our opinion, the clinical applicability and good tolerance of IORT has been sufficiently tested and proven. It is necessary at this time to investigate the influence of IORT on pain reduction and life expectancy by means of prospective randomized studies. We proposed such a trial at the IORT symposium at the Medical College of Ohio.

We plan to include primarily unresectable rectal cancers in our IORT program.[13] Following preoperative radiation (45 to 50 Gy), IORT is applied during resection.*

Experience in other centers lead us to expect positive results, especially in preventing local recurrence.[13]

We are proud to be able to host the IORT symposium for 1988 in Innsbruck. In the meantime, further experience (including that of centers in Germany now beginning with IORT) will increase our knowledge of this method. We are confident that our symposium will uphold the high scientific standard presented at the First International Meeting in Toledo at the Medical College of Ohio.

REFERENCES

1. **Oesterreichische Krebsstatistik,** Statistische Nachrichten, *Heft,* 3, 172, 1984.
2. **Moossa, A. R.,** Pancreatic cancer. Approach to diagnosis selection for surgery and choice of operation, *Cancer,* 50, 2689, 1982.
3. **Tepper, J., Nardi, G., and Suit, H.,** Carcinoma of the pancreas-review of MGH experience from 1963—1973. Analysis of surgical failure and implications for radiation therapy, *Cancer,* 37, 1519, 1976.
4. **Herter, F. P., Cooperman, A. M., Ahlborn, T. N., and Antinori, C.,** Surgical experience with pancreatic and periampullary cancer, *Ann. Surg.,* 195, 274, 1982.
5. **Levin, P. L., Counelly, R. R., and DeVesa, S. S.,** Demographic characteristics of cancer of the pancreas: Mortality, incidence and surgical, *Cancer,* 47, 1456, 1981.
6. **Shipley, W. U., Wood, W. C., Tepper, J. E., Warshaw, A. L., Orlow, E. L. et al.,** Intraoperative electron beam irradiation for patients with unresectable pancreatic carcinoma, *Ann. Surg.,* 200, 289, 1984.
7. **Tepper, J. and Sindelar, W.,** Summary on intraoperative radiation therapy, *Cancer Treat. Rep.,* 65, 911, 1981.
8. **Wood, W. C., Shipley, W. U., Gunderson, L. L., Cohen, A. M., and Nardi, G. L.,** Intraoperative irradiation for unresectable pancreatic carcinoma, *Cancer,* 49, 1272, 1985.
9. **Abe, M. and Takahashi, M.,** Intraoperative radiotherapy: the Japanese experience, *Int. J. Radiat. Oncol. Biol. Phys.,* 7, 863, 1981.
10. **Goldson, A. L., Ashaveri, E., Espinoza, M., Roux, V., Cornwell, E. et al.,** Single high dose intraoperative electrons for advanced stage pancreatic cancer: Phase I pilot study, *Int. J. Radiat. Oncol. Biol. Phys.,* 7, 869, 1981.
11. **Nishimura, A., Nakano, M., Otsu, H., Nakano, K., Iida, K. et al.,** Intraoperative radiotherapy for advanced carcinoma of the pancreas, *Cancer,* 54, 2375, 1984.
12. **Hiraoka, T., Watanabe, E., Mochinaga, M., Tashiro, S., Miyauchi, Y. et al.,** Intraoperative irradiation combined with radical resection for cancer of the head of the pancreas, *World J. Surg.,* 8, 766, 1984.
13. **Tepper, J., Cohen, A. M., Wood, W. C., Hedberg, S. E., and Orhow, E.,** Intraoperative electron beam radiotherapy in the treatment of unresectable rectal cancer, *Arch. Surg.,* 121, 421, 1986.
14. **Aufschnaiter, M.,** Sonographische Kriterien zur Therapiewahl bei malignen Pankreastumoren, *Zentralbl. Chir.,* 108, 979, 1983.
15. **Bodner, E. and Lederer, B.,** Intraoperative fine needle biopsy with tumors of the pancreas and the periampullary region, *J. Abdom. Surg.,* 18, 194, 1976.
16. **Burlefinger, R., Voeth, C., Ottenjann, R., and Kutane, H.,** Implantationsmetastase nach Feinnadelpunktion eines Pankreascarcinomas, *Leber Magen Darm,* 15, (5), 217, 1985.
17. **Caturelli, E., Rapaccini, G. L., Anti, M., Fabiano, A., and Federli, G.,** Malignant seedings after fine-needle aspiration biopsy of the pancreas, *Diagn. Imag. Clin. Med.,* 54, 88, 1985.

* Our first IORT rectal cancer patient was treated while preparing this chapter.

18. **Smith, I. E., Courienay, V. D., Mills, J., and Peckham, M. J.,** *In vitro* radiation response of cells from four human tumours propagated in immune-suppressed mice, *Cancer Res.,* 38, 390, 1978.

19. **Sindelar, W. F., Kinsella, T., Tepper, J., Travis, E. L. Rosenberg, S. A., and Glatstein, E.,** Experimental and clinical studies with intraoperative radiotherapy, *Surg. Gynecol. Obstet.,* 157, 205, 1983.

20. **Gunderson, L. L., Shipley, W. U., Suit, H. D., Epp, E. R., Nardi, G. et al.,** Intraoperative irradiation: a pilot study combining external beam photons with "boost" dose intraoperative electrons, *Cancer,* 49, 2259, 1982.

21. **Gunderson, L. L., Tepper, J. E., Biggs, P. J., Goldson, A., Martin, J. K., McCullough, E. C., Rich, T. A., Shipley, W. U., Sindelar, W. F., and Wood, W. C.,** Intraoperative and/or external beam irradiation *Curr. Probl. Cancer,* VII (11), 1983.

22. **Fortner, J. G.,** Regional pancreatectomy for cancer of the pancreas, ampulla, and other related sites, *Ann. Surg.,* 199, 418, 1984.

Chapter 31

INTRAOPERATIVE RADIATION THERAPY IN SPAIN: CLINICAL EXPERIENCES AT THE UNIVERSITY CLINIC OF NAVARRA

Felipe A. Calvo, Luis Escude, and Carlos Dy

TABLE OF CONTENTS

I. INTRODUCTION

The International Symposium on Intraoperative Radiation Therapy (IORT), (Toledo, OH)[1] emphasized the enthusiasm for the application of this treatment to a variety of tumor types and anatomic locations. The effort, in our institution, has been primarily directed toward the following general objectives:

1. Feasibility of IORT as a combined treatment
2. Exploration of the utility of IORT in tumors of different anatomic areas
3. Assessment of patient tolerance and treatment toxicity
4. Integration of IORT into multidisciplinary treatment protocols

An analysis of 96 patients treated for a variety of tumor types and locations during the period from September 1984 to May 1986 is reported. All treatments were performed at the Clinic of the University of Navarra (CUN) in Pamplona, Spain, utilizing a Siemens® Mevatron 77 linear accelerator (electron energies — 6, 9, 12, 15, 18, or 20 meV). Computed tomography (CT)-assisted computerized dosimetry was modified and used for IORT treatment planning. The technical details of the IORT applicators, patient transportation, and the preliminary physics data has been previously published.[2]

This report will describe the preliminary information obtained in the sites shown in Table 1. The results will be assessed in terms of control within the treated volume (local control), preliminary follow-up data, and complications.

II. CLINICAL EXPERIENCE IN VARIOUS TUMOR TYPES AND LOCATIONS

A. INTRACRANIAL TUMORS

Several reports[3-6] have described IORT in supratentorial malignant tumors. The important principles appear to be the potential for accurate delineation of residual malignant disease during the surgical procedure and the potential for delivering high-dose electron beam therapy to tumor tissue following removal of major hypoxic areas.

Technically, intracranial IORT was most often accomplished utilizing 5- to 9-cm-diameter treatment applicators. Bolus was necessary in the surgical cavity following tissue removal. Depending upon the depth of the tumor, the electron beam energies were in the range of 12 to 20 meV. A preoperative CT scan of the brain is imperative for proper treatment planning and for anticipating the beam direction.

Goldson, et al.[3] suggested 15 Gy as a safe dose of IORT in brain neoplasms. The treatment protocol activated at CUN combined maximal possible tumor resection, IORT (15 Gy), and external beam radiation therapy (50 Gy in 5 weeks), whole brain in *de novo* patients. In two patients, the external beam radiation therapy component of the program was combined with weekly intracarotid infusion of cisplatinum as a radiosensitizer. Patients whose disease had recurred after previous definitive brain irradiation were treated to a dose of 20 Gy only by IORT without subsequent external beam irradiation. A total of eight patients have been analyzed. The patient characteristics are shown in Table 2. Malignant glioma comprises the predominant histology. At the time of this analysis, the median follow-up time (MFT) was approximately 12 months. Six of the eight patients are still alive at 11+, 12+, 13+, 14+, and 15+ months following IORT. Two patients died with tumor progression at 7 and 10 months following IORT.

None of the patients developed febrile episodes in the postoperative, post-IORT period. However, one patient who had recurrence of glioblastoma multiforme after radical external beam radiation therapy and chemotherapy and who was retreated by partial tumor resection

TABLE 1
Major Sites of Tumors Treated by IORT in
96 Patients

Tumor location	Number of patients
Intracranial	8
Head and neck	8
Intrathoracic	9
Upper abdominal	32
Pelvic	18
Bone and soft tissues	21

TABLE 2
Characteristics of Patients with Intracranial
Primary Neoplasms Undergoing IORT

Characteristics	Number of patients
Age	
>40	3
<40	5
Sex	
Male	2
Female	6
Karnofsky score	
>60	7
<60	1
Tumor location	
Fronto-temporal	2
Parietal	5
Optic nerve	1
Histology	
Glioblastoma multiforme	2
Anaplastic astrocytoma	3
Neuroblastoma	1
Low-grade glioma	1
Previous radiotherapy	
Yes	3
No	5
Type of surgery (IORT)	
Partial resection	8

and IORT (20 Gy) developed acute cerebral edema within 48 h following surgery and IORT. A postoperative CT scan of the brain revealed massive edema in the surgically manipulated area and within the IORT volume. The clinical and radiological picture was reversed within 1 week on intensive antiedema therapy. An evident tumor response was documented in this patient lasting for 10 months.

The preliminary results suggest that IORT for intracranial malignant neoplasma is feasible, well tolerated, and may produce long-term survivors, especially when combined with adequate surgery and external beam radiation therapy. The risk of infection does not appear, from this data, to be a major barrier to the use of IORT for intracranial malignant primary disease. Retreatment of recurrent disease by surgical resection and IORT may provide significant palliation. Still, careful postoperative examination for edema should be undertaken.

TABLE 3
Characteristics of Patients Treated by
IORT for Recurrent Head and Neck
Cancer

Characteristics	Number of patients
Age	
<40	8
>40	0
Sex	
Male	6
Female	2
Tumor stage	
III/IV	8
Previous therapy	
Surgery	7
Radiotherapy	5
Type of surgery (IORT)	
Complete resection	2
Partial resection	6

B. RECURRENT HEAD AND NECK CANCER

The management of early head and neck cancer is well established. Many excellent centers are now adopting a conservative approach to the management of early-stage disease, utilizing sophisticated external beam and brachytherapy radiation techniques. This is an effort to avoid major surgical procedures and preserve function and cosmesis.[7] Surgery is often reserved for salvage. Advanced-stage disease, however, is often approached with a combination of surgery and radiation therapy.[8] Presently, there is an ongoing investigational effort to determine whether chemotherapy should be sequenced into the multimodal approach to advanced head and neck cancer.

Recurrent disease after radical therapy remains a major challenge for salvage therapy.[9] Depending upon the size and location of the lesion, as well as upon the previous treatment history, surgery and/or interstitial brachytherapy may be employed. If surgery is to be considered, its combination with IORT has a very attractive rationale. Such an approach may better enable critical definition of residual disease (such as the spinal cord), making any toxicity to critical anatomic structures avoidable with the selection of the appropriate electron beam energies. The major head and neck vasculature (carotid artery, jugular vein) cannot be protected from IORT; however, large vessels have been reported to have a high tolerance to single-dose IORT.[10] Unfortunately, there is no adequate information regarding the IORT dose required to control microscopic or macroscopic recurrent head and neck disease. Thus, it is particularly difficult to establish a treatment program for these patients.

Table 3 describes the eight patients who have been treated at the CUN. All patients had advanced-stage disease. Seven patients had previous radical surgery, and four of these had additionl radiation therapy. One patient had recurrent disease following radical radiation therapy alone.

Seven of the eight patients were treated by IORT for neck recurrence. Surgical resection was considered complete in only two of the eight patients.

Six patients received 10 Gy, and the remaining two patients received 20 Gy of IORT. Treatment applicators ranged from 5 to 10 cm in diameter, and the electron energies used varied from 6 to 12 meV. In four of our patients, the surgical area was covered with a vascularized myocutaneous flap and an additional course of external beam radiation therapy was delivered (40 to 50 Gy in 5 weeks).

At the time of present analysis, the MFT is 8 months. Four patients remain alive with follow-up at 4 + , 6 + , 8 + , and 12 + months following IORT. Two patients died of distant metastatic disease with the local area being controlled, and the remaining two patients died from locally recurring disease.

The sole complication observed in this group of patients was the development of a pharyngostoma in an area partially including the treated volume. This fistula resolved with conservative management in 4 months.

The above data are a collection of patients considered for individualized therapy programs in an effort to provide effective salvage therapy for recurrent disease. IORT remains attractive as a potential salvage or palliative modality combined with surgery. It is anticipated that many patients could become candidates for such a program, facilitating systematic trials. It is still premature to consider using IORT as an integrated part of a primary therapeutic regimen. However, its use in recurrent head and neck cancer appears well tolerated with a few short-term complications.

It is of interest to note that both patients dying with local recurrence after IORT did not have excision of the skin adjacent to the tumor site removed. We hypothesize the potential for residual tumor in the dermal or subdermal structures as the most likely cause of this local failure and are encouraging wider skin excision and the use of skin flaps to avoid this potential type of failure.

C. INTRATHORACIC TUMORS

The tolerance of normal mediastinal structures to IORT has been studied in animals. Doses of 10 to 20 Gy appear to have acceptable acute and chronic toxicity.[11] However, caution is advised in treating the bronchial suture line following pneumonectomy.[12] Some early clinical information is available regarding IORT used for intrathoracic tumors,[13] but the lack of any recent literature would appear to indicate that this effort might have been abandoned.

Tumor size and location are important parameters for determining resectability in non-small-cell carcinoma of the lung. Central lesions with involvement of hiliar and/or mediastinal structures are difficult to control surgically.[14] Radical external beam radiation therapy has produced some long-term survivors, but often at the price of significant respiratory compromise. IORT may offer a less toxic alternative in the multidisciplinary treatment of lung cancer. The areas of tumor involvement can be easily defined at surgery; the mediastinum and chest wall can be treated by IORT fields, and normal structures can be protected, if desireable, with lead shielding.

At the CUN, all patient candidates for IORT were subjected to lateral thoracotomy; the exact level of the incision depended upon tumor location. The incision was in the third and fourth intercostal space for upper lobe lesions and in the fifth intercostal space for hiliar and lower lobe lesions. Treatment applicators ranged from 5 to 12 cm in diameter. The electron energies used varied from 6 to 20 meV. Left-sided tumors were more difficult to treat due to the continuous pulsations of the heart. The CUN protocol consisted of surgical resection, if technically possible, and 10 Gy IORT to positive nodal sites, the tumor, and/or areas of suspected residual disease such as the chest wall. This was subsequently followed by external beam radiation therapy (46 Gy in 5 weeks).

To date, nine patients with primary intrathoracic malignant disease have been treated. These patients are reviewed in Table 4. All the patients were male. Five of the patients had no attempt at surgical extirpation of their disease. The histologies varied as shown in Table 4. IORT was directed at the primary lesions in these patients. In the remaining four patients, in whom surgical extirpation of the primary site was attempted, IORT was used to treat the mediastinal nodes.

The MFT was 6 months. In this small group there were two postoperative deaths: the one patient undergoing pneumonectomy subsequently developed a bronchopleural fistula

TABLE 4
Characteristics of Lung Cancer Patients
Treated by IORT

Characteristics	Number of patients
Age (range 44—62 years)	
Sex	
Male	9
Female	0
Karnofsky score	
>60	7
<60	2
Tumor location	
Left hiliar mass	4
Right hiliar mass	1
Mediastinal	2
Pleural and chestwall	2
Histology	
Squamous cell CA	3
Adenocarcinoma	1
Small cell CA	1
Mixed cell CA	2
Mesothelioma	2
Type of surgery	
Pneumonectomy	1
Lobectomy	3
Tumor exposure	5

(the bronchial stump sutures may have received 1 Gy at most); the second died with uncontrolled fungal pneumonia (confirmed by autopsy). The additional patients died with disseminated disease and questions of local recurrence. Thus, four of the seven evaluable patients achieved local control. These patients have survived, at the time of this analysis, 6 + , 7 + , 18 + , and 20 + months. Three of these patients, including the two with the longest survivals, had no effort made to resect their tumor. These patients show radiologic evidence of fibrosis in the area treated by combined IORT and external beam radiation therapy.

An interesting observation was the development of acute pneumonitis 2 to 3 weeks following IORT in patients treated through normal pulmonary parenchyma for unresectable disease. This was observed in asymtomatic patients, and the radiographs clearly defined the volume included in the IORT treatment. This pneumonitis resolved without specific therapy. Two of our patients developed mild esophagitis during the external beam component of their radiation therapy.

Our experience would suggest that IORT should be considered in a multimodal approach to the therapy of non-small-cell lung cancer. It appears well tolerated, especially if the bronchial stump is avoided in patients undergoing pneumonectomy. The fact that our two longest survivors did not have their primary lung lesions resected at surgery is certainly of preliminary encouragement. It must be recognized that long-term fibrosis will occur in lung treated by IORT and external beam radiation therapy.

D. GASTRIC CANCER

Remarkable information relative to the rationale and results of IORT in gastric cancer have been reported by Abe et al.[15,16] At CUN we have treated 13 patients with this diagnosis with IORT. Our treatment has always been directed to the celiac axis and nodal area delivering 15 Gy. Technical factors of the therapy include electron energies ranging from 9 to 12 meV and applicator sizes from 6 to 10 cm in diameter. IORT is followed by external beam

TABLE 5
Characteristics of Patients with Gastric Carcinoma Treated by IORT

Characteristics	Number of patients
Age (range 34—82 years)	
Sex	
Male	10
Female	3
Karnofsky score	
>60	11
<60	2
Tumor stage	
T_{1-2}	2
T_{3-4}	11
N_0	3
N_+	10
Type of surgery	
Partial gastrectomy	4
Total gastrectomy	9

radiation therapy (46 Gy in 5 weeks) to a volume covering the tumor bed and the draining nodal area.

The characteristics of this group of patients are given in Table 5. It is evident that the vast majority of our patients had advanced-stage primary disease and also positive celiac nodes. Most of these patients underwent total gastrectomy.

At the time of this analysis, the MFT was 9 months. Follow-up shows 11 of 12 patients alive. One patient died from hepatic metastases, but had apparent local celiac axis control. The single patient who did not achieve local control had N_3 nodal disease pretreatment. This patient remains alive on 5-fluorouracil and cisplatinum 5-days infusion chemotherapy.

Celiac axis IORT appears to be well tolerated. Only a single toxicity was observed, that being fibrosis of the celiac axis with the development of associated liver hemangiomas, simulating liver metastasis.

E. PANCREATIC CANCER

Pancreatic cancer, along with gastric cancer and rectosigmoid recurrences, has provided the major impetus for IORT.[17-19] The rationale for IORT in pancreatic cancer has been written about extensively.[20-22]

The patients with pancreatic cancer treated at the CUN have all received 20 Gy IORT, followed by external beam radiation therapy via a four-field technique utilizing CT scan-aided treatment planning. The IORT technical factors have included electron energies ranging from 18 to 20 meV delivered through applicators of 6 to 10 cm diameters (Figure 1). Careful attention should be paid to the location of the duodenum in relation to the tumor mass. Surgical diversion of the biliary tree and gastroenteric anastomosis was performed.

Table 6 clearly presents the characteristics of the patients, and, as expected, it was unlikely that any major surgical excision was attempted. At the CUN, IORT is delivered prior to major diverting surgery. Of interest is the fact that two of three of our cases were in the head of the pancreas, and two of these cases partially involved the duodenum. Moreover, all of our cases were of large-size primary lesions (>6 cm), which can be considered at the worst end of an already poor prognosis.

The MFT was 7 months at the time of this analysis. Six patients are alive, most at early times after IORT, but we have one survivor at 18 + months. Of the three patients who have died, two died with hepatic metastases. The other patient who died was the only one to

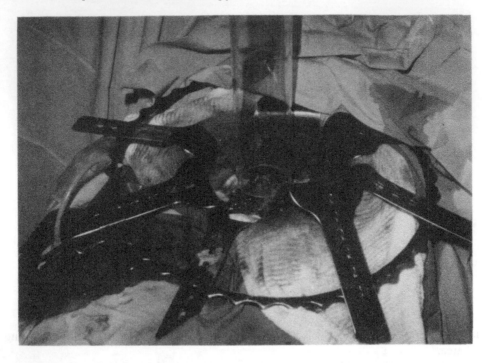

FIGURE 1.   IORT for an unresectable pancreatic cancer. The tumor mass is exposed to the treatment applicator and other intra-abdominal structures are mobilized from the treatment field.

TABLE 6
Characteristics of Patients with Pancreatic
Cancer Treated by IORT

Characteristics	Number of patients
Age (range 54—69 years)	
Sex	
Male	4
Female	5
Karnofsky score	
>60	4
<60	5
Tumor location	
Head (2 cases partially included duodenum)	6
Body	2
Tail	1
Additional liver metastases	2
Tumor size	
>6 cm	9
<6 cm	0
Type of surgery	
Pancreatectomy	1
Tumor exposure	8

undergo surgical removal of the tumor. This was attempted by total pancreatectomy. The patient died postoperatively following dehiscences of the esophagojejunal anastomosis (outside of the IORT field as assessed at autopsy).

Seven patients had pretreatment complaints of significant pain, and all of these exhibited major reduction or disappearance of the pain within 48 h of IORT.

TABLE 7
Characteristics of Patients with
Miscellaneous Extrapelvic Retroperitoneal
Tumors Treated by IORT

Characteristics	Number of patients
Age (range 3—77 years)	
Sex	
Male	5
Female	5
Karnofsky score	
>60	7
<60	3
Tumor location	
Retroperitoneum	3
Lumbar fossa	7
Histology	
Soft tissue sarcomas	3
Wilm's tumor	2
Neuroblastoma	2
Pheochromocytoma	1
Renal cell carcinoma	2

We observed one severe toxicity in this group of patients. One patient, in whom the duodenum was in the IORT field, developed upper gastrointestinal bleeding 4 months after treatment. This responded to conservative therapy.

For pancreatic cancer, IORT plus external beam radiation therapy appears to be well tolerated. Long-term survival appears possible, even in a group of patients with lesions larger than 6 cm. Rapid and effective palliation of pain was constantly observed.

F. MISCELLANEOUS NEOPLASMS OF THE UPPER ABDOMEN

A mixed group of ten patients with malignant extrapelvic retroperitoneal disease was analyzed. Table 7 describes these patients. This group of patients included all the pediatric cases treated with IORT except for those children with sarcoma of the bone and those with sarcoma of the pelvic bones. These children comprise those cases of Wilm's tumor, neuroblastoma, and pheochromocytoma, shown in the table. Treatment consisted of surgical resection and IORT (10 Gy) to the tumor bed area. Electron beam energies ranged from 6 to 9 meV, and treatment applicators from 6 to 9 cm in diameter.

Although there is no way of providing even preliminary survival data on such an heterogenous group of patients, it can be said that treatment was well tolerated. This is extremely important in pediatric patients, where the role for radiation therapy is being minimized for fear of late toxicities.[23] Theoretically, IORT with its major advantage of sparing the normal tissues outside of the critical treatment volume, in contrast with external beam techniques which must deliver a dose to superimposed structures outside of the critical treatment volume, may prove that a continuing effort should be made to assess the potential for IORT in pediatric oncology,[24] especially in these difficult-to-treat tumors of the extrapelvic retroperitoneum.

G. RECURRENT RECTOSIGMOID CARCINOMA

The rationale and results of IORT for recurrent rectosigmoid lesions has been established with the pioneering experience of the Massachusetts General Hospital group.[25,26]

At CUN, the following protocol is used for previously unirradiated patients. All patients receive 46 Gy in 5 weeks by external beam, utilizing three- or four-field techniques. This is followed in 4 to 6 weeks by surgical resection and IORT (10 to 20 Gy). Two patients

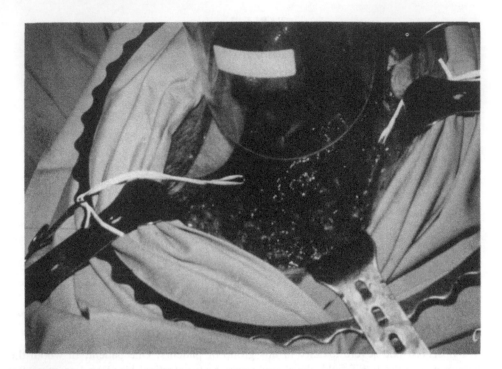

FIGURE 2.   Pelvic area exposed for IORT of a presacral recurrence of rectosigmoid carcinoma. A beveled applicator is moved into the pelvic area, while ureters and other structures are mobilized out of the IORT field.

have been treated in this manner. Our previous protocol utilized postoperative and post-IORT external beam therapy (46 Gy in 5 weeks). However, at the time of surgery it was noted that recurrence was extremely difficult to remove. Changing the external beam component to precede surgery and IORT has impressed the surgeons by making the surgical resection often easier. In the unusual case we treated who had previously been irradiated prior to recurrence, 30 Gy IORT was delivered at the time of surgery as the sole radiation therapy. Technical factors include electron energies of 9 to 12 meV and treatment applicators of 6 to 10 cm diameter. Anterior abdominal or transperitoneal approaches were used depending upon the tumor location. Beveled applicators were most useful in the pelvic area (Figure 2).

The characteristics of the 11 patients treated are given in Table 8. The majority of the patients had presacral relapses, and three of our patients had known hepatic metastases at the time of pelvic recurrence.

These patients have been followed now with an MFT of 8 months. Two of the three patients with liver metastases prior to treatment have died: one showing local control of the pelvic disease, one with pelvic progression. The third patient to have died had a presumably unrelated pulmonary embolus and died with his pelvic disease in control. Of the remaining eight patients, three have failed locally, including the single patient who had no attempt at tumor resection. Of these five remaining patients, four have no evidence of disease at 2+, 3+, 7+, and 8 + months after IORT. One patient's lesion remains questionable. Thus, local control was achieved in 7 of 11 patients.

Of the 11 patients, 4 had infection of the abdominoperineal resection wound. These slowly healed with antibiotic therapy and are thought to be surgical rather than radiation complications. Four patients developed a pain syndrome beginning about 1 month after IORT and spontaneously resolving by 5 to 6 months after the onset. They were refractory to antinflammatory analgesics.

TABLE 8
Characteristics of Patients Treated for
Recurrent Rectosigmoid Carcinoma by IORT

Characteristics	Number of patients
Age (range 24—80 years)	
Sex	
Male	8
Female	3
Karnofsky score	
>60	6
<60	5
Site of relapse	
Presacral	9
Pelvic walls	2
Additional liver metastases	3
Type of surgery	
Complete resection	3
Partial resection	7
Tumor exposure	1

H. ADVANCED BLADDER CANCER

Preliminary information has suggested that IORT is an attractive modality for the treatment of bladder cancer.[27-29] An integrated approach for the management of advanced bladder carcinoma at the CUN was developed; we integrated IORT into the surgical and radiotherapeutic sequence. The patient is initially taken to surgery for ureteroileal diversion and lymph node dissection, at which time 15 Gy IORT is administered. This is subsequently followed by external beam radiation therapy (46 Gy in 5 weeks). After an appropriate rest interval, definitive radical cystectomy is performed and the excised specimen is then carefully studied in the pathology laboratory.

Technical details in IORT included the use of electron energies in the range of 9 to 12 meV; treatment applicators varied between 5 to 8 cm in diameter. The bladder was filled with water and placed within the applicator. The rectum can be protected with lead. Pelvic areas with macroscopic fixed nodes were treated with IORT at the same time.

Table 9 defines the patient population. All the patients treated were male. All had advanced primary disease (T_3 or T_4) and six of seven had positive nodes prior to IORT. One of the seven patients had bone metastases at time of diagnosis and had no further therapy after his external beam treatment (15 Gy IORT plus 46 Gy external beam therapy).

The MFT was 6 months. Four patients remain alive with no evidence of diseae at 5^+, 5^+, 7^+, and 9^+ months after therapy. One patient died 2 d postoperatively of a cerebral infarct. Two other patients have died with extra pelvic progression, including the patient with bone metastases at diagnosis. Local control of the bladder disease was achieved in six of seven cases. Most interesting to note is the six patients undergoing cystectomy after IORT and 46 Gy external beam radiation therapy; five of their six surgical specimens contained no evidence of tumor on pathologic examination ($_pT_0$).

Although more patients are required before any recommendations can be made, it is certainly interesting to speculate that IORT and subsequent external beam radiation therapy, as delivered at the CUN, may alleviate the need for subsequent radical cystectomy in a proportion of patients.

I. BONE AND SOFT TISSUE SARCOMAS

An attempt to integrate IORT into the multimodal management of patients with bone and soft tissue sarcomas has been piloted. In general, at the time of surgery, we have treated the tumor bed with IORT delivering 10 to 20 Gy.

TABLE 9
Characteristics of Patients with Advanced
Transitional Cell Carcinoma of the Bladder
Treated by IORT

Characteristics	Number of patients
Age (range 54—63 years)	
Sex	
Male	7
Female	0
Karnofsky score	
>60	5
<60	2
Tumor stage	
T_3	3
T_4	4
N_0	6
N_+	1
Distant metastasis (bone)	1

Osteosarcoma has been successfully managed at the CUN because of the close cooperation of the Pediatric Oncology, Medical Oncology, and Orthopaedic Surgery Departments, using a multidisciplinary program that includes preoperative intra-arterial cisplatinum, "en block" surgical resection, and prosthesis implantation, followed by systemic alternating adjuvant chemotherapy.[30] IORT of 20 Gy to the tumor bed was recently incorporated in the program with no additional radiation therapy (Figure 3).

IORT of 20 Gy in Ewing sarcoma was initially explored to treat the tumor bed of recurrent local disease during bone salvage surgery. Recently it has been integrated into the treatment of new cases in which surgery was considered a part of the multidisciplinary approach. In this situation, 10 Gy IORT is delivered to the tumor bed area, followed with 40 to 50 Gy in 4 to 5 weeks external beam radiation therapy. The first case treated at the CUN (September 1984) was an 18-year-old male with Ewing sarcoma involving the 12th dorsal vertebrae. He presented with paraplegia and was treated with surgical fixation of the dorso-lumbar vertebras, laminectomy, curettage of the soft tissue mass and vertebral body, IORT of 10 Gy (with lead protection of the spinal cord), postoperative external beam radiation therapy 40 Gy in 4 weeks, and systemic adjuvant chemotherapy. The patient remains alive, free of disease, and able to walk.

IORT was initially employed for the treatment of central location soft-tissue sarcomas (neck, chest wall, etc.), and, after assessing feasibility and tolerance, the modality was moved to the integrated radical treatment of sarcoma of the extremities. The program includes maximal tumor resection, IORT of 10 to 20 Gy to the tumor bed, and postoperative radiation therapy (40 to 50 Gy in 4 to 5 weeks).

Table 10 summarizes the characteristics of the 21 patients we have treated. Of most interest is that almost half of our treated patients had primary disease sites in the extremities, but the rest had central tumor locations.

The MFT was 10 months in this group. Seven patients have died, five of which with distant metastases without local recurrence. One patient died with local failure and distant metastatic disease. The remaining patient died postoperatively of an arterial anastomosis rupture, demonstrated at autopsy to be outside of the IORT field. Of the 21 patients, 2 are alive with locally recurrent disease. Thus, 18 of 21 patients achieved local control.

Two patients developed treatment toxicity. Three patients exhibited delayed wound healing. Another patient developed a skin recall reaction with subsequent administration of high-dose methotrexate. This recall phenomenon did not prevent completion of the adjuvant chemotherapy.

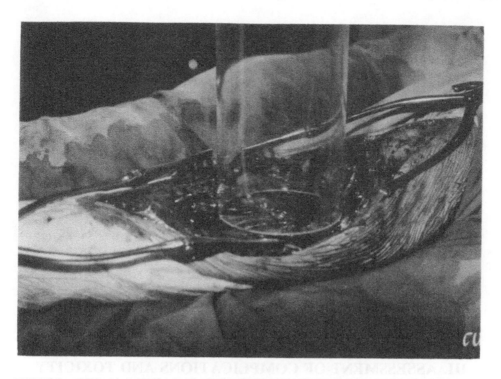

FIGURE 3.   IORT of the tumor bed of a resected osteosarcoma of the tibia before prosthesis implantation.

TABLE 10
Characteristics of Patients with Bone or Soft
Tissue Sarcomas Treated by IORT

Characteristics	Number of patients
Age (range 4—55 years)	
Sex	
Male	9
Female	12
Karnofsky score	
>60	17
<60	4
Tumor location	
Extremities	10
Central	11
Histology	
Soft tissue sarcoma	11
Osteogenic sarcoma	5
Ewing's sarcoma	5
Previous treatment	
Surgery	7
Surgery + radiotherapy	5
Surgery + chemotherapy	2
Type of surgery at time of IORT	
Complete resection	10
Partial resection	10
Tumor exposure	1

TABLE 11
Complications in IORT Patients

Surgical complications
  Suture dehiscence
    Gastro-esophageal or gastrojejunal anastomosis (3); out of IORT field
    Arterial anastomosis (1); out of IORT field
    Bronchial stump (1); out of IORT field
  Infections
    Wound infection (9); includes 4 infections in A-P resections
    Postoperative pneumonia (12)
Radiation complications
  Pelvic pain (4)
  Acute pneumonitis (4)
  Delayed healing (3)
  Brain edema (1)
  Recall phenomenon (1)
  Proctitis (1)
  Salivary fistula (1)
  Celiac axis fibrosis (1)
  Upper GI bleeding (1)
  Severe pelvic bleeding during IORT procedure (1)
  Hypotension; compression of inferior vena cava by the treatment applicator (1)

III. ASSESSMENT OF COMPLICATIONS AND TOXICITY

A constellation of IORT-related complications and toxicities have been previously described, including most of the findings in the CUN experience.[31-33] When consideration is given to the potential toxicity of combined modality therapy, it is often difficult to separate complications relative to each component of that therapy. When IORT is considered, it is important to know what complications can be ascribed to that therapy, separate from the surgical intervention. Since the IORT field is so strictly delineated, it is often possible to separate surgical from radiation complications. With this understanding, the summarized results are shown in Table 11. Whenever it has been not possible to separate surgical from radiation complications, the toxic event has been included as a radiation complication.

The data show that surgical complications occur in two clearly defined categories: suture dehiscence (anastomotic sites) and infection. There were 110 patients in all: 5 of 110 anastomotic ruptures, and 21 of 110 infection episodes. Infections were nearly evenly divided between wound infection and postoperative pneumonia.

However, in the case of radiation complications, no such sharp definition is available. There were 18 of 110 patients who developed radiation toxicity. Of these 18 patients, 4 developed pelvic pain syndrome and 4 developed an asymptomatic acute pneumonitis. These toxicities appear self-limiting. The remaining ten instances of complication run the gamut, ranging from a mechanically induced transient hypotension at the time of the treatment IORT application, to severe cerebral edema requiring intensive therapy.

IV. CONCLUSIONS

At the CUN, it has been shown that IORT is certainly feasible as a combined therapeutic modality and can be successfully integrated into multidisciplinary therapeutic protocols. IORT also appears feasible in a variety of anatomic sites and directed against a variety of tumor types, either for recurrent or advanced primary disease. The patients analyzed appeared to have an acceptable tolerance to IORT.

Obviously, the experience with IORT in Spain is young. Further experience and longer patient follow-up with this emerging modality are needed before we can carefully decide where IORT may be applied most effectively. For the present, we will continue to accumulate and follow patients treated by IORT in order to make such conclusions. National (with the IORT program activated at the Instituto Oncologico de San Sebastian and many other groups interested in this modality across the Spanish geography) and international cooperation should be encouraged and expected in the coming years.[34,35]

ACKNOWLEDGMENTS

The authors wish to express their gratitude to all the oncology, surgical, anesthesiology, and nursing staff involved in IORT for the professional excellence to develop this program.

A special acknowledgment to Dr. Arnie E. Markoe for his comments and assistance with this manuscript.

REFERENCES

1. Intraoperative Radiation Therapy, First Int. Symp., Medical College of Ohio, Toledo, May 15 and 16, 1986.
2. **Calvo, F. A. and Escude, L. L.,** Radioterapia intraoperatoria, *Rev. Med. Univ. Navarra,* 29, 110, 1985.
3. **Goldson, A. L., Streeter, O. E., Ashayeri, E., Collier-Manning, J., Barber, J. B., and Fan, K.,** Intraoperative radiotherapy for intracraneal malignancies, *Cancer,* 54, 2807, 1984.
4. **Abe, M., Fukuda, M., and Yamono, K.,** Intraoperative irradiation in abdominal and cerebral tumors, *Acta Radiol.,* 10, 408, 1971.
5. **Matsuda, T.,** Intraoperative Radiotherapy and Confirmation of Radiotherapy with Special Emphasis on the Treatment of Pancreatic Cancer and Glioblastoma, Abstr. 4th Asian Oceanian Congr. of Radiology, 1983, 452.
6. **Matsutani, M., Matsuda, T., and Nagashima, T.,** Surgical treatment and radiation therapy for glioblastoma multiforme with special reference to intraoperative radiotherapy, *Jpn. J. Cancer,* 30, 201, 1984.
7. **Wang, C. C.,** *Radiation Therapy for Head and Neck Neoplasms,* John Wright, Boston, 1983.
8. **Million, R. R., Cassisi, N. J., and Wittes, R. E.,** Cancer in the head and neck, in *Cancer: Principles and Practice of Oncology,* DeVita, V. T., Hellman, S., and Rosenberg, S. A., Eds., J. B. Lippincott Co., Philadelphia, pp 304—386, 1982.
9. **Marcial, V. A., Hanley, J. A., Ydrach, A., and Vallecillo, L. A.,** Surgery after radical radiotherapy of carcinoma of the oropharynx, *Cancer,* 46, 1910, 1980.
10. **Sindelar, W. F., Morrow, B. M., Travis, E. L., Tepper, J., Merkel, A. B., Kranda, K., and Terrill, R.,** Effects of intraoperative electron irradiation in the dog on cell turnover in intact and surgically anastomosed aorta and intestine, *Int. J. Radiat. Oncol. Biol. Phys.,* 9, 523, 1983.
11. **Barnes, M., Pass, H., Tochner, Z., Deluca, A., Terrill, R., Sindelar, W., and Kinsella, T.,** Response of the mediastinal and thoracic viscera of the dog to intraoperative radiation therapy, *Int. J. Radiat. Oncol. Biol. Phys.,* 11 (Suppl. 1), 113, 1985.
12. **Hoekstra, H.,** Personal communication.
13. **Abe, M. and Takahashi, M.,** Intraoperative radiotherapy: the Japanese experience, *Int. J. Radiat. Oncol. Biol. Phys.,* 7, 863, 1981.
14. **Shields, T. W.,** Treatment failures after surgical resection of thoracic tumors, *Cancer Treat. Rep.,* 2, 69, 1983.
15. **Abe, M.,** Intraoperative radiation therapy for gastrointestinal malignancy, in *Clinical Management of Gastrointestinal Cancer,* DeCosse, J. J. and Sherlock, P., Eds., Martinus Nijhoff, Boston, 1984, 327.
16. **Abe, M.,** Intraoperative radiotherapy — past, present and future, *Int. J. Radiat. Oncol. Biol. Phys.,* 10, 1987, 1984.
17. **Abe, M.,** Intraoperative Radiotherapy for Carcinoma of the Stomach and the Pancreas, XVI Int. Congr. of Radiology, Hawaii, July 8 to 12, 1985.
18. **Nishimura, A., Nakano, M., Otsu, H., Nakano, K., Iida, K., Sakata, S., Iwabuchi, K., Maruyama, K., Kihara, M., Takao, O., Todoroki, T., and Iwasaki, Y.,** Intraoperative radiotherapy for advanced carcinoma of the pancreas, *Cancer,* 54, 2375, 1984.

19. **Gunderson, L. L., Shipley, W. U., Suit, H. D., Epp, E. R., Nardi, G., Wood, W., Cohen, A., Nelson, J., Battit, G., Biggs, P. J., Russell, A., Rockett, A., and Clark, D.,** Intraoperative irradiation: a pilot study combining external beam photon with 'boost' dose intraoperative electrons, *Cancer,* 49, 2259, 1982.

20. **Goldson, A. L., Ashaveri, E., Espinoza, M. C., Roux, V., Cornwell, E., Rayford, L., McLaren, M., Nibhanupudy, R., Mahan, A., Taylor, H. F., Hemphil, N., and Pearson, O.,** Single high dose intraoperative electrons for advanced stage pancreatic cancer. Phase I pilot study, *Int. J. Radiat. Oncol. Biol. Phys.,* 7, 869, 1981.

21. **Matsuda, T.,** Radiotherapy for Pancreatic Carcinoma, Combination of Intraoperative Radiotherapy and Conformation Radiotherapy, Department of Radiotherapy, Tokyo Komagome Hospital, presented at the U.S.-Japan Semin., October 2 to 5, 1982.

22. **Wood, W. C., Shipley, W. U., Gunderson, L. L., Cohen, A. M., and Nardi, G. L.,** Intraoperative irradiation for unresectable pancreatic carcinoma, *Cancer,* 49, 1272, 1982.

23. **Teft, M.,** Radiation related toxicities in National Wilm's Tumor Study Number 1, *Int. J. Radiat. Oncol. Biol. Phys.,* 2, 455, 1977.

24. **Kaufman, B. H.,** Intraoperative irradiation: a new technique in pediatric oncology, *J. Pediatric Surg.,* 19, 861, 1984.

25. **Gunderson, L. L., Cohen, W. C., Dosoretz, D. D., Shipley, W. U., Hedberg, S. E., Wood, W. C., Rodkey, G. V., and Suit, H. E.,** Residual, unresectable or recurrent colorectal cancer. External beam irradiation and intraoperative electron beam boost resection, *Int. J. Radiat. Oncol. Biol. Phys.,* 9, 1597, 1983.

26. **Tepper, J. E., Wood, W. C., Cohen, W. C., Shipley, W. U., Hedberg, S. E., Warshaw, A. L., Nardi, G. L., and Biggs, P. J.,** Intraoperative radiation therapy, in *Important Advances in Oncology,* DeVita, V. T., Hellman, S., and Rosenberg, S., Eds., Lippincott, Philadelphia, 1984, 226.

27. **Matsumoto, K., Kakizoe, T., Mikuriya, S., Tanaka, T., Kondo, I., and Umegaki, Y.,** Clinical evaluation of intraoperative radiotherapy for carcinoma of the urinary bladder, *Cancer,* 47, 509, 1981.

28. **Martinez, A. and Gunderson, L. L.,** Intraoperative radiation therapy for bladder cancer, *Urol. Clin. North Am.,* 11, 643, 1984.

29. **Shipley, W. U.,** Radiation therapy in the management of patients with bladder carcinoma, *Int. J. Radiat. Oncol. Biol. Phys.,* 1 (Suppl. 9), 62, 1983.

30. **Sierrasesumaga, L., Martinez, de Negri, J., Calvo, F. A., Dy, C., Gil, A., Cañadell, J., and Villa, I.,** Preoperative Intra-Arterial Cisplatinum, Bone Resection and Functional Prosthesic Implant in Osteosarcoma, in XVII SIOP Meet., Venice, October 1985, 231.

31. **Sindelar, W. F., Kinsella, T. J., Hoekstra, H., Tochner, Z., Smith, R., and Maher, M.,** Duodenal hemorrhage as a complication of IORT for unresectable carcinoma of the pancreas, *Proc. Am. Soc. Clin. Oncol.,* 4, 277, 1985.

32. **Tepper, J. E., Gunderson, L. L., Orlow, Cohen, A. M., Hedberg, S. E., Shipley, W., Blitzer, P. H., and Rich, T.,** Complications of intraoperative radiotherapy, *Int. J. Radiat. Oncol. Biol. Phys.,* 10, 1831, 1984.

33. **Sindelar, W. F., Kinsella, T. J., Hoekstra, H., Schneider, P., Tochner, Z., Maher, M., Smith, R., and Glatstein, E.,** Treatment complications in intraoperative radiotherapy, *Int. J. Radiat. Oncol. Biol. Phys.,* 11 (Suppl. 1), 117, 1985.

34. **Irigaray, J. M.,** Personal communication.

35. **Calvo, F. A., and Hanks, G. E.,** International clinical trials in intraoperative radiation therapy, *Int. J. Radiat. Oncol. Biol. Phys.,* in press.

Chapter 32

THE ECONOMICS OF INTRAOPERATIVE RADIATION THERAPY

Harvey B. Wolkov

TABLE OF CONTENTS

I. INTRODUCTION

Radiation therapy in the U.S. has dramatically progressed since World War II. Major technological advances have included development of the medical linear accelerator, computerized treatment planning, heavy ion therapy, and the use of radiation sensitizers and hyperthermia in conjunction with radiation.

Paralleling the rapid technologic advances in radiation therapy was an upward trend in family income and a major expansion in hospital insurance. Government financing became available for the first time (Hill-Burton Act, 1946) to assist voluntary hospitals; funding from the National Institute of Health increased the budgets of academic health centers, and private sector and government programs financed the rapidly expanding costs of medicine through patient reimbursement.

Congressional approval of Title XVII (Medicare) and Title XIX (Medicaid) provided medical services to a segment of the population which was not under the umbrella of personal or employer-supported insurance.

During the 1970s, society became aware of the steep inflation in health care prices fueled by rising malpractice premiums, improved outlook for professional earnings, and new sources of government and private funding. This resulted in a bold emphasis on cost containment which has changed the major goal of health care from quality of care regardless of cost to a philosophy of cost-controlled care. Recent federal legislative changes in the Medicare and Medicaid programs, specifically the 1982 Tax Equity and Fiscal Responsibility Act (TEFRA) and the Social Security Amendment, have been the catalysts behind cost containment.

Intraoperative radiation therapy (IORT) has developed during the recent era of increasing cost consciousness. If radiation oncologists are to remain fiscally responsible, IORT will require economic evaluation while clinical trials are proceeding.

II. IORT FINANCIAL SURVEY

Two independent surveys were conducted in early 1986 to identify IORT facilities in the U.S. which were either in the final stages of establishing IORT or already had ongoing programs.[1,2] With the aid of the information provided by these surveys, as of March 1986, 33 facilities were identified which could provide financial data for analysis.

In March, 1986, a financial survey was conducted to review the total start-up cost, procedure charges, and reimbursement data for the various IORT programs.[3] Financial data, updated in October 1986, was obtained from 9 dedicated and 23 nondedicated IORT facilities.[4] The survey demonstrated a wide variation in billing charges ranging from no charge to approximately $3000. The average billing charge for 25 institutions which submitted gross revenue data by the various CPT codes is shown in Table 1. The sum of the individual components was approximately $2000. which is consistent with the charge for many other radiation boost techniques (i.e., interstitial implants). The majority of institutions which responded to a reimbursement question on the IORT Financial Survey indicated a current reimbursement rate of 80 to 100% of billed charges.

In most centers, the major cost associated with the establishment of IORT were construction and radiation therapy equipment costs. New construction costs averaged $23,000 for a nondedicated facility and $128,000 for dedicated facilities. The average cost for radiation therapy equipment was $17,000 for nondedicated facilities and $332,000 for dedicated facilities. Median costs were significantly lower for both construction costs and radiation therapy equipment (Figures 1 to 4).

The total start-up costs averaged $57,000 for nondedicated facilities and $466,000 for dedicated facilities (median costs of $20,000 and $200,000, respectively; Figures 5 and 6).

TABLE 1
IORT Financial Survey Gross Revenue

Billing charges	CPT code	Avg. charge ($)
Treatment plan	77263	350
Basic physics	77300	180
Other physics	77370	200
Treatment charge	77499	630
Prof. physician fee	77799	600
Total		1960

The financial survey data probably underestimates the true total cost of establishment of an IORT program owing to hidden costs not appreciated by the radiation oncologists and radiation therapy administrators who completed the questionnaires.

A proforma income statement and a break-even analysis was performed based on the results of the IORT financial survey including equipment cost, equipment and leasehold depreciation, personnel salaries and overtime, and capital cost (Table 2).[3,4,6] The analyses were performed comparing various treatment practices in a nondedicated facility with a dedicated facility which employed either mega- or orthovoltage equipment. Both analyses demonstrated that the economic risk to a radiation therapy department for the development of a nondedicated IORT facility is acceptable, but that the risk is greatly increased for dedicated facilities, depending on the type of equipment purchased and the cost of lease-hold improvements (Tables 3 and 4). It is self evident to the radiation therapist that a dedicated IORT facility is unable to exist without the support of an ongoing organizationally integrated outpatient radiotherapy department in spite of sufficient financial reserves.

A. COST EFFECTIVENESS

Cost effectiveness analysis and cost benefit analysis are common techniques used to identify and quantify the costs of alternate therapeutic means of achieving a given goal. These costs can vary from quantifiable negative costs, such as working time saved by performing a given medical therapy, to economic evaluations which assign a dollar value to life. Well-designed clinical studies reflecting the basic efficacy of IORT have not been conducted prior to dissemination of IORT, and it is therefore not known if IORT can reduce health care cost by replacing more costly therapeutic procedures and what these negative costs may be to society. To establish the true cost effectiveness of IORT, extensive clinical comparison with other modalities will need to be performed. Unfortunately, this approach has many obvious inherent problems.

B. REIMBURSEMENT

Until recently, hospital reimbursement by public and private health insurance under-writers has been based on paying actual costs per day. This approach has provided the financing for increasingly elaborate technologies and hospital services. Hospitals in turn have been able to attract a full range of specialty services, even with duplication of these services in a given area. At the same time, insurance companies have provided financial access to a major portion of the population. Because of the inflationary nature of the reimbursement system, there has been impetus to shift costs to other insurance underwriters. This impetus has created inequities regulating limits on insurance expenditures which in turn have led to a prospective payment system. Currently, hospitals are reimbursed on a per case basis, with payment adjusted for complexity through the Diagnostic-Related Group (DRG) which is also adjusted annually for inflation.

Hospitals continue to have an incentive to encourage admissions through increasing

FINANCIAL SURVEY

New Construction Costs
for
Non-Dedicated IORT Facilities

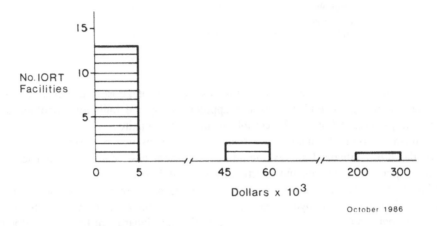

FIGURE 1. IORT Financial Survey — new construction costs — nondedicated facility (16 facilities).

FINANCIAL SURVEY

New Construction Costs
for
Dedicated IORT Facilities

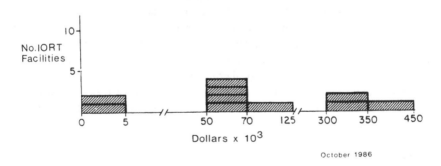

FIGURE 2. IORT Financial Survey — new construction costs — dedicated facility (ten facilities).

public relation techniques, but emphasis will be placed on minimizing the length of hospital stay and the applications of costly technologies provided by the physician and hospital in the inpatient setting. Scant data are available regarding additional costs created by IORT and the resulting impact on reimbursement. Two analyses were conducted in conjunction with the Radiation Oncology Center in Sacramento, CA, to address this question. The first analysis compared average billed charges before the introduction of IORT with IORT procedures for the same DRG category. This analysis suggested the average billed charges for an IORT case significantly exceeded the cost of a non-IORT case. Due to a wide variation of medical acuity within a DRG group, a second analysis was performed to review cases

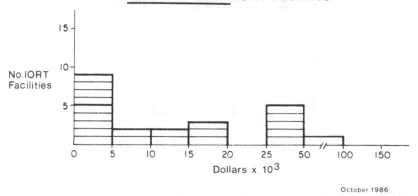

FIGURE 3. IORT Financial Survey — radiation therapy equipment costs — dedicated facility (nine facilities).

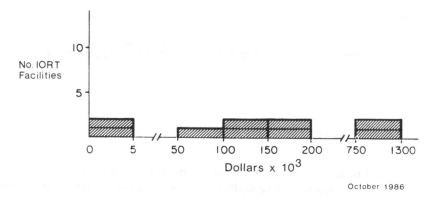

FIGURE 4. IORT Financial Survey — radiation therapy equipment costs — dedicated facility (nine facilities).

of the predominant oncologic surgeon involved in IORT before and after introduction of IORT with cases matched by sex, age, and medical condition, in addition to diagnosis. While not conclusive, this analysis suggested that additional costs associated with IORT were not significant from the standpoint of length of hospital stay, supplies, or other special procedures used.[5,6]

Recently, there has been an increasing share of the marketplace captured by prospective payment systems. These include health maintenance organizations (HMO), which are basically a per capita prospective payment system, and preferred provider organizations (PPO), which represent independent practicing physicians or hospitals that agree to provide care to

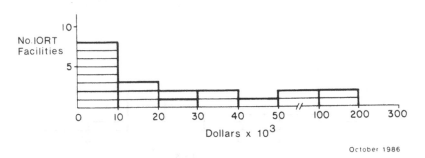

FIGURE 5.   IORT Financial Survey — total start-up costs — nondedicated facility (20 facilities).

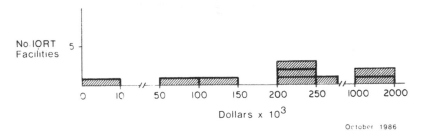

FIGURE 6.   IORT Financial Survey — total start-up costs — dedicated facility (nine facilities).

an insured group at negotiated and often discounted rates. In either scenario, the main focus is one which limits nonmandatory procedures and may eventually limit consultations in efforts to decrease costs. The impact these organizations may have on the application of unproven procedures and treatments is uncertain.

In recent years, there has developed increasing concern regarding the rising costs of medical care, which has led to federal and private sector policies which are changing the health care delivery system in the U.S. Current health care payment systems include the DRG method, contracting for services with insurance companies on a per diem basis, discount per case basis, and by capitation. This will result in increased competition among tertiary providers, which will reduce the profitability of innovative, clinically accepted procedures.

III. CONCLUSION

To date, the true cost effectiveness for IORT has not been determined. If IORT is not

TABLE 2
Considerations: Proforma Income Statement

Direct expenses
   Personnel costs
   Fringe benefits
   Supplies
   Professional services
Indirect expenses
   Facilities costs
   Leasehold improvement depreciation
   Equipment depreciation
   Capital costs
   Lost contribution to overhead[a]

[a] Lost contribution to overhead refers to a nondedicated facility where IORT is performed during the day and routine external beam patients cannot be treated.

TABLE 3
Proforma Income Statement

30 Cases/Year

| | Nondedicated IORT ($) | | Dedicated IORT ($) | |
| | Performed | | Equipment | |
	After hrs.	During hrs.	Ortho (used)	Megavoltage
Net revenue	49,200	49,200	49,200	49,200
Direct expenses	26,729	25,866	24,866	24,866
Indirect expenses	7,787	17,357	28,016	184,444
Total expenses	34,516	42,223	52,882	209,310
Contribution to O/H	14,684	6,977	[3,682]	[160,110]

60 cases/Year

Net revenue	98,400	98,400	98,400	98,400
Direct expenses	53,457	49,731	49,731	49,731
Indirect expenses	9,017	28,157	29,246	185,674
Total expenses	62,474	77,888	78,977	235,405
Contribution to O/H	35,926	20,512	[19,423]	[137,005]

proven to be more efficacious than current state of the art techniques, then funding restrictions may prevent application of IORT in the future. If the procedure is clinically accepted and proven to be more efficacious than current state of the art patient management, then funding will most likely be available, but with decreased profitability per procedure due to competition.

In an era of cost consciousness, it is inevitable that further financial analysis of IORT will be expected of physicians. Discrete measurable indices of both cost and relative efficacy will need to be established to enable fiscally responsible evaluation of this evolving technology.

TABLE 4
IORT Break-Even Analysis

Nondedicated IORT after hours	10 patients/year
Nondedicated IORT during hours	15 patients/year
Dedicated	
Used — orthovoltage	35 patients/year
New — orthovoltage	75 patients/year
Megavoltage	238 patients/year

Note: Nondedicated facility assumes $7000 lease-hold improvement. Dedicated facility (used orthovoltage) assumes $50,000 lease-hold improvement and $50,000 equipment purchase price (new orthovoltage — $250,000 purchase price). Dedicated facility megavoltage assumes $175,000 lease-hold improvement and $750,000 equipment purchase price.

REFERENCES

1. **Hanks, G.,** Personal communication, January, 1986.
2. **Dobelbower, R. R.,** Personal communication, May, 1986.
3. **Wolkov, H.,** The economics of intraoperative radiation therapy, presented at the First Int. Symp. on Intraoperative Radiation Therapy, Medical College of Ohio, Toledo, May 15 to 16, 1986.
4. **Wolkov, H.,** The intraoperative radiation therapy financial survey and its implications, presented at the American Society of Therapeutic Radiology and Oncology, Los Angeles, November, 1986.
5. **Stenberg, S.,** Personal communication, February, 1986.
6. **Wolkov, H., Wright, W., McPeek, C., and Dunlap, K.,** The intraoperative radiation therapy financial survey and its implications, in preparation.

Chapter 33

SYNOPSIS AND FUTURE DIRECTIONS

Ralph R. Dobelbower, Jr.

Intraoperative radiation therapy (IORT) is a rapidly developing treatment modality with ancient roots in the speciality of radiation oncology. As of this writing, it is estimated that less than 3000 patients have been treated with IORT worldwide. Most of these patients have been treated in Japanese IORT centers; however, there are now at least 30 IORT centers in the U.S., and a global proliferation of such facilities is being observed.

As documented in the prior chapters in this work, considerable useful information has been gained over the course of the last 24 years; however, an enormous amount of work remains to be done. There are clear indications that IORT enhances local control of gross, and especially microscopic, disease in various clinical situations. It is hoped that this will translate into improved survival.

It should be noted here that early results have been relatively disappointing for treatment of cancer of the pancreas and retroperitoneal sarcomas — both disease entities for which IORT was initially felt to hold great promise. It is important that clinical investigators not be unduly swayed by such results. A recent report from the Japan National Cancer Center indicates a 1-year survival of 86% for patients with pancreatic cancer treated with external resection, 30 Gy IORT, and local infusion of Mitomycin-C.[1]

Encouraging results have been seen in the adjuvant use of IORT in gastric cancer, initially unresectable rectal cancer, and several other specific disease entities. It must be noted, however, that at present we have not been able to clearly establish indications and contraindications for IORT for most tumor sites and stages of disease. This remains to be accomplished via prospective study. Attempts to collect such data are currently underway in the U.S. under the ageis of the Radiation Therapy Oncology Group (RTOG) that has undertaken five prospective (nonrandomized Phase I and II) studies of cancer of the stomach (Figure 1), bile ducts (Figure 2), pancreas (Figure 3), rectum (Figure 4), uterine cervix (Figure 5), and sarcomas (Figure 6). The survival result of the pancreas study (now terminated) has been disappointing and the cervix study has been closed because of poor accrual. Accrual of patients onto the remaining studies has been disappointedly slow; however, it is expected to improve as the use of IORT becomes more routine and as more facilities with IORT capability come on line.

It is worthy of note that at the present time, little or no clinical information exists regarding the use of IORT for a wide variety of tumors: tumors of the orbit, sinuses, and nasal cavity; mediastinal tumors; tumors of the lung, esophagus, and mediastinum; tumors of the gall bladder and kidney; bone tumors; and pediatric tumors, to list a few. There is a great need for further definition of the tolerance of certain normal tissues to the high single doses employed with IORT. There is a definite need for information regarding the tolerance of normal tissues to IORT when combined with heat, chemotherapy, external beam radiation therapy, and radiation sensitizers. The problems of combining high single doses with conventional fractionated external beam radiation therapy have been outlined by Milligan, Horton, and others in this work. Kiel has assumed an RBE of 2 for IOEBT. It remains to be seen whether such approaches can be justified. The volume factor has been largely ignored to date as regards IORT local toxicity.

The question of safety of transportation of anesthetized patients has been only superficially addressed. Some feel that such practice constitutes an accident waiting to happen that may cast a bad light over the entire practice of IORT. The use of dedicated IORT radiotherapy equipment remains to be fully studied. The role of superficial and orthovoltage

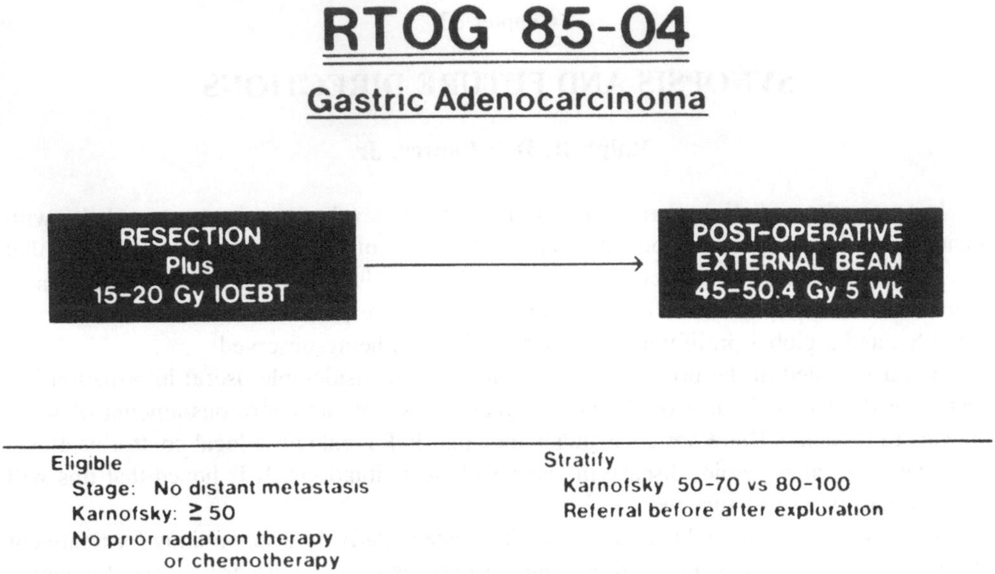

RTOG 85-04

Gastric Adenocarcinoma

RESECTION Plus 15-20 Gy IOEBT	→	POST-OPERATIVE EXTERNAL BEAM 45-50.4 Gy 5 Wk

Eligible
  Stage: No distant metastasis
  Karnofsky: ≥ 50
  No prior radiation therapy
      or chemotherapy

Stratify
  Karnofsky 50-70 vs 80-100
  Referral before after exploration

FIGURE 1.   Schema for RTOG Study 85-04, gastric adenocarcinoma.

RTOG 85-06

Extrahepatic Biliary Cancer

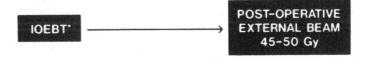

IOEBT*	→	POST-OPERATIVE EXTERNAL BEAM 45-50 Gy

*IOEBT dose 12.5-20 Gy according to extent of disease

Eligible
  Age: 18-80
  Karnofsky: ≥ 70
  Life Expectancy: ≥ 3 Mo
  Serum Creatinine: < 2.0
  Demonstrable left renal function
  No chemotherapy

FIGURE 2.   Schema for RTOG Study 85-06, extrahepatic biliary cancer.

radiation therapy units for use in IORT also deserves further study. The precision with which IORT must be delivered will undoubtedly lead to the development of new IORT devices and improved IORT patient support assemblies. Such developments are now in relatively embryonic phases.

One point has become quite clear: each IORT system must be individually calibrated in conjunction with the machine on which it will be used. One cannot simply purchase an IORT device and commence treatment without detailed careful measurements of beam characteristics, as these will vary from machine to machine and with various applicator sizes and shapes. Radiation oncologists must not be cavalier in these regards

RTOG 85-05

Unresectable Localized Adenocarcinoma Pancreas

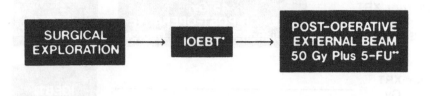

'IOEBT dose 12.5-20 Gy according to extent of disease
''5-FU 500 mg m^2 1st 3 days of post-operative external beam treatment

Eligible
 Age: ≥ 18
 Karnofsky: ≥ 50
 No prior radiation therapy, chemotherapy

FIGURE 3.   Schema for RTOG Study 85-05, unresectable localized adenocarcinoma of the pancreas.

RTOG 85-08

Advanced, Unresectable or Recurrent Rectal Adenocarcinoma

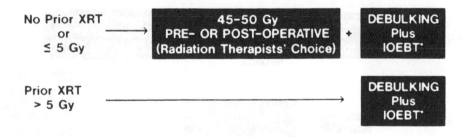

'IOEBT dose 12.5-20 Gy according to extent of disease

Eligible
 Age: 18-75
 Karnofsky: ≥ 60

FIGURE 4.   Schema for RTOG Study 85-08, advanced unresectable or recurrent rectal adenocarcinoma.

Although it is now clear that IORT is a feasible treatment modality that can be employed in both academic and community radiation therapy centers, the experience to date has raised more questions than it has answered. We have just begun to scratch the surface of the body of knowledge regarding the applicability of this modality to the treatment of malignant disease. The remainder of the 20th century is expected to provide a wealth of new IORT data. One hopes that these will be generated by facilities that not only have the technologic

RTOG 85-09

Recurrent Carcinoma Cervix

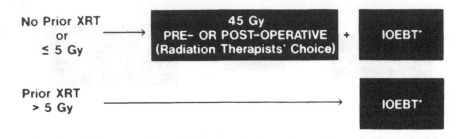

'IOEBT dose 12.5-20 Gy according to extent of disease

Eligible
  Age: 18-75
  Karnofsky: ≥ 50
  No prior radiation therapy, chemotherapy
      or heat within 4 weeks

Stratify
  Karnofsky 50-70 vs 80-100

FIGURE 5.   Schema for RTOG Study 85-09, recurrent carcinoma of uterine cervix.

RTOG 85-07

Localized Retroperitoneal/Intra-Abdominal Sarcomas

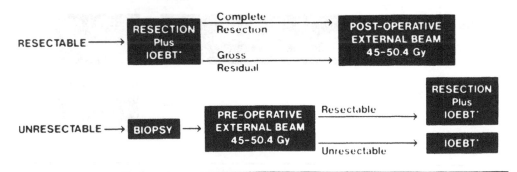

'IOEBT dose 12.5-20 Gy according to extent of disease

Eligible
  Age: ≥16
  Karnofsky: ≥ 60
  No prior radiation therapy,
      chemotherapy

Stratify
  T Stage: 1.2.3
  Grade: 1.2.3
  Residual: none. micro. gross
  External Beam: preoperative. postoperative

FIGURE 6.   Schema for RTOG Study 85-07, localized retroperitoneal intra-abdominal sarcomas.

capacity to embark on an IORT program, but that can also cooperatively collect meaningful data in a prospective fashion and interpret same.

REFERENCE

1. **Ozaki, H., Kinoshita, T., Egawa, S., and Kisi, K.,** Combined treatment for resectable pancreatic carcinoma, in *New Trends in Gastroenterology* Sugahara, K., Ed., Japanese Society of Gastroenterology, Kofu, 1987, 215.

INDEX

A

Abdominal tumors, 6, 385
Accelerated fractionation, 26
Acute brain swelling, 134
Adenocarcinomas, 282, see also Cancer; specific types
   types
  pancreatic, see Pancreatic cancer
  rectal, see Rectal cancer
Administration of IORT, 117
Advantages of IORT, 14—15
Anal cancer, 335, see also Rectal cancer
Anaplastic astrocytoma, 124, 148
Anesthesia, 75—81
  in brain tumors, 140—141, 148
  choice of, 80
  concurrent therapy and, 81
  control of, 81
  equipment for, 15, 78, 251—252
  facilities for support of, 76—79
  in gastric cancer, 167
  in gynecological malignancies, 251—252
  holding area for, 76—77
  logistics of, 81
  management alternatives in, 76
  patient transport during, 80
  remote monitoring area for, 79
  thermal control during, 80—81
  types of, 80
Antineoplastic drugs, see Chemotherapy
Applicator systems, 50—53, 61—62, see also specific types
   specific types
Astrocytomas, 124, 126, 138, 148, 347, 348, see also specific types
   specific types
Austria, 363—375
  complications in, 369—371
  external beam therapy in, 368
  history of IORT in, 6, 364
  methods in, 365—368, 372—374
  pancreatic cancer in, 364
  patient selection in, 365—367
  surgery in, 367
  survival in, 370—371
  tumor morphology in, 372

B

Beam profile, 53—54, 68—70, 108
Betatron, 141
Biliary tract cancer, 4, 12, 307—308, 334—335
Bladder cancer, 3, 96
  brachytherapy for, 230—232
  complications in, 221
  dose in, 218
  electron beams in, 228—230
  indications for IORT in, 222
  intraoperative irradiation techniques in, 218
  location of tumors in, 219
  at Medical College of Ohio Hospital, 349
  number of deaths from, 228

patient selection in, 218—219
  recurrence of, 220, 224, 225
  in Spain, 387, 388
  survival in, 219
  tumor size in, 219
Bleeding, see Hemorrhage
Bone absorption, 109
Bone sarcoma, 387—389
Brachytherapy, 230—232
Brain carcinoma, 124
Brain edema, 134, 347
Brain tumors, 118, 133, see also specific types
  anesthesia and, 140—141
  complications of, 148
  glioblastoma multiforme type, see Glioblastoma multiforme
   multiforme
  IOEBT for, 128
  at Medical College of Ohio Hospital, 346—348
  metastatic, 153—156
  patient selection in, 142—143, 347
  patient transport and, 140—141
  pilot studies of, 143—145
  surgery for, 140
  treatment protocols in, 142—143, 155—156
Breast cancer, 118, 343—345
Bremsstrahlung X-ray contamination, 49—50

C

Cancer, 84, see also Carcinomas; Sarcomas; Tumors; specific types
   specific types
  anal, 335
  biliary tract, 4, 12, 307—308, 334—335
  bladder, see Bladder cancer
  breast, 118, 343—345
  cervical, 249, 259, 335—341
  colon, 331—333
  colorectal, see Colorectal cancer
  duodenal, 335
  gastric, see Gastric cancer
  gastrointestinal, see Gastrointestinal cancer
  lung, see Lung cancer
  mammary, see Breast cancer
  ovarian, 341—343
  pancreatic, see Pancreatic cancer
  prostatic, see Prostatic cancer
  pulmonary, see Lung cancer
  radioresistant, 138
  rectal, see Rectal cancer
  skin, 18
  stomach, see Gastric cancer
  uterine, 5
  uterine cervical, 335—341, 401
  vaginal, 345
Carcinomas, see also Cancer; specific types
  adeno-, see Adenocarcinomas
  biliary tract, see Biliary tract cancer
  brain, 124
  breast, see Breast cancer
  cerebral, see Brain; Cerebral malignancies

Verification, 57

W

Whipple's procedure, 317
Wound infections, 119, 134—135

X

X-ray equipment, 107—111, see also specific types
X-rays vs. electrons, 87
  safety, 108—109, 401
  sarcomas, 40